Medical LLMs for Clinical Safety Assessment

Fernando Ortiz-Rodriguez
https://orcid.org/0000-0003-2084-3462
Tamaulipas Autonomous University, Mexico

Mrignainy Kansal
https://orcid.org/0009-0005-2610-040X
Netaji Subhas University of Technology (NSUT), Delhi, India

Rajesh Kumar Dhanaraj
https://orcid.org/0000-0002-2038-7359
Symbiosis International (Deemed to be) University, India

Firoz Khan
Ball State University, USA

IGI Global
Scientific Publishing
Publishing Tomorrow's Research Today

Vice President of Editorial	Melissa Wagner
Director of Acquisitions	Mikaela Felty
Director of Book Development	Jocelynn Hessler
Production Manager	Mike Brehm
Cover Design	Jose Rosado

Published in the United States of America by
IGI Global Scientific Publishing
701 East Chocolate Avenue
Hershey, PA, 17033, USA
Tel: 717-533-8845 | Fax: 717-533-7115
Website: https://www.igi-global.com E-mail: cust@igi-global.com

Library of Congress Cataloging-in-Publication Data

Names: Ortiz-Rodriguez, Fernando, 1974- editor | Kansal, Mrignainy, 1993- editor | Dhanaraj, Rajesh Kumar editor | Khan, Firoz, 1974- editor
Title: Medical LLMs for clinical safety assessment / edited by: Fernando Ortiz-Rodriguez, Mrignainy Kansal, Rajesh Kumar Dhanaraj, Firoz Khan.
Description: Hershey PA : IGI Global Scientific Publishing, [2026] | Includes bibliographical references. | Summary: "This book examines the safe and ethical use of large language models in healthcare, providing frameworks, methodologies, and case studies for clinical evaluation. It integrates technological, medical, and regulatory perspectives to guide responsible AI adoption, ensuring patient safety and advancing evidence-based practices in medical LLM deployment"-- Provided by publisher.
Identifiers: LCCN 2026002860 (print) | LCCN 2026002861 (ebook) | ISBN 9798337378626 hardcover | ISBN 9798337378633 paperback | ISBN 9798337378640 ebook
Subjects: LCSH: Artificial intelligence--Medical applications | Natural language processing (Computer science) | Medical informatics--Technological innovations
Classification: LCC R859.7.A78 M4285 2026 (print) | LCC R859.7.A78 (ebook)
LC record available at https://lccn.loc.gov/2026002860
LC ebook record available at https://lccn.loc.gov/2026002861

British Cataloguing in Publication Data
A Cataloguing in Publication record for this book is available from the British Library.

Table of Contents

Detailed Table of Contents

Large Language Models (LLMs) play a complex and ever-evolving role in medicine. LLMs, in general, can help medical professionals identify patients by giving them fast, data-driven information. They are able to analyse patient data, compare it with a comprehensive medical history, and make recommendations for potential diagnoses or identify issues that need more research. This chapter examines the threats that prompt injection attacks, perfect overturn, and data leak could pose to PHI and offers solutions to lessen these risks through federated learning, secure model design, and privacy-preserving AI methods. These models are very decent at comprehending and producing human language and are built on deep learning and natural language processing technologies. LLMs have developed exceptional skills in vocabulary, grammar, semantics, and specialized knowledge, particularly in medicine, thanks to the extensive training on vast amounts of textual material. A proposal for an ethical framework to safeguard that medical LLMs operate within the bounds of patient trust closes the chapter.

Large Language Models (LLMs) are being deployed in clinical and healthcare systems, which requires serious consideration of their safety, reliability. This chapter

This chapter, per the authors, provides a comprehensive evaluation of Large Language Models (LLMs) within safety-critical healthcare environments, moving beyond traditional performance benchmarks toward a reliability-centered paradigm. The purpose of this chapter is to identify core clinical risks—including hallucinations, bias, uncertainty mismanagement, and privacy leaks—that can compromise patient safety despite high accuracy on standardized tests. Systematic principles for safety-critical assessment are established, emphasizing robustness, uncertainty awareness, and human-in-the-loop validation as essential for clinical trust. Furthermore, the authors discuss technical methods for stress testing and bias mitigation alongside the necessity of continuous monitoring, auditability, and lifecycle evaluation to handle model drift. By aligning these technical frameworks with emerging international regulatory standards, the chapter outlines a path for integrating clinical language models as dependable medical aids.

Conversational large language models (LLMs) are increasingly used in healthcare for triage, patient education, documentation, and decision support. Safety debates often emphasize accuracy, bias, and privacy, but overlook how these systems shape trust and decision-making through communication. This chapter proposes a communication-centered framework to assess clinical safety in medical LLMs. It defines dialogic safety across three layers: Linguistic Safety (expression of uncertainty, evidence, and sensitive topics), Interactional Safety (clarification, error recovery, escalation), and Institutional Safety (auditability, role clarity, and alignment with guidance from World Health Organization, Food and Drug Administration, and European Union). The framework provides checklist-style indicators for red-teaming, simulations, and human oversight. By treating safety as a property of clinical dialogue rather than isolated outputs, it supports stronger governance, clinician supervision, and patient trust.

The rise of Medical Large Language Models (LLMs) has brought significant new possibilities in healthcare. They enable effective clinical reasoning, automate documentation, interpret data in real time, and improve patient communication. However, their use in high-stakes medical settings also raises important concerns about safety, ethics, transparency, and following regulations. This chapter suggests a governance framework that ensures the trustworthy, safe, and ethical use of Medical LLMs throughout the AI lifecycle. The framework focuses on main areas: data governance, clinical safety validation, ethical oversight, and regulatory alignment. It includes structured processes like dataset quality audits, demographic bias checks, human-in-the-loop oversight, and ongoing monitoring after deployment. This work positions governance as the key foundation for responsibly scaling Medical LLMs.

It ensures that AI-driven innovations support clinical expertise, adhere to ethical and legal standards, and foster a safer, fairer, and more reliable future for digital healthcare.

Large Language Models (LLMs) are becoming an important part of today's healthcare system, especially in helping doctors with clinical documentation and routine tasks. While these tools can save time, reduce workload, and improve the quality of medical records, their use also brings important safety and ethical questions. This chapter takes a practical look at what it means to use LLMs responsibly in healthcare. It explains why human oversight is essential, how errors like hallucinations or bias can affect patient care, and why protecting patient privacy must remain a top priority. The chapter also describes simple and effective ways to reduce risks—through proper validation, transparent workflows, data security, and continuous monitoring. Overall, the chapter highlights that LLMs can be powerful partners in healthcare, but only when used carefully, ethically, and with the patient's well-being at the center of every decision

Despite tremendous advancements in text creation, large language models (LLMs) are still not sufficiently advanced to be applied on their own in mission-critical fields such as medical, finance, and law. The current solutions require professional assistance or human support, which makes them less scalable. As the application of Generative Artificial Intelligence (GAI) increases, it is only reasonable that concerns about security and other problems would soon arise. Large language models, or LLMs, have been widely used in many therapeutic domains, such as establishing individualised treatment plans, speeding up diagnosis, and aiding in radiological diagnostics. In hepatology and gastroenterology, doctors are having a harder time making decisions. Large language models (LLMs), a subset of generative artificial intelligence (AI), are creating new opportunities in CDSS by providing more adaptive and flexible support that better reflects the situation's complexity.

The fast adoption of Large Language Models (LLMs) in the field of healthcare has new opportunities of transformative power in clinical safety measurement, diagnostic aid, and patient treatment. Nevertheless, the increased privacy in data, information security, as well as the safety of Protected Health Information (PHI), are associated with this progress. The chapter discusses the core values, standards, and best practices required to guarantee data confidentiality and regulatory standards in medical AI systems. It describes some of the privacy-saving tools, like anonymization of data, differential privacy, federated learning, and secure multi-party computation. Also, the chapter addresses ethical and legal issues of the deployment of LLM in healthcare, such as compliance with standards, such as HIPAA, GDPR, and ISO/IEC 27701. The paper ends with the discussion of recent issues and suggests effective approaches to developing privacy-aware LLMs that will not only support the trust of patients but also clinical accuracy.

Medical LLMs are increasingly used for diagnosis support, triage, documentation, and patient interaction, yet traditional validation methods often fail to detect unsafe reasoning hidden behind fluent clinical language. This chapter introduces Cognitive Hazard Mapping, a framework designed to identify and prevent reasoning-level risks such as diagnostic hallucination, premature closure, causal misalignment, and guideline divergence. By analyzing inference pathways, applying multi-layer checks, and integrating clinician review, the model uncovers subtle hazards that may lead to patient harm despite seemingly accurate outputs. The chapter presents a taxonomy of cognitive hazards, real-world case studies, and methods for monitoring,

Preface

Large Language Models (LLMs) have moved from research prototypes to influential actors in clinical workflows, patient communication, and health systems. Medical professionals now routinely encounter LLM-powered decision support, summarisation tools, chatbots, and image text systems, often before there is a clear, shared understanding of how safe and trustworthy these systems truly are. This book has been conceived to bridge the gap. This brings together foundational concepts, methodological advances, and practice-oriented perspectives on how to evaluate, govern, and deploy medical LLMs.

Safety shouldn't be something you think about only after a model is finished. Instead, it must be a core part of the plan from the very beginning—guiding how models are made, tested, and used in healthcare. The chapters reflect this philosophy. They move from conceptual foundations of LLMs in healthcare through formal frameworks for risk and governance to application-specific evaluations. In doing so, the book aims to serve as both a reference text and a practical guide for researchers, clinicians, regulators, and industry professionals who are navigating the rapidly evolving landscape of medical AI.

CHAPTER OVERVIEW

The first two chapters establish formal safety-assessment perspectives. Clinical Safety Evaluation Frameworks for Medical Large Language Models reviews existing safety taxonomies, harm typologies, and regulatory concepts and proposes structured frameworks for assessing clinical risk across different types of LLM-enabled applications. Fuzzy Neural Framework for Clinical Safety Evaluation of Medical Large Language Models: Risk, Governance, and Trust in Healthcare AI introduces a more technical, hybrid approach that combines fuzzy logic and neural methods to quantify safety-related uncertainty and to link these measures to governance and trust requirements at system and organisational levels. Together, these chapters demonstrate how safety assessment can be operationalised in both conceptual and computational terms.

Several contributions focus on conversational systems and their role in clinical education, communication, and patient-facing interactions. Safety and Reliability Evaluation of Medical Chatbots Powered by Large Language Models: A Review of Clinical Education and Recommendation Systems synthesises evidence on how chatbots perform when providing educational content or recommendations to clinicians and patients, with particular attention to harmful hallucinations, misleading reassurance, and inappropriate advice.

The book also recognises that safety assessment must be tightly coupled with information security and ethics. Information Security and Clinical Ethics in LLM-based Healthcare Systems examines vulnerabilities related to data leakage, model inversion, prompt injection, and unauthorised access, and it articulates the ethical duties of developers and institutions to prevent misuse and protect sensitive health information. Evaluating LLM safety and reliability requires sound methodology. Evaluation Methods for LLM Safety and Reliability in Clinical and Healthcare Applications provides a structured overview of quantitative and qualitative methods, from benchmark-based assessment and scenario testing to simulation, expert review, and in-situ clinical validation. Evaluating the Safety of Medical LLMs for Patient Use narrows the focus to patient-facing scenarios, discussing risk thresholds, usability and comprehension, misinterpretation hazards, and cultural and linguistic factors that affect safe use. Beyond Performance Benchmarks: A Safety-Critical Evaluation Paradigm for Reliability and Trust in Clinical Language Models argues for evaluation regimes that move beyond accuracy-centric leaderboards, incorporating calibration, robustness, out-of-distribution behaviour, and system-level impact on clinical workflows as core dimensions of trust. Dialogic Safety: A Communication-Centered Framework for Clinical Risk Assessment of Conversational Medical LLMs then reframes safety as an inherently dialogic property, proposing analytic tools and metrics that account for turn-taking, clarification, uncertainty communication, and the dynamics of shared decision making in clinician–patient–AI interactions. Trust and governance are recurring themes. Trustworthy Medical LLMs: A Governance Framework for Clinical Safety, Ethical Validation, and Regulatory-Aligned Deployment synthesises organisational, ethical, and regulatory requirements into a governance framework that spans model selection, validation, deployment, and ongoing monitoring. Ensuring Safe and Ethical Use of LLMs in Healthcare translates these principles into practical guidelines for clinicians and institutions, including documentation, disclosure, and accountability practices. Expert Consensus on LLM Safety in Clinical Decision Support reports expert-driven guidance on acceptable use, oversight mechanisms, and escalation pathways for AI-assisted decision support. Complementing this, Data Privacy, Security, and PHI Protection discusses technical and organisational safeguards for handling protected health information (PHI), including de-identification, access control, and privacy-preserving training techniques, and relates these mechanisms to emerging regulatory expectations. Cognitive Hazard Mapping: A New Framework for Predicting and Preventing Unsafe Reasoning in Medical LLMs proposes a structured way to identify patterns of unsafe or misleading reasoning within LLM outputs, anticipating potential failure modes before they manifest in practice. Dialogic Safety (as discussed earlier) and related chapters emphasise that safe AI-supported care is inseparable from communication quality, shared understanding, and clearly defined roles for human oversight.

Ethical and legal questions are addressed in depth in a cluster of chapters. Safety Assurance Through Red-Teaming, MLOps, and Continuous Monitoring for Medical LLMs complements this with an operational perspective, detailing how red-teaming, robust MLOps practices, and continuous surveillance can identify and mitigate safety regressions over time.

Collectively, these contributions seek to move the discussion of medical LLMs beyond technological optimism or simple performance claims. They argue for a safety-critical, ethically grounded, and clinically embedded approach to design, evaluation, and governance. It is our hope that this volume will support clinicians in asking better questions about AI tools, guide researchers in developing methods that meaningfully address safety and trust, assist regulators and policymakers in shaping proportionate oversight, and help industry partners to design products that are not only powerful, but also responsible and aligned with the fundamental aims of medicine.

Acknowledgment

We express our sincere gratitude to all the contributors, researchers, and practitioners whose chapters and insights have shaped this book on the safety, governance, and ethical deployment of medical large language models in healthcare. Their commitment to improving clinical practice, protecting patients, and advancing trustworthy AI has made this volume possible.

We are thankful to the editorial and review teams for their careful guidance, constructive feedback, and support throughout the development of this manuscript. Their efforts helped refine the ideas presented here and ensured that the book can serve as both a practical guide and a reference for clinicians, researchers, regulators, and industry professionals.

Our heartfelt thanks also go to the institutions and organizations that encouraged and supported this work, fostering a collaborative environment in which diverse perspectives on safety, risk, and ethics in medical AI could be brought together. Finally, we acknowledge our family, friends, and colleagues for their constant encouragement and understanding during the writing and compilation of this book.

Chapter 1
Clinical Safety Evaluation Frameworks for Medical Large Language Models

P. Umamaheswari
http://orcid.org/0000-0003-2007-697X
SASTRA (Deemed to be) University, India

Jeyapandian Munisamy
http://orcid.org/0000-0001-8422-6557
SASTRA (Deemed to be) University, India

R. Sujarani
SASTRA (Deemed to be) University, India

G. Loganayaki
http://orcid.org/0000-0002-5944-1420
SASTRA (Deemed to be) University, India

A. Sumathi
http://orcid.org/0000-0003-4700-5573
SASTRA (Deemed to be) University, India

ABSTRACT

The introduction of Large Language Models (LLMs) in the medical sector is a new epoch in healthcare technology. These are models that are trained with huge amounts of biomedical literature, clinical notes and interactions with patients and have shown abilities in decision support, clinical documentation, patient communication and disease diagnosis. The immediate release of medical LLM, like Med-PaLM, BioGPT, and GatorTron have demonstrated possibilities and threats of applying AI

DOI: 10.4018/979-8-3373-7862-6.ch001

in healthcare. The lack of accurate recommendations, prejudices in the interpretation of the data, and the possibility of information confidentiality have marked the necessity of developing robust clinical safety assessment systems as an urgent need. These frameworks can provide a mediating role between AI innovation and medical governance, as well as make sure that the LLMs comply with regulatory, ethical, and technical requirements before they reach patient care. The chapter covers the current gaps, solutions, and a multidisciplinary approach

1. INTRODUCTION

Large Language Models (LLMs) are increasingly being used as useful devices in the medical field, assisting doctors, patients, and hospitals by comprehending human-like language and producing it. They are able to read and summarize medical reports, provide clinical answers, aid in prescription writing or discharge summaries and help the patient communicate using chatbots or virtual assistants. Since LLMs are able to process large volumes of medical knowledge and respond in a relatively brief period of time, they can ease the workload of clinicians and enhance the efficiency of medical services. They also assist in decision-making through evidence-based information even when it should be applied carefully to prevent mistakes or misconceptions. Altogether, LLMs create new prospects of smarter, faster, and more accessible healthcare and streamline the understanding of medical information and raise the quality of patient care.

2. BACKGROUND: EVOLUTION OF AI AND LLMS IN HEALTHCARE

Artificial Intelligence in healthcare (Raeini, 2023) is developed based on three large directions: Rule-Based Systems, Machine Learning, and Large Language Models all of them make a specific contribution to enhancing medical care as shown in Figure. 1 Rule-Based Systems are based on predetermined rules and expert knowledge to imitate clinical decision-making; they direct diagnosis or treatment recommendations using if-then logic and not based on data. Machine Learning systems, on the contrary, are trained on large sets of medical data, and thus they can perform tasks such as disease prediction, analyze medical images, and provide tailored treatment suggestions and only get better as they learn over time. Large Language Models are the latest development in AI that is able to comprehend and create natural language to facilitate tasks connected to communication, such as summarization of medical reports, aiding in documentation, responding to patient questions, and improving the communication between doctors and patients. These three types of AI are powerful in healthcare delivery and can help hospitals(Kao & Kao, 2025) to enhance diagnostic support, work more efficiently, communicate more effectively, and use data-driven decision-making in clinical and administrative environments.

Figure 1. Artificial Intelligence in healthcare based on three large directions

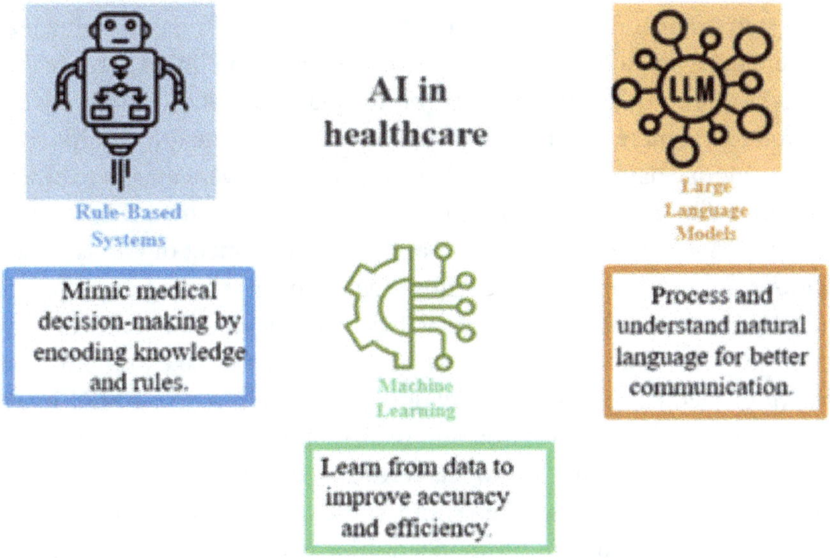

2.1 Early Use of AI in Medicine

The first implementation of artificial intelligence in the field of healthcare was rule-based expert systems such as MYCIN and INTERNIST-I (Drăgoi & Neme , 2023) that were created in the 1970s and 1980s. The systems operated based on preset medical logic drawn up by specialists with an if-then logic helping physicians to diagnose diseases. MYCIN was created to detect bacterial infections and prescribe antibiotics whereas INTERNIST-I specialized in the diagnosis of complicated internal medicine. Even though these systems were not able to learn and adapt to new information, they proved that computers could aid in clinical reasoning. They put in place organized clinical bases of knowledge, decision trees and rule based inference mechanisms. Their application demonstrated the opportunities as well as the difficulties of applying AI in the actual medical practice. The early systems allowed researchers to learn that accuracy, transparency, and domain expertise are important to AI. They have also introduced the way to more advanced techniques such as machine learning. Finally, through MYCIN and INTERNIST-I, there were stepping stones towards the current data-driven AI and large language models of healthcare.

2.2 From Machine Learning to Deep Learning

The transition between the traditional machine learning and deep learning is a significant step towards the development of healthcare AI. Initial machine learning systems were designed to perform well on simple tasks and failed in more difficult medical tasks due to their high reliance on manually derived features by domain experts. Due to the increased rate of growth of electronic health records, medical images and genomic datasets, machine learning methods were unable to effectively process the high dimensionality and complexity of the modern medical data. With the accessibility of massive amounts of data and the development of GPUs to perform computations, a new category of algorithms called deep learning appeared, which automatically acquires patterns in the raw data. The convolutional neural networks (CNNs) as deep learning models(Li et al., 2026) proved to be extremely useful in the problem of medical image classification, including tumors in MRI images or tumors in X-rays. Transformer-based and recurrent neural networks improved the field of clinical text mining as the models were able to extract information based on unstructured clinical notes, discharge summaries, and patient narratives. Genomic prediction was another domain of application of deep learning, through the discovery of more intricate patterns in DNA sequences and the assistance of finding disease-related genetic markers. Deep learning was much more accurate than the traditional ML, less manual feature engineering is needed, and the performance of deep learning was almost human or even superhuman in some diagnostic tasks. The effectiveness of deep learning models in the healthcare sector hastened the process of creating automated diagnostic systems, precision medicines and clinical decision support systems. Altogether, the shift towards deep learning is a pivotal technological breakthrough that was still propelling the advancement of the healthcare ecosystem.

2.3 The Emergence of Large Language Models

The emergence of Large Language Models like GPT, PaLM, and LLaMA(T-soutsanis & Tsoutsanis, 2024) is a significant step towards using AI in healthcare applications. The models are constructed on the transformer architectures that are better at contextual understanding, comprehending long-range dependencies, and producing fluent and human-like text. The fact that they are able to handle large volumes of medical knowledge, clinical notes and communication with patients makes them useful in most tasks in the clinical setting. When used in healthcare,

LLM may be able to summarize long electronic health records so that clinicians can easily understand the history of a patient. Another quality they can possess is the ability to answer patient questions using language that is easy to understand to enhance health literacy and facilitate virtual care. The application of LLMs by researchers is in creating research hypotheses, investigating medical questions, and reviewing scientific evidence in a speedy fashion. Since they are trained on large-scale datasets, LLMs can generalize on a large variety of tasks without task-oriented programming. This same generality, however, is dangerous: LLMs can generate false or untrue information - also known as hallucination - and this information can be harmful in clinical decision-making. Their productions can also differ with phrasing, context or uncomplete inputs. Reliability is achieved through careful assessment, reinforcement learning as well as clinical management. Nevertheless, LLMs are an innovative development that promises highly valuable assistance in the medical knowledge processing, communication, and automation. They can be extremely valuable instruments of contemporary healthcare with proper protection.

3. ETHICAL AND SAFETY CONCERNS IN MEDICAL LLMs

3.1 Bias and Fairness

Fairness and bias are the key issues (Lu et al., 2025)in the application of Large Language Models in healthcare, as such models are trained on data that is commonly representative of the inequality in the real world. When the training data is not balanced in terms of race, gender, age, socioeconomic status, or geographic background, that data may be used to unconsciously reproduce the biases in the medical outputs of the model. Whereas, when some of the demographic groups are underrepresented in the clinical datasets, the LLM will be less precise in making recommendations to the same groups. Such biased results may affect the diagnosis, treatment recommendations, or risk evaluation, which may result in unfair healthcare delivery. The bias can be implicit i.e. when the reason given to the patient is different when the identity is different, or more serious i.e. omission of crucial symptoms in minority groups. Inequality of history which is inherent in medical texts can also support the development of negative stereotypes. This is particularly dangerous in clinical decision-support systems, where biased advice may slow down the treatment process or misinform medical practitioners. Some social biases amplified by LLLMs are also assumptions regarding pain tolerance, mental health, or lifestyle of specific groups. Diverse, representative and curated datasets are essential to ensure the fairness. In order to detect and rectify imbalances, continuous auditing, bias detection algorithms as well as human oversight are necessary. Ethics should provide transparency in development and reviewing of models. In addition, clinicians ought to receive training in knowing the constraints of AI-generated outputs. Finally, the issue of bias is not only a technical problem but also an ethical issue, which is necessary to maintain equitable and inclusive healthcare across all patients.

3.2 Hallucinations and Misinformation

The most severe problems associated with the use of Large Language Models in healthcare are hallucinations and misinformation(Sun et al., 2025). Hallucination is a propensity of an LLM to create information that appears to be accurate but which is actually incorrect, unfinished, or even entirely fake. Due to the fact that these models generate the most likely word that follows the trends in data, sometimes they come out with medically unsafe sentences without realizing they are false. LLMs lack actual clinical reasoning, medical judgment, and a concept of consequences that human clinicians have. They are unable to check the facts, compare laboratory findings, or take into consideration the background of the patient, unless it is explicitly given. This exposes them to giving wrong diagnosis, wrong doses of drugs, or wrong explanations in case the input is ambiguous or vague. They also might not give similar responses to the same question depending on the phrasing and, thus, their responses are not constant. Because the information is said with confidence in the LLMs, users can trust it wrongly with false suggestions on medicine. Hallucinations may lead to harmful clinical consequences in situations with high risks, like emergency care or drug prescriptions. When deployed in patient-facing applications, misinformation can also go viral and strengthens myths or wrong health behaviors. In order to minimize risk, the results of LLM should be sent to trained clinicians and embedded into a controlled workflow instead of implementing it as a decision-maker. Some methods, like retrieval-augmented generation (RAG) (Matthew & Hicks, 2025), rule-based constraints, and fine-tuning using verified clinical data can be used to enhance reliability. Constant observation, guard rails and rigorous testing criterion are also required. Finally, it is essential to reduce the rate of hallucinations in the cards of establishing trust and safe implementation of LLMs in healthcare.

3.3 Privacy and Data Protection

The issue of privacy and data protection are fundamental conditions under Large Language Models use in medical care, as medical information has highly sensitive and individually identifiable data. Patient records consist of information regarding such diseases, medication, genetic profiles, mental health, and other lifestyle information, so they are one of the most confidential types of data. The outcome of any abuse or leakage may cause discrimination, stigma, economic damages, or mistrust of the healthcare facilities. Hence, before implementing LLMs, it is necessary to adhere to the legal frameworks, including the HIPAA in the United States, GDPR in Europe(Mohammed & Malhotra, 2025), national health data regulations in other countries of the world. These legislations provide stringent requirements in regards to data storage, data processing, control of access and consent. LLMs should be built in a way that preserves patient identities and this may involve de-identification, anonymization and encryption. During development of models or fine-tuning, developers will need to make sure that the raw patient data is not ever leaked or retained in the model. The other threat is inadvertent disclosure, which is when an LLM can recreate sensitive data on its training data. To ensure confidentiality, there is a need to have secure data pipelines, audit logs, and role-based access. Another risk that hospitals need to evaluate is the process of using AI tools based on the cloud and making sure that data is transferred and stored safely. Also, the use of their data should be explained to the patients, and a right to opt-out must be offered where needed. Privacy-by-design techniques assist in making the protection mechanisms more embedded instead of being added as post-hacks. Finally, stringent privacy control is essential to not only conduct business in accordance with the law but also uphold the principles of ethics and citizen confidence in AI-based healthcare systems.

3.4 Accountability and Transparency

Acquiring AI systems, particularly the Large Language Models, into healthcare should be done with accountability and transparency to achieve a safe integration. Among the most significant issues, it is necessary to identify a person who will be responsible in case an AI model will provide the wrong diagnosis, dangerous recommendation, or dangerous medical guidance. AI models cannot be responsible legally or ethically as opposed to human clinicians. This puts hospitals, developers and regulators in doubt. In case the patient is hurt, it cannot be easily determined who is responsible, model creators, the healthcare institution, the clinician using the AI output, or the data providers. Clear audit trails are therefore necessary in order to overcome these fears. The audit trails are documentation of the process through which the AI system came to a decision, the data it utilized, and the time and the person who accessed it. This type of records aids in the adherence to the law and assists investigators in the direction of where the error originated. Explainable AI (XAI)(Jung et al., 2024) schemes also make model decisions more transparent to clinicians. XAI can assist physicians in comprehending why an AI made the particular diagnosis or treatment, therefore, allowing them to identify possible mistakes and establish a trust toward the system. Clinicians might be reluctant to trust AI-made recommendations without an explanation. Regulatory bodies across the globe insist on the importance of accountability systems, risk evaluation systems, and safety follow-ups during the AI lifecycle. Easy to understand measures are necessary to establish human oversight, legal obligations and safe deployment in the clinical setting. Finally, trust and responsibility ensure patient safety, boost trust, and facilitate responsible adoption of AI technologies in healthcare.

4. THE NEED FOR CLINICAL SAFETY EVALUATION FRAMEWORKS

The healthcare industry is subject to strict protocols regarding safety, organized clinical trials, and evidence-based recommendations to ensure that every instrument or treatment is tested prior to receiving it. Nevertheless, large language models present new obstacles because they do not behave like medical devices. The results produced by these tools are probabilistic, not deterministic. The answers can differ slightly for changing the wording of the sentence-prompt. The unpredictability of LLM-generated recommendations makes it challenging for clinicians to fully rely on them without standard evaluation. The typical validation processes we use for things like drugs or medical equipment won't work for AI models that evolve, learn with data and are constantly changing. Consequently, the demand for a Clinical Safety Evaluation Framework (CSEF), specifically addressing the distinctive risks and behaviors of LLMs, is increasing rapidly.

A strong CSEF will provide a primary approach to assess the safety of the model prior to its deployment, and assess its safety post deployment. First, the frameworks need to validate the model's performance against clinical milestones, such as assessing the gold-standard datasets, expert answers, or clinical exam questions at a benchmark-level. This ensures that the model is performing at a level that is justifiable as clinically useful. Second, the framework must discern stability, transparency, and consistency. This ensures that the model is predictable across different patients, is stable during high workloads, and provides adequate explanations that the clinician is able to understand. Especially with the clinical datasets that may be highly variable, testing for stability is very critical, as the model must be able and respond in a clinically safe manner.

Lastly, a CSEF must assess ongoing performance after LLM deployment, with the understanding that LLMs may experience degradation, novel concept drift, or novel situations. Continuous monitoring is necessary to detect and address hallucinations, biases, drifts, or safety failures before serious consequences occur. This may involve log auditing, monitoring for negative outcomes, and timely model updates to address deficiencies. Further, the framework (Parish et al., 2020)must include Human Factors to stipulate the circumstances and mechanisms by which the clinician can intervene. There must also be ethical and medical compliance safeguards. In the end, within clinical safety evaluation frameworks, LLMs may be high performing, and easily and readily integrated into clinical workflows; however, LLMs will also be safe and trustworthy, and aligned with all pertinent clinical safety standards.

5. EXISTING FRAMEWORKS AND STANDARDS

5.1 Regulatory Perspectives

When it comes to large language models in healthcare, it is crucial considering the impact of various regulations. Agencies, including the FDA in the United States, European Medicines Agency (EMA)(Palomo et al., 2023) in the European Union, and WHO, face such challenges and develop policies aimed at mitigating risk, safeguarding patient wellbeing, and ensuring the accountability of relevant health care services. These institutions understand and appreciate the differences between the automated intelligence and traditional medical equipment, and thus, the need for unique regulatory controls in these devices.

In the USA, the FDA considers and controls LLMs as Software as a Medical Device(Ajmera et al., 2025). SaMD guidelines delineate the parameters within which such software providing a medical service will be tested, validated, and monitored. When it comes to AI model, the FDA prioritizes analytical and clinical validations, as well as ongoing surveillance of the model postmarket. The FDA is also thoughtful in delineating use of models, the need for active human control over the models to avoid undesirable outcomes, and transparency in how the models function. The FDA has been considering postmarket surveillance within a proactive regulatory framework of adaptive AI systems. Adaptive AI systems update their operating algorithms, and thus, the FDA is mainly concerned with the potential compromise of safety with updates. The EMA emphasizes ethical AI, algorithmic transparency, and data protection more than the rest of Europe. Their regulations require explainability, fairness, traceability, and adherence to privacy regulations like the GDPR(Mourby et al., 2021). The EMA states that AI in decision making needs to be auditable, and developers need to be transparent about risks, data used, and limitations. The AI Act that is coming to Europe classifies medical AI as 'high risk', and that comes with strict documentation, mandatory human supervision, and risk control procedures.

Through the Guidance on Ethics and Governance of Artificial Intelligence for Health, the WHO is able to provide a global viewpoint. WHO's pillars are equity, patient rights, inclusiveness, and global access to AI for Health. They point to the need to ensure that AI is closing the health equity gap, rather than widening it, particularly in low-resource settings. WHO demands transparency, accountability and responsibly applied data to promote healthcare equity. They argue for robust governance, ethical evaluations, and international collaboration to provide harmonized safety. With all agencies, a consistent pattern arises: medical AI must be open, responsible, secure, and within the bounds of morality. LLMs bring extra complications because of their erratic behaviour, supposed hallucinations and reliance on very large data sets. Thus, there is a greater emphasis on the need for continuous monitoring. This collection of regulatory viewpoints is a pillar for the responsible integration of AI in healthcare systems around the world.

5.2 Technical Frameworks

Technical frameworks are crucial to advancing the safety of the development, assessment, and deployment of AI, and more specifically, of LLMs within healthcare. They allow for AI transparency, traceability, and governance across the lifecycle of the AI through structured documents and frameworks. Three of the most popular and established technical frameworks, Model Cards, Datasheets for Datasets, Continuous Learning Systems, are essential to the design and development of trustable medical AI.

Model Cards are a standard practice to capture building and training details of an AI model, intended purposes and limitations, and training dataset a standard practice for all AI. Model Cards also require health care AI to contain a performance model stratified across demographic groups to facilitate equity assessments and bias identification. Model Cards addresses the transparency of a model to health care providers by clarifying its clinical reliability, intended use, clinical scenarios to caution its use, emission of certain clinical factors, and design assumptions. This transparency promotes confidence and compliance to regulations.

Datasheets for Datasets prioritize documenting the origin, contents, quality, and ethical principles guiding the collection, the data validation and training, and the prediction. Primary data collection, data representation, data cleaning, and overall available data limitations are discussed. In the medical field, where data are under-specified, and the range of data needed is diverse, Datasheets assist in making sure the range of datasets are representative and gathered ethically, while preventing the unintentional use of low-quality data or sensitive information. Datasheets assist with data provenance as a means of ensuring reproducibility, oversight, and more accurate risk assessments.

Continuous Learning Systems is the term given to AI systems that are meant to adapt and grow as more and more data are fed to them. In contrast to static systems, LLMs and Medical AI tools are designed with the expectation that they will, and in fact, require updates in order to preserve their usefulness and accuracy. Continuous learning introduces a number of risks should the model behave in unexpected and unanticipated manners. A technical framework for continuous learning includes self-regulation, monitoring tools, drift detection algorithms, version control mechanisms, and validation checkpoints. In relation to Healthcare, Continuous Learning Systems ensure that Adaptive AI systems remain safe, stable, and clinically aligned.

The combined efforts of these technical frameworks foster the development of a reliable system for recording, assessing, and overseeing the multi-dimensional aspects of AI. Model Cards, Datasheets, and Continuous Learning Systems facilitate the responsible and trustworthy deployment of LLMs and artificial intelligence systems into healthcare settings by increasing transparency, improving the governance of information, and enabling adaptive governance.

5.3 Institutional Frameworks

Configuring institutional frameworks has become critical for the deployment of Artificial Intelligence, including Large Language Models for clinical and administrative purposes, in hospitals, medical facilities, and research institutes. Such technology has implications for how clinical information is processed, how communication is conducted with patients, and how data are manipulated. Hence, sceptical institutional oversight is needed for responsible deployment. One of the most visible and promising outcomes in these are the dedicated AI oversight functions being set up in many health care facilities is of significant interest.

These committees assemble, in a collaborative model, representatives of several fields including the clinical, data science, ethics, law, IT, patient safety, and regulatory domains. The committees pre-market the AI tools and assess them for safety, harm mitigation, and regulatory compliance, including data protection and privacy provisions. For instance, the AI tool is evaluated for clinical accuracy, its performance equity for the different demographics the health institution serves, and whether its use is in alignment with the clinical governance frameworks of the health institution. They also review compliance with the frameworks of the tools including Model Cards and Datasheets in order to appreciate the risk associated with the tool and the areas in which its deployment would add no value to the outcomes.

Beyond the pre-deployment evaluation AI oversight committees are responsible of the evaluation of the tool while it is being used. These committees monitor adverse incidents, system performance changes (inexplicably, unexpectedly, improperly), and propose system safety during updates, retraining and model drift. The committees also help streamline compliance to administrative safeguards such as HIPAA, GDPR, and national health regulations.

How problems of ethics such as obtaining patient consent, the opacity of AI recommendations, and the effect on marginalized groups are handled, is also crucial.

To promote uniformity in the evaluation of AI, organizations may have internal guidelines, frameworks for stratified/ tiered approaches, and processes for gaining approvals. Some hospitals opt for "AI registries" to monitor the AI applications in their facilities, much as they do for medical devices. Part of the educational and training programs for clinicians provided by organizations also help health workers to understand AI and its responsible applications. In academic settings, ethics review boards may be responsible for AI in addition to their usual tasks related to AI in the clinical sphere.

With the adoption of frameworks that create system oversight, health institutions are able to prevent themselves from adopting AI in a haphazard manner. These frameworks provide AI systems the transparency and trust the clinicians and the patients require and most importantly, address the legal and ethical dilemmas. In the end, institutional AI governance allows the system to be efficient by integrating innovations in technologies to healthcare, while preserving fundamental values of safety and accountability.

6. PROPOSED CLINICAL SAFETY EVALUATION FRAMEWORK (CSEF-LLM)

CSEF-LLM is the first step in establishing the groundwork for dependable, secure, and ethically sound AI systems in healthcare. LLMs function differently from traditional software and medical devices, posing distinct challenges. This framework provides a comprehensive and stratified approach to guiding the development, validation, deployment, and ongoing surveillance of LLMs. The framework is composed of four interrelated and distinct layers: Data Governance, Model Development, Clinical Validation, and Post-Deployment Monitoring. This multi-layered approach to the framework in Figure. 4 provides accountability and transparency in addressing some of the most complex challenges associated with medical AI.

Figure 2. The four-layer clinical safety evaluation framework for medical LLMs

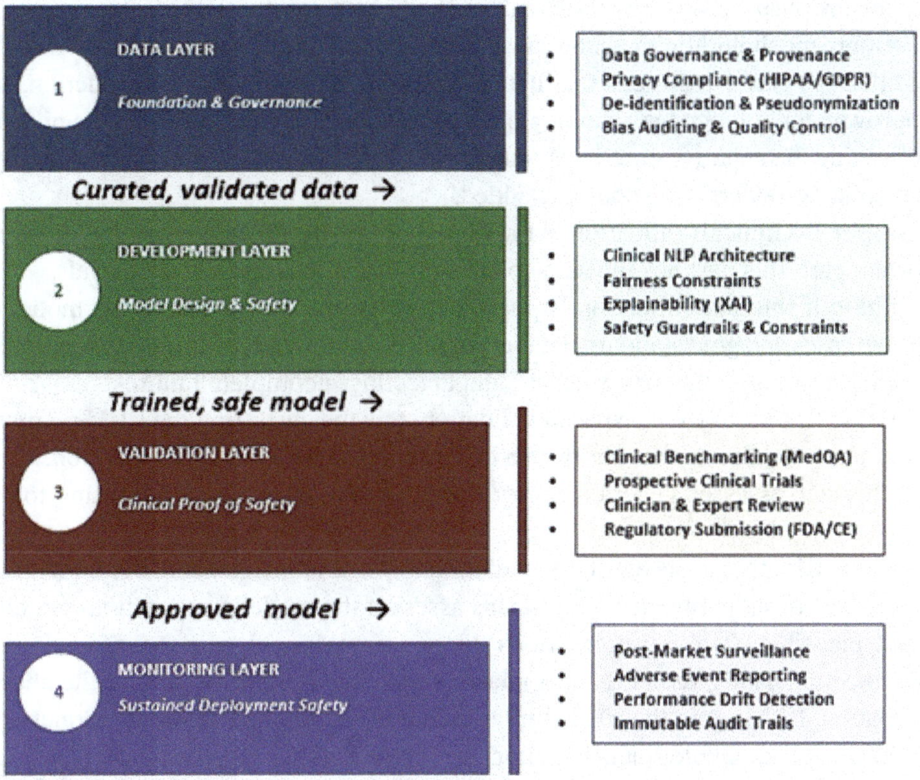

Layer 1: Data Governance considers the quality, variety, and safety of the data to be incorporated to train the LLMs. The data sets to train models need to be of high quality, devoid of biases, completeness, and noise, as these parameters drive the model to unsafe behaviors. To ensure model performance is generalizable to the target patients (including those from minor and underrepresented cohorts), diversity in data sets is needed to train the model. Robust de-identification protocols need to be incorporated to ensure the model never sees sensitive and potentially identifiable patient data or reproduces it in the model outputs. Dataset use needs to be authorized from ethics review boards or Institutional Review Boards (IRBs) so they ensure compliance with HIPAA, GDPR, and other health legal regulations. That level serves as a base for trustworthy AI growth because of the ethically sourced and safe training data.

Layer 2: Building and refining the long and short-term memory model, the second layer of the structure, is called model development. In this step, developers should embed tools of bias, fairness, and demographic performance adjacently.

Weaknesses and vulnerabilities can be uncovered through adversarial testing, where models are purposefully given difficult and ambiguous prompts. Furthermore, model development should be in accordance with medical ontologies like SNOMED CT and ICD-10 because this can facilitate interpretability, hallucination reduction, and improvement of language accuracy from the medical domain. Also, for the purpose of limiting the negative outcomes, safety layers like guardrails, rule-based filtering, and content moderation should be added.

Layer 3: Clinical Validation is the third layer of the structure and the most important part, this part has the same pattern as that of the clinical drug trials.

Phase I: Internal validation is phase one and comes with testing the model on known cases and gold standard data sets of the development institution. The purpose here is checking for accuracy, safety and detecting incomplete failures.

Phase II: Phase two is external validation, this means testing the LLM on previously unseen datasets that are from a different hospital or a different region.

This step assesses generalizability and limits the chances of overfitting to one dataset.

Phase III: Human-in-the-loop validation is when clinicians collaborate with the model within set parameters. Clinicians assess if the model's suggestions are clinically plausible, flag any suggestions that are unreasonably dangerous, and make sure the model aids, rather than supplants, clinical judgment. Thanks to the phased validation, LLMs gain the trust similar to that of recognized medical products.

Layer 4: Post-Deployment Monitoring is about making sure the model is still safe after it is deployed in the real world. Since LLMs can deteriorate with time or can be confronted with data they have not seen before, ongoing performance audits are a must. Hospitals have to gather and analyze user feedback, monitor safety reports, and look for any patterns of hallucinations or bias.

These four layers join to provide a holistic structure that guarantees LLMs are established, endorsed, and released safely across medical care. The CSEF-LLM boosts trust, guarantees patient safety, and makes the responsible use of sophisticated AI tools in the clinical environment more seamless. Beyond basic model training, ensuring that medical LLMs behave safely and helpfully in clinical contexts requires advanced alignment and augmentation strategies. Two techniques are particularly relevant: Reinforcement Learning from Human Feedback (RLHF) is a training paradigm in which clinicians and domain experts evaluate model outputs and provide preference rankings. These rankings are used to train a reward model, which then guides the LLM to generate responses that align with clinical standards, safety norms, and professional judgment. In medical settings, RLHF enables (Singhal et al., 2024) the model to learn not just factual accuracy but appropriate tone, risk communication, and escalation behaviour — qualities that cannot be captured by standard loss functions alone.

Retrieval-Augmented Generation (RAG)(Steybe et al., 2025) addresses a fundamental limitation of LLMs: their knowledge is frozen at the point of training. In clinical environments where guidelines, drug interactions, and protocols are frequently updated, a purely parametric model risks providing outdated advice. RAG architectures address this by connecting the LLM to a live, curated knowledge base — such as clinical guidelines from NICE or the WHO, pharmacological databases, or institution-specific protocols. At inference time, the model retrieves the most relevant, current documents and incorporates them into its response generation, substantially reducing hallucination rates and improving factual currency

7. EVALUATION METRICS

A thorough evaluation framework is necessary to understand the risk, trustworthiness, as well as ethical implications of using LLMs in the medical domain. Differently from traditional models, LLMs generate text outputs in a probabilistic manner, thus complicating the assessment of correctness, reasoning, and fairness. Therefore, evaluation metrics must reflect the combination of technical and ethical aspects of responsibility to ensure clinical relevance.

7.1 Accuracy and Reliability

In order to determine how well the LLM performs in the area of healthcare, we must consider the metrics of accuracy and reliability. Sensitivity assesses whether a machine learning algorithm can detect a phenomenon (e.g. a disease) when it actually exists, and thus correctly identifies positive cases. In contrast, specificity assesses whether a machine learning algorithm correctly identifies the absence of a phenomenon (e.g. a disease), thus reducing the chances of false positive outcomes that lead to an unnecessary workup. In healthcare, it is common for datasets to be highly imbalanced; the F1-score offers a balanced evaluation. The AU_ROC (Area Under the Receiver Operating Characteristic Curve) is standard for measuring discrimination ability at an array of different cut points. The model's reliability needs to be consistent; it should yield the same results after numerous repetitions, worded in different ways, or presented with variations of the same clinical scenario. Other reliability assessments are likely to be calibration scores issued for the model, and they reflect whether the model made predictions are actual probabilities, and if so, did they actualize. Collectively, these metrics help inform whether a model is clinically safe enough to be used in the real world.

7.2 Explainability and Interpretability

Explainability is very important in parts of the health care field, especially when clinicians must trust and verify AI insights. Some techniques, like SHA P(Ukwuoma et al., 2025), try to explain, in a precise way, the contribution of each input to a specific output of a model in order to offer transparency, risk score assessments, and/or suggestions of the potential diagnosis(s). Other techniques, like LIME, offer specific explanations at a point of interest, thereby giving the healthcare provider explanations of the decisions made for particular patients. With LLMs that have attention, we can visualize which pieces of the input text were deemed more important during the 'reasoning' process. This can help surface a model's potential faults, like hallucinations or biases, which were present during the mental 'processing' of the input. Being able to explain a model's reasoning is a fundamental need in healthcare and regulatory requirements of AI will necessiate healthcare systems to adopt 'explainable' AI. As a result, in high-stakes cases like prescribing a medication or determining a diagnosis when a patient has complex symptoms, healthcare professionals will need to see more reasonable pathways before trusting the AI. For that reason, explainability will look at the accuracy and completeness of a model's reasoning.

7.3 Ethical Compliance Indicators

Medical AI systems must guarantee fairness and equity across all patient populations. Ethical compliance considers whether the model exhibits differential performance along the demographic axes of sex, race, age, region, and socio-economic status. Metrics related to fairness may include demographic parity, equalized odds, or predictive parity. These calculations identify potential and unfair biases in the model's training data and/or the model's behavior. For instance, a model that underperforms relative to the majority population can result in the inequitable provision of care, exacerbate health disparities, or result in the misdiagnosis of individuals. Ethical compliance also considers the integration of privacy-preserving techniques, informed consent, and the fundamental tenets of medicine—beneficence and nonmaleficence. Keeping track of social performance metrics ensures that the model does not reinforce inequities and that the model's potential biases are kept in check. Most importantly, these metrics make sure that LLMs not only do their tasks in a timely and appropriate manner, but that they do so with the socio-legal conscience of equity, fairness, and respect for the dignity of the patient.

8. CASE STUDIES

Examples from the real world show the integration of Large Language Models into Healthcare workflows and describe advantages and disadvantages of such deployments. These events show the function of LLMs in improving clinical work and research, as well as the importance of efficiency, support in clinical decision-making and research, and the need for safety measures, bias mitigation, and constant monitoring. These examples provide insights for creating more advanced and ethically balanced Clinical Safety Evaluation Frameworks.

8.1 Clinical Documentation Assistant

Documenting patient information affects the quality of patient care due to extended time spent documenting patient information in the hospital (Alboksmaty et al., 2025). Documentation time has been improved with the help of an LLM that was trained on thousands of patient summaries. Discharge summaries created by LLMs allow hospital workers to gain patient history and other information faster which has improved overall efficiency by 35%. Clinicians gain the ability to interact and make more decisions in the during patient meetings.

Despite the early improvements in efficiency gained by LLMs, summaries produced were subpar and required reviewing by staff. Lapses which resulted in missing content were common. These omitted medications which were prescribed interventions that did not result in improvement and follow-ups which were required to assess the patient's status. Leaving out these details illustrates the complexity that LLMs suffer from: LLMs do not understand even lower components of health care. Because of this, the case shows that systemic LLMs needs human input supervision and needs to be explained to the staff participating in focused LLM technology health care.

8.2 AI-Based Triage System

Emergency departments (EDs) (Xompero et al., 2025) are regularly faced with intense operational strain and have to make quick decisions to allocate cases effectively in order to manage a case backlog. An AI triage system utilizing a large language model (LLM) (Lindner & Ravioli, 2025) was created to manage and evaluate a patients' presenting complaints, vital signs, and medical history to determine risk levels (high, medium and low). The model was effective in recognizing and differentiating high-priority patients (e.g., patients with sepsis and/or patients in cardiac distress). This aide and/or delegation for identifying large volumes of high-risk patients allowed for improved medical staff workload prioritization and was of particular value during busy, staffed, peak shifts.

Though effective, post-installation reviews found evidence of risk assessment bias in that the AI triage system was assigning younger patients similar clinical profiles risk assessment tiers that were disproportionately higher than older patients. This bias was due to the historical triage dataset that was used to design the model. Younger patients were more often marked as high risk in historical triage data and skewed the model. The model's bias was corrected with fairness reengineering of historical triage data, and the dataset was augmented (in many cases, by oversampling older patient profiles) to create a more reflective historical triage dataset. Hospitals are encouraged to create Balance Bias Monitoring frameworks. This case demonstrated one of the many use cases of AI, Bias Balance Monitoring and Bias Mitigation frameworks in action in high-stakes, time-critical environments in this case, emergency healthcare.

8.3 Med-LLM in Oncology Research

In oncology, professionals treat and study adults with cancer and its related disorders(Tan et al., 2024), where new studies and guidelines, new ways to treat and new ways to track progress come out routinely. To help with this new specialized LLM (Med-LLM-Onco) was created to summarize literature with oncology. It helped oncologists to track and trace literature related to their filed developed over the years, and determine and connect the treatments with the therapy actionable to the patients based on their marker status.

Oncologists appreciated this design to assist with tumor boards and to report on new medications. The LLM squired sample improvement opportunities within a collection of literature, and for reviewing available scientific literature on a subject less. Clinicians reviewing LLM summaries to confirm findings relevance, accuracy, and overall fit into current medical practice was a given. The LLM experienced challenges with some of oncology literature's contradictory and/or specialized word choices. This exemplifies the importance of LLM to describe their support of clinical work. When used with professional clinical practice LLMs can facilitate research and help clinicians make decisions based on literature in complex areas of cancer care.

9. INTEGRATING HUMAN OVERSIGHT

AI models cannot understand or have the same clinical experience, contextual thought, and ethical consideration that are the hallmarks of trained healthcare professionals, so the presence of human oversight is paramount when implementing

Large Language Models in healthcare. While LLMs are trained to process and analyze content in large data sets, offer summaries, and formulate recommendations, LLMs do not have the experience, clinical intuition and responsibility that are vital in patient care. Thus, the foundation of building patient care systems with LLMs and other AI models is the collaboration of humans and machines.

Such models have physicians in supervisory roles, allowing AI-generated recommendations to be validated by the physician before engaging with patients. Outputs of an LLM are, by that rationale, considered not as recommendations, but as auxiliary comments. This approach provides an LLM with accountability and mitigates risks of hallucinations, false interpretations, or biased recommendations.

AI integration without human oversight is deemed irresponsible, and it further enhances the building of trust. Knowing AI is not a replacement, but an adjunct, helps healthcare professionals incorporate AI tools seamlessly. This integration offers a unique mix of efficiency and responsiveness.

A vital part of oversight frameworks is the human-in-the-loop system that consists of clinicians analyzing the outputs from the AI system, making updates, and providing comments. This type of feedback acts as a protective barrier from AI system malfunctions and assists in the continuous improvement of the model. Over the years of engagement, the LLMs become more precise and contextually aware, in part, because of their engagement in genuine clinical scenarios. Feedback loops also facilitate the discovery of new biases and slippage in performance, thus enabling continued systems safety.

In volatile scenarios like emergency care, radiology, and chronic disease management, human supervision aids in the analysis of the subtleties that AI is likely to overlook, including slight indicators, patient affect, and peculiar presentations. Moreover, clinicians are in a position to account for the patients' values, ethical issues, and socio-cultural elements which LLMs lack the competence to comprehend fully.

10. FUTURE DIRECTIONS AND POLICY IMPLICATIONS

The future of Large Language Models (LLMs) in healthcare hinges on strong, responsive, and harmonized governance systems ensuring safety, transparency, and accountability across the entirety of the AI Value Chain. With the advancement of LLMs, integrated into clinical workflows, the balance between technological advancement and policy innovation becomes pivotal. Developing global governance systems is undoubtedly the most critical of these. Harmonizing standards and enabling the safe, regulatory, cross-border implementation of medical AI systems is a critical step necessitating the collaboration of AI developers, healthcare professionals, and regulators with the general public.

One of the most pertinent obstacles to the clinical deployment of LLMs is the technical challenge of unlabeled data hallucinations, bias, and the unreliable, unpredictable responses generated in a shifting clinical context. Transdisciplinary studies of federated learning suggest promising avenues whereby models are trained on distributed datasets without data transfers, preserving the integrity of private data, and optimizing the broader training data to improve model performance. Closely related is the generation of synthetic data - a constructive means of creating datasets that preserve the statistical characteristics of a distribution of real data but without compromising privacy.

Future AI pipelines should seek to incorporate mechanisms that allow for the tracking and auditing of data use, prediction generation and error correction, thereby improving traceability and risk mitigation. Such traceability will facilitate anomaly detection, compliance monitoring, and accountability across AI systems by regulators.

Many medical device regulations jurisprudentially were designed for immutable software systems, and thus, display a critical gap for use with adaptive AI. This gap mandates that legislation be modified to include evolving AI LLM systems and adaptive systems certification. The formation of AI Safety Boards (akin to drug approval boards or ethics committees) to establish clinical safety, fairness, risk management, and the other key attributes of AI tool use in medicine is one such proposed innovation.

Policies must also relieve existing liability frameworks to ensure that clinicians will always be the final decision-makers, and as such, will establish who is responsible for AI's erroneous decision(s). Ethical transparency will be key to maintaining public trust and will include explainability, informed consent for the use of AI, and fairness.

LLMs in healthcare will only progress if complex technologies are paired with foundational policy structures that allow for the safe, equitable, and responsible use of such systems on a global scale. The predicted benefits to the system are key.

11. CONCLUSION

Large Language Models are cutting-edge technology in the healthcare industry, affecting improvements in diagnosis, documentation, triage, research, and clinical decision support. In processing significant amounts of unstructured data and generating insights, LLMs offer tremendous healthcare innovation, particularly in an era of advanced data technology. However, LLMs' capabilities are tempered by safety, ethical, and regulatory issues.

LLMs are the first clinical tools to operate within a different paradigm. Rather than operating deterministically, LLMs function probabilistically, producing confident outputs that can be wrong, biased, or hallucinated. Such risks reinforce the need for clinical tools to be supported by custom and standardized Clinical Safety Evaluation Frameworks. These frameworks help in building medically usable LLMs that address deficiencies in precision, consistency, equity, and explainability. Such tools can sustain clinical practice without endangering patients.

An evaluation framework should encompass the entire lifecycle of AI, covering data governance and model building, clinical validation, and monitoring after the system is live. This oversight facilitates transparency, and early detection of bias, and ensures models continue to meet medical and ethical standards. During this LLM process, human oversight is important. LLMs should not substitute providers; trained clinicians, with contextual, ethical, and patient reasoning AI cannot replicate, should make all clinical decisions. The thoughtful integration of LLMs into clinical practice should strike a balance between innovation LLMs afford and the ethical obligations clinicians must meet. Forethinked policies, institutional governance, and safety-minded developers should all converge to enable the efficient and equitable access to quality medical knowledge embedded LLMs are capable of providing. As discussed, patient welfare must remain paramount when incorporating AI in medicine. As we harness the potential of AI, patient safety, a strong evaluation framework, and responsible human collaboration must remain closely aligned, allowing AI to augment rather than replace the clinician, ultimately providing a smarter and more equitable approach to healthcare.

REFERENCES

Ajmera, P., Dillard, R., Kline, T., Missert, A., Korfiatis, P., & Khandelwal, A. (2025). FDA-approved artificial intelligence products in abdominal imaging: A comprehensive review. *Current Problems in Diagnostic Radiology, S0363018825000829*. Advance online publication. DOI: 10.1067/j.cpradiol.2025.04.011 PMID: 40287285

Alboksmaty, A., Aldakhil, R., Hayhoe, B. W. J., Ashrafian, H., Darzi, A., & Neves, A.-L. (2025). The impact of using AI-powered voice-to-text technology for clinical documentation on quality of care in primary care and outpatient settings: A systematic review. *EBioMedicine, 118*, 105861. DOI: 10.1016/j.ebiom.2025.105861 PMID: 40694861

Drăgoi, A.-L., & Neme , R.-M. (2023). The "Electronic Pediatrician (EPed®)" – A clinically tested prototype software for computer-assisted pathophysiologic diagnosis and treatment of ill children. *International Journal of Medical Informatics, 178*, 105169. DOI: 10.1016/j.ijmedinf.2023.105169 PMID: 37562316

Jung, J., Kang, S., Choi, J., El-Kareh, R., & Kim, H. (2024). *Evaluating the Impact of Explainable Ai on Clinicians' Decision-Making: A Study on Icu Length of Stay Prediction. SSRN*. DOI: 10.2139/ssrn.5017467

Kao, J.-P., & Kao, H.-T. (2025). Large Language Models in radiology: A technical and clinical perspective. *European Journal of Radiology Artificial Intelligence, 2*, 100021. DOI: 10.1016/j.ejrai.2025.100021

Li, D., Jin, Z., Guan, C., Ji, L., Zhang, Y., Xu, Z., & Zhang, J. (2026). KACNet: Enhancing CNN feature representation with Kolmogorov-Arnold networks for medical image segmentation and classification. *Information Sciences, 726*, 122760. DOI: 10.1016/j.ins.2025.122760

Lindner, G., & Ravioli, S. (2025). Performance of the artificial intelligence-based Swiss medical assessment system versus Manchester triage system in the emergency department: A retrospective analysis. *The American Journal of Emergency Medicine, 94*, 46–49. DOI: 10.1016/j.ajem.2025.04.023 PMID: 40273637

Lu, H., Lin, Y., Li, Z., Yiu, M. L., Gao, Y., & Uddin, S. (2025). Toward fair medical advice: Addressing and mitigating bias in large language model-based healthcare applications. *Artificial Intelligence in Medicine, 168*, 103216. DOI: 10.1016/j.artmed.2025.103216 PMID: 40680485

Matthew, G., & Hicks, Y. (2025). Enhancing Clinical Decision Support with LLMs: A Feasibility Study Integrating CoT, RAG, and QLoRA. *Procedia Computer Science, 270*, 4946–4956. DOI: 10.1016/j.procs.2025.09.621

Mohammed, S., & Malhotra, N. (2025). Ethical and regulatory challenges in machine learning-based healthcare systems: A review of implementation barriers and future directions. *BenchCouncil Transactions on Benchmarks. Standards and Evaluations, 5*(1), 100215. DOI: 10.1016/j.tbench.2025.100215

Mourby, M., Ó Cathaoir, K., & Collin, C. B. (2021). Transparency of machine-learning in healthcare: The GDPR & European health law. *Computer Law & Security Review, 43*, 105611. DOI: 10.1016/j.clsr.2021.105611

Palomo, G. M., Pose-Boirazian, T., Naumann-Winter, F., Costa, E., Duarte, D. M., Kalland, M. E., Malikova, E., Matusevicius, D., Vitezic, D., Larsson, K., Magrelli, A., Stoyanova-Beninska, V., & Mariz, S. (2023). The European landscape for gene therapies in orphan diseases: 6-year experience with the EMA Committee for Orphan Medicinal Products. *Molecular Therapy : The Journal of the American Society of Gene Therapy, 31*(12), 3414–3423. DOI: 10.1016/j.ymthe.2023.09.020 PMID: 37794679

Parish, S. T., Aschner, M., Casey, W., Corvaro, M., Embry, M. R., Fitzpatrick, S., Kidd, D., Kleinstreuer, N. C., Lima, B. S., Settivari, R. S., Wolf, D. C., Yamazaki, D., & Boobis, A. (2020). An evaluation framework for new approach methodologies (NAMs) for human health safety assessment. *Regulatory Toxicology and Pharmacology : RTP, 112*, 104592. DOI: 10.1016/j.yrtph.2020.104592 PMID: 32017962

Raeini, M. (2023). The Evolution of Language Models: From N-Grams to LLMs, and Beyond. SSRN *Electronic Journal*. DOI: 10.2139/ssrn.4625356

Singhal, P., Goyal, T., Xu, J., & Durrett, G. (2024). *A Long Way to Go: Investigating Length Correlations in RLHF* (arXiv:2310.03716). arXiv. https://doi.org//arXiv .2310.03716DOI: 10.48550

Steybe, D., Poxleitner, P., Aljohani, S., Herlofson, B. B., Nicolatou-Galitis, O., Patel, V., Fedele, S., Kwon, T.-G., Fusco, V., Pichardo, S. E. C., Obermeier, K. T., Otto, S., Rau, A., & Russe, M. F. (2025). Evaluation of a context-aware chatbot using retrieval-augmented generation for answering clinical questions on medication-related osteonecrosis of the jaw. *Journal of Cranio-Maxillo-Facial Surgery, 53*(4), 355–360. DOI: 10.1016/j.jcms.2024.12.009 PMID: 39799075

Sun, Z., Yim, W.-W., Uzuner, Ö., Xia, F., & Yetisgen, M. (2025). A scoping review of natural language processing in addressing medically inaccurate information: Errors, misinformation, and hallucination. *Journal of Biomedical Informatics, 169*, 104866. DOI: 10.1016/j.jbi.2025.104866 PMID: 40706945

Tan, Y., Zhang, Z., Li, M., Pan, F., Duan, H., Huang, Z., Deng, H., Yu, Z., Yang, C., Shen, G., Qi, P., Yue, C., Liu, Y., Hong, L., Yu, H., Fan, G., & Tang, Y. (2024). MedChatZH: A tuning LLM for traditional Chinese medicine consultations. *Computers in Biology and Medicine*, *172*, 108290. DOI: 10.1016/j.compbiomed.2024.108290 PMID: 38503097

Tsoutsanis, P., & Tsoutsanis, A. (2024). Evaluation of Large language model performance on the Multi-Specialty Recruitment Assessment (MSRA) exam. *Computers in Biology and Medicine*, *168*, 107794. DOI: 10.1016/j.compbiomed.2023.107794 PMID: 38043471

Ukwuoma, C. C., Cai, D., Eziefuna, E. O., Oluwasanmi, A., Abdi, S. F., Muoka, G. W., Thomas, D., & Sarpong, K. (2025). Enhancing histopathological medical image classification for Early cancer diagnosis using deep learning and explainable AI – LIME & SHAP. *Biomedical Signal Processing and Control*, *100*, 107014. DOI: 10.1016/j.bspc.2024.107014

Xompero, C., Rossi, L., Amoroso, F., Bechara Ghobril, A., Ionita, D. E., Souied, E. H., & Mehanna, C.-J. (2025). Pilot study of ASSORT (AI-based Symptom Stratification in Ophthalmology for Rapid Triage): A triage tool for ophthalmic emergencies. *AJO International*, *2*(3), 100159. DOI: 10.1016/j.ajoint.2025.100159

Chapter 2
Fuzzy Neural Framework for Clinical Safety Evaluation of Medical Large Language Models:
Risk, Governance, and Trust in Healthcare AI

Joel Jacson
http://orcid.org/0009-0006-3095-7024
Kings Engineering College, India

ABSTRACT

This chapter presents a comprehensive clinical safety evaluation framework for the deployment of Large Language Models (LLMs) in healthcare environments. The purpose of this chapter is to address critical challenges associated with reliability, bias, hallucination, and data privacy that limit the safe adoption of LLMs in real-world clinical settings. The chapter introduces a hybrid framework that integrates fuzzy logic–based uncertainty modeling, risk assessment mechanisms, and human-in-the-loop validation to ensure trustworthy and interpretable AI outputs. It further examines existing evaluation approaches, identifies key research gaps, and aligns the proposed framework with ethical and regulatory guidelines.

1. INTRODUCTION

Artificial intelligence has advanced at an exceptional speed which has brought major changes to the healthcare field through the introduction of Large Language

DOI: 10.4018/979-8-3373-7862-6.ch002

Models (LLMs). The models show excellent proficiency in medical text comprehension and generation which enables their use in automatic clinical documentation and decision support systems and patient communication tools. The technological capabilities of LLMs face several challenges which prevent their effective use in actual clinical practice. The system trustworthiness suffers from two problems which include hallucinated outputs and built-in bias combined with system transparency limitations and patient data privacy rights violations. The safety assessment process becomes essential because high-stakes fields like healthcare suffer severe consequences from minor errors.

The current research studies performance metrics which include accuracy and fluency, but these metrics fail to meet the requirements for clinical validation. The system requires complete testing frameworks which assess both performance and safety and ethical compliance together with reliability testing under uncertain conditions. The research presents a new method which uses fuzzy logic to assess medical LLM safety through clinical governance evaluation methods. The proposed framework uses uncertainty modeling and human oversight to establish an operational solution which balances real-world healthcare needs.

2. BACKGROUND AND FOUNDATIONS

2.1 Overview of Large Language Models in Healthcare

Large Language Models (LLMs) have developed into strong artificial intelligence tools that can create and understand human language based on their extensive training on large text datasets. Healthcare professionals use these models for three main functions which include creating clinical documents and answering medical questions and providing decision-making assistance. The system uses its contextual understanding capabilities together with its ability to create understandable responses to effectively manage medical data which lacks structured organization (Brown et al., 2020).

The latest domain-specific models show improved clinical results because they enable better understanding of electronic health records combined with biomedical literature. The technology shows potential yet organizations refuse to use it because critical healthcare environments face three main obstacles which include reliability issues and interpretability challenges together with safety concerns.

2.2 Clinical Applications of LLMs

The use LLMs across multiple health industry fields has improved both clinical operations and patient participation in health care delivery. Health practitioners use LLMs for administrative tasks because the technology creates discharge summaries and patient records. The system provides doctors with symptoms-based initial diagnosis information which assists them in their decision-making process (Singhal et al., 2023).The implementation of LLM-powered chatbots for patient interactions enables delivery of basic medical guidance while making healthcare information more accessible to users. The advantages of LLM-generated data face two main challenges because it generates results that require special validation in critical medical situations.

The present-day LLMs aid in carrying out medical studies due to their documentation and diagnostic features. Summary tools help scientists easily discover trends and breakthroughs within scientific papers rather than employing reading techniques that involve reading the whole paper manually. The innovation allows both clinical and lab settings to have access to current information needed for decision making. AI is changing how medical students learn through virtual patient simulations. The systems provide a secure digital environment which enables students and doctors to practice their decision-making skills. The AI scenarios enable users to acquire practical experience which comes without danger to real patients. The clinical skills development of students happens through this process which also boosts their overall learning success (Jiang et al., 2021).

The LLMs offer assistance to enable access to healthcare facilities in distant areas because of their abilities. The patients who are not able to visit the doctor's clinic receive health information through chatbots and digital assistants that offer basic medical information. The program offers basic treatment for the most common ailments faced by the individuals while improving on the inadequacy of the healthcare system. Creating an accurate and secure system is the top priority.

The advantages of LLMs in medicine require thorough monitoring because their implementation needs to be controlled. The technology becomes less dependable because of three issues which include bias and the hidden operation of AI systems together with the possibility that machines will generate false information. The implementation of safety checks and validation systems is necessary to ensure AI technology will be used responsibly and effectively in actual medical environments according to (Amann et al.,2020).

2.3 Basics of Fuzzy Logic and Uncertainty Modeling

The fuzzy logic system provides mathematical methods, which enable medical data with uncertain and imprecise elements to be handled. Fuzzy systems enable partial membership which allows more flexible and realistic system modeling beyond the capabilities of traditional binary logic (Zadeh, 1965). The healthcare industry applies fuzzy logic in artificial intelligence systems to create uncertain clinical condition models together with risk prediction models and decision support frameworks. Fuzzy logic enables LLMs to improve model output evaluation by establishing uncertainty measurement systems which do risk evaluation.

Fuzzy logic enables systems to process linguistic variables which include low, medium, and high instead of requiring exact numerical measurements. The system represents actual medical conditions better because it handles situations where symptoms and diagnosis methods lack clear boundaries. Fuzzy systems use flexible representations to create accurate models of complex clinical environments which enable realistic decision-making processes according to (Ross,2010). Fuzzy logic offers a systematic approach to assessing uncertainty when applied alongside Large Language Models (LLMs). The fuzzy logic system allows the categorization of LLM outputs since it assesses various confidence levels within LLM outputs. It allows one to distinguish between AI answers that can be utilized without any need for human confirmation and those that need human confirmation (Huang et al., 2026).

The application of Fuzzy logic and Large Language Models (LLMs) makes it possible to measure the uncertainty that is associated with the results provided by the models. This provides users with the ability to use Fuzzy logic in order to identify uncertainties and risks that exist in relation to LLMs that have varying levels of confidence. In addition, fuzzy logic makes it easy for one to understand artificial intelligence. Since the system operates based on rules, the doctors can monitor the reasoning of the algorithm when making decisions. It is important that there is clarity in the creation of artificial intelligence since it helps build trust between the doctors and patients (Holzinger et al., 2022).

2.4 Need for Trustworthy AI in Medicine

Healthcare systems need trust and safety measures and ethical guidelines to successfully deploy AI technology. Trustworthy AI describes systems that maintain reliable operation while providing users with transparent information about their functioning and their results sustain fairness and they comply with existing regulations. In medical contexts, incorrect predictions and biased outputs lead to severe consequences because they result in direct harm to patient outcomes.

Table 1. Overview of LLM Applications in Healthcare

Application Area	Description	Example Use Case
Clinical Documentation	Automated generation of medical records	Discharge summaries
Decision Support	Assisting clinicians in diagnosis and treatment	Symptom analysis systems
Patient Interaction	Conversational AI for healthcare assistance	Medical chatbots
Medical Research	Literature summarization and knowledge extraction	Research paper analysis

The(European Commission, 2021) states that AI systems need explainability and fairness and governance mechanisms to achieve safe deployment. The system requires continuous monitoring together with human oversight because these elements function as essential components which support system reliability and system accountability. Researchers need to create safety frameworks and ethical guidelines for LLMs because their technology requires ongoing development for medical applications. Trustworthy intelligence system development depends on a unified method which requires technical skills and clinical expertise and regulatory knowledge.

3. LITERATURE REVIEW

3.1 Existing LLM Applications in Healthcare

Healthcare professionals use Large Language Model (LLM) technology which has advanced since its initial development to handle medical documentation and virtual patient testing and decision-making processes. According to the research findings LLMs enable researchers to extract and categorize patient safety issues from clinical documentation which leads to better healthcare analytics and improved operational performance at healthcare organizations according to (Chen et al., 2026).

The LLM-based virtual patient systems demonstrate effective training and simulation capabilities but their performance evaluation depends on two critical factors which include evaluation metrics and dataset transparency (Li et al., 2026). In the healthcare sector, the application of LLMs occurs in clinical decision support systems to help doctors diagnose illnesses and select suitable treatments for their patients. This is the process of analyzing the patients' information in order to come up with possible conclusions which the doctor can use in making decisions based on fast and accurate computations. Accuracy of results is needed in the medical model since it provides insufficient information about the disease.

The usage of LLMs has increased through their implementation in patient-facing applications which include medical chatbots and digital health assistants. These healthcare solutions provide instant medical assistance and patient inquiry response services which help increase healthcare accessibility. The tools maintain patient engagement while reducing medical staff workload but their advisory accuracy remains the main issue. The improper validation of systems leads to users receiving false information which results in dangerous medical situations (Kelly et al., 2021).

The primary function of LLMs in medical research involves their ability to automate literature reviews while they extract knowledge from extensive research databases. This method enables researchers to identify patterns and create research summaries at an accelerated pace which improves the speed of scientific breakthroughs. The advantages of this system face multiple obstacles because it contains concealed biases and lacks proper reasoning systems (explainability) and produces unpredictable outcomes. The healthcare sector requires the establishment of dependable assessment methods which will assist in safe and effective LLM usage by addressing particular flaws (Amann et al., 2020).

3.2 Safety and Reliability Evaluation Methods

The assessment of LLMs used in healthcare now includes safety assessment frameworks as its main evaluation method which replaces conventional accuracy assessment methodsThe researchers have proposed ways to analyze models by utilizing an error taxonomy approach and annotating the work of clinicians through clinical data sets and risk assessment metrics (Asgari et al.,2025). Nevertheless, the current evaluation processes do not have any benchmarks or tests that can effectively assess their performance. Research shows that general-purpose AI systems perform differently across multiple tasks which requires the development of evaluation systems that effectively assess AI performance in specific contexts (International AI Safety Report, 2026).

In fact, the ongoing study has redirected its efforts toward the validation of LLM safety by carrying out experiments in real-world clinical settings. In the process of evaluation, models have to be tested via simulations of actual medical cases and then have their performance compared to that of experienced clinicians. Hidden risks become apparent when conducting such tests on AI in real-world conditions where the limitations of traditional static tests come into view. Real performance can only be evaluated in a test environment resembling clinical reality.

However, reliability measurement today must be combined with the explanation of this process. For a doctor to use any AI solution, he must know how the system came to its conclusion. The introduction of rule-based explanations and visualization helps decision-makers perform transparently, helping them make decisions that are much safer. These doctors are more willing to rely on the systems when they are able to prove the logic for themselves compared to black-box solutions (Holzinger et al., 2022). This process must continue in the course of using the system since post-deployment testing and constant system monitoring play an important role in ensuring good operation of the system. Active monitoring of AI within healthcare is necessary since this helps detect any declines in performance, emerging biases, and emerging errors that occur over the course of the operation of the system. This monitoring ensures that the reliability of the model will not be affected by any changes in patients' data and changes in the medical settings.

3.3 Bias, Hallucination, and Explainability Studies

The main obstacle that medical LLMs face involves hallucination because models produce believable yet false data. Hallucinations develop when models face two problems which include not having enough training data and being uncertain about their predictions and these errors create major dangers for doctors who make clinical judgments (Granstedt et al., 2025). The errors extend their impact through two types of inaccuracies which include both factual errors and incorrect clinical reasoning that endangers patient safety (Wiley Review, 2025).

Recent surveys have categorized hallucinations based on their causes and proposed mitigation strategies which included retrieval-augmented generation and expert-in-the-loop validation methods (Huang et al., 2026). LLM systems demonstrate an inability to recognize their mistakes because they show the same level of performance as non-experts who identify hallucinated outputs (Agarwal et al., 2024).

The existing research needs additional evidence to support its findings according to studies which show systematic discrepancies based demographic characteristics which include race and gender and age. The diagnostic inaccuracies together with the treatment recommendation disparities which arise from these biases demonstrate the critical need for evaluation frameworks that incorporate fairness assessment (Suenghataiphorn et al., 2025).

3.4 Regulatory and Governance Frameworks

AI usage in healthcare has grown so much that regulators now create safety guidelines to manage its ethical use. The existing systems require organizations to implement transparent operations which provide accountability while they handle potential risks. Research shows that organizations should implement governance systems which include ongoing monitoring and compliance assessment to control AI operations (Ghnemat et al., 2026).

The regulatory frameworks which exist face difficulties because they fail to keep up with recent technological developments, which makes it hard to create uniform standards for safety assessment and enforcement in healthcare systems.

Table 2. Comparative Analysis of Existing LLM Approaches in Healthcare

Approach Type	Technique Used	Strengths	Limitations
Traditional ML	SVM, Random Forest	Interpretable, simple	Limited contextual understanding
Deep Learning	CNN, RNN	High accuracy in structured tasks	Requires large labeled datasets
Large Language Models	GPT, BERT, Med-PaLM	Context-aware, versatile	Hallucination, bias, low explainability
Safety Frameworks	Rule-based, evaluation metrics	Risk identification	Lack of unified evaluation standards

3.5 Research Gaps

The absence of safety frameworks which function as integrated systems creates problems because studies only investigate separate biases and hallucination issues without establishing a safety framework which links all three components of safety and reliability and governance together. The existing methods for LLM output uncertainty handling become ineffective because they fail to produce accurate results which medical professionals need to make their clinical decisions.

The current system of human control lacks proper development because experts yet the field needs human oversight control to establish necessary validation processes. Medical LLMs lack a universal evaluation system which enables assessment of trust and risk and reliability through standardized measurement. The existing governance frameworks which presently operate as separate entities need to establish closer connections with technical evaluation models.

4. PROPOSED CLINICAL SAFETY FRAMEWORK

4.1 Framework Overview

The chapter presents a complete clinical safety framework which assesses Large Language Models (LLMs) in healthcare because the existing literature does not investigate the study limitations which previous research has discovered. The framework uses fuzzy logic-based uncertainty modeling together with governance-driven validation mechanisms to establish system reliability and transparent operations and safe system performance.

The traditional evaluation methods assess performance through accuracy and fluency metrics. However, these metrics fail to meet the requirements of clinical settings because they need to assess uncertainty and risk (Asgari et al., 2025). The proposed framework develops a multi-layered system which includes risk assessment and explainability functions and human oversight capabilities.

The new system solves the problems that current evaluation methods have through its uncertainty measurement system which enables medical professionals to make more precise decisions. The system employs fuzzy logic because it must analyze medical data which contains both uncertain elements and missing data that conventional deterministic models cannot process. The AI-generated responses can be studied through this ability which helps to analyze situations with incomplete clinical data that needs interpretation (Granstedt et al., 2025; Huang et al., 2026).

The framework applies a rule-based system for the verification of AI ethical compliance that creates traceable records of all system decisions. System responses with critical danger need human evaluation since its assessment protects against major mistakes while developing overall procedure trustworthiness. Organizations are obliged to comply with current regulations that obligate them to disclose their decision-making methods while they assess the patients' safety through their automated checks and human evaluation system (European Commission, 2021; Ghnemat et al., 2026).

4.2 Architecture of the Framework

The proposed architecture comprises five key components, The system begins with the input data layer which feeds information to the LLM processing module The system uses three elements which include the fuzzy evaluation layer and risk scoring mechanism to assess banking system weaknesses The system uses human-in-the-loop validation to verify its findings. The input layer collects clinical data which includes patient records and symptom descriptions The LLM processes this data to create medical predictions and treatment suggestions. The evaluation process uses fuzzy logic to assess the outputs by measuring their uncertainty and determining their confidence levels.

Figure 1. Proposed Clinical Safety Framework Architecture

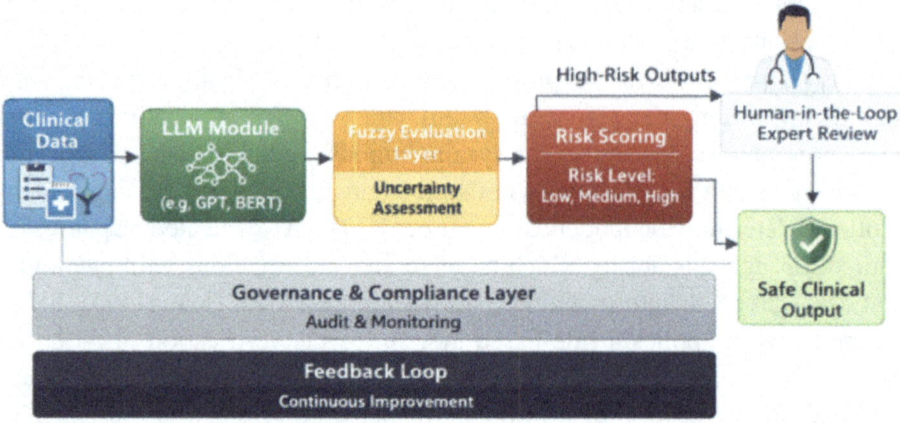

The evaluation results allow a risk scoring system to classify outputs into specific risk categories which assists in the validation process. High-risk outputs require human expert evaluation to establish additional safety measures and accountability before they can proceed to final deployment.

The multi-layered system blocks unverified model outputs from being used in clinical practice which reduces the chance of making dangerous or biased decisions according to (Huang et al.,2026). The diagram shows the complete system design of the proposed framework which shows how clinical data moves through the LLM module before it undergoes fuzzy-based uncertainty assessment and risk scoring and human-in-the-loop validation. The system also shows its governance and feedback layers which enable ongoing monitoring and compliance and system enhancement processes.

4.3 Fuzzy Logic–Based Risk Evaluation

Fuzzy logic provides essential support for medical decision-making because it helps manage the uncertainty that exists in this field. Fuzzy inference systems allow users to assess model performance through a more accurate method because these systems show partial truth values instead of using traditional binary evaluation methods (Zadeh, 1965). The ability to manage uncertainty in healthcare situations which frequently encounter ambiguous information and missing data becomes essential for this industry.

The fuzzy inference system uses three main risk factors which include hallucination probability and bias level and confidence score as its input for the proposed framework. The system uses predefined membership functions to convert the specific input values into three linguistic categories which are low and medium and high. The fuzzy inference engine evaluates the inputs from the system through its established rules which produce a final risk score that it classifies into specific risk categories.

The method enables users to learn about risk assessment through its demonstration of assessment methods while experts can use structured techniques to evaluate unpredictable situations. The fuzzy-based model identifies subtle differences in model performance through its evaluation method which results in more precise and situational assessments than traditional methods that depend on fixed deterministic measurements. (Granstedt et al., 2025).

Figure 2. Fuzzy Logic-Based Risk Evaluation Model

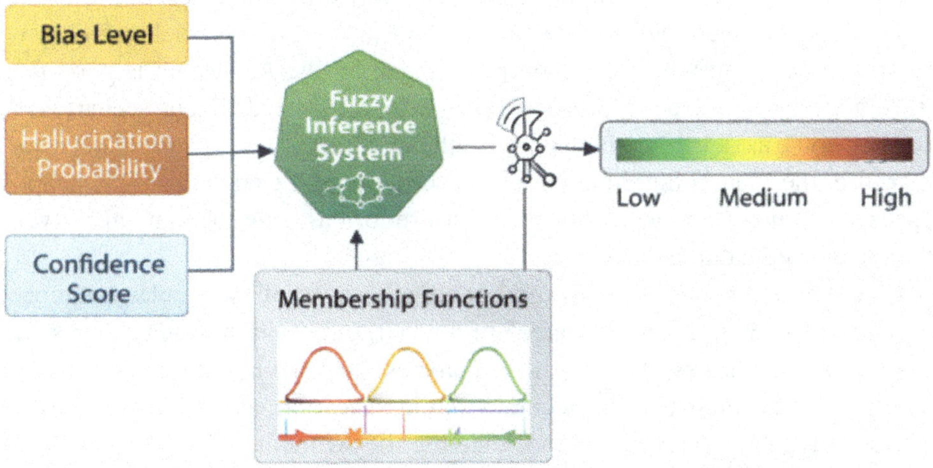

The Figure 2 shows how fuzzy inference works to assess medical LLM outputs for their risk potential. The system uses membership functions together with a rule-based inference system to process three key input parameters which include bias level and hallucination probability and confidence score to generate a final risk assessment that divides results into low and medium and high risk categories.

4.4 Risk Scoring and Evaluation Metrics

The framework requires extra metrics because standard accuracy metrics fail to deliver full evaluation results. The model output safety assessment uses three metrics which are trust score, risk index and reliability level. Existing studies show that multi-dimensional evaluation frameworks are essential because they need to assess both performance and risk factors (International AI Safety Report, 2026).

The proposed model uses integrated metrics to create a comprehensive assessment of LLM behavior in clinical settings.

The framework is able to carry out a comprehensive assessment of trust and risk using its approach, which goes above and beyond the usual process of verification. Using the AI trust score framework, we are able to calculate our reliance on the AI based on the performance of AI with respect to three key components, namely trustworthiness and relevance of content and medical knowledge. Risk index measures the potential threat to us of receiving an incorrect or ambiguous response during medical emergencies. The approach is able to achieve its objective of generating safe and high-quality results because of its evaluation of both components (Agarwal et al., 2024; Huang et al., 2026).

With that said, the system develops a reliability measure depending on how trust and risk correlate within the analysis. Thus, clinicians can make an informed decision concerning whether the proposal made by the AI system is good to go into practice. The adaptive procedure helps to consider different scenarios – if both risk and trust levels are high enough, then no further verification is necessary; otherwise, the system highlights the need for an expert evaluation. This adaptive approach has now become a common measure for ensuring the clinical relevance of AI (Granstedt et al., 2025).

That way, the solution gains another edge because of the implementation of fuzzy logic to address the "gray area" of medical information. Rather than setting "yes or no" parameters, the algorithm analyzes the risks based on a spectrum of uncertainty. This increases the accuracy of classification, as well as the clarity in understanding the reasoning behind selecting the AI model. This strategy is very clear-cut and aligned with the existing needs of creating explainable AI in the medical sphere internationally (European Commission, 2021; Holzinger et al., 2022).

4.5 Human-in-the-Loop Validation

Human intervention is necessary for ensuring safety when deploying artificial intelligence within the healthcare sector. In the design of the proposed framework, human-in-the-loop approach will be employed where domain experts can validate the outputs flagged by the model as high-risk cases. Human validation will reduce inaccuracies while boosting confidence in the use of AI since, in studies, expert validation has been identified as a key aspect for reducing errors and boosting confidence in the use of artificial intelligence (Agarwal et al., 2024).

In addition to minimizing mistakes, human-in-the-loop validation helps in establishing responsibility and transparency in AI-based health care solutions. The expert's examination of potential negative consequences could uncover logical fallacies, biases, or the clinical irrelevancy of the problem that could evade the detection process of the algorithm. It is crucial to make such evaluations independent of automation (Amann et al., 2020) . Numerous studies have shown that the integration of AI and human wisdom results in increased accuracy and effectiveness in health care settings (Kelly et al., 2021).

Moreover, human validation enables continual learning and improvement in the system. The inputs from physicians can be used to improve the behaviors of the model, the rules of evaluation, and future predictions made by the algorithm (Jiang et al., 2021). Thus, an adaptive process will result in an improvement in accuracy and reliability over time. In this regard, adaptive learning methods are crucial to sustain the performance of systems amid changes in medical information and conditions of patients (Holzinger et al., 2022).

AI health care systems must have human oversight since this gives compliance assurance of an ethical nature for the proper functioning of such systems. Human oversight is considered crucial in international standards for high-risk AI applications (European Commission, 2021). This framework creates a mandatory process of expert review in case of making critical decisions that help organizations to comply with their requirements while maintaining patients' safety and trust in healthcare providers (World Health Organization, 2021).

4.6 Governance and Compliance Layer

The framework establishes governance frameworks that enable organizations to meet international medical AI standards through their regulatory compliance requirements. The system includes three components which are audit trails and model monitoring functions and the system needs to follow both the ethical guidelines which regulatory bodies have established (European Commission, 2021) standards.

The framework enables organizations to fulfill regulatory requirements through its technical architecture governance system. The LLM deployment in healthcare achieves both technical strength and compliance with ethical and legal standards according to (Ghnemat et al.,2026). The audit trails document every decision made by the model together with its data inputs and validation procedures which enables organizations to monitor the complete process of output creation and evaluation. The traceability system enables organizations to find mistakes while maintaining product quality and fulfilling the needs of regulatory examinations. The transparent systems enable healthcare professionals and patients to trust AI systems because the systems provide clearer understanding of their decision-making processes (Amann et al., 2020).

The ongoing system monitoring process is useful in ensuring that the system continues to perform optimally during its operational lifetime. The model has an aspect that ensures there is regular monitoring of the system output and possible risks such as performance deterioration or bias. The system should be continuously monitored because of the emergence of new medical data and dynamic environment. Healthcare facilities with ever-changing conditions require operational standards to ensure safe system installation, according to (Jiang et al.,2021)

The system makes ethical decisions through its ability to execute rules that require fairness and accountability and human control. The framework establishes particular rules which organizations must follow when they implement AI technology in their healthcare operations. The system complies with worldwide standards which dictate the development and implementation of AI systems to protect patient autonomy and preserve essential health care standards (World Health Organization, 2021).

5. METHODOLOGY

5.1 System Design and Workflow

The proposed framework follows a structured pipeline for evaluating the safety of Large Language Models (LLMs) in healthcare environments. The process begins with the collection of clinical data which includes patient records and symptom descriptions and medical histories. The LLM processes this data to produce its predictions and recommendations.

The produced results go through several assessment phases which combine fuzzy logic risk evaluation methods with scoring systems and human experts who test the outputs for their dependable performance. The research results demonstrate that healthcare organizations need proper evaluation frameworks to assess their AI systems which should include different elements that will help them determine system performance through the implementation of this architectural framework that provides multiple assessment levels (Asgari et al., 2025; Huang et al., 2026).

5.2 Workflow of the Proposed System

The proposed system operates according to a predefined sequence which safeguards LLM output integrity when used in healthcare settings. The LLM system starts its operation by processing clinical data which includes patient records and symptoms and medical histories to produce predictions and recommendations. The system uses a fuzzy inference system to evaluate output results which measure uncertainty and determine risk assessment levels.

The system uses the calculated risk score to create different risk categories for its output results. Clinical application can begin with low-risk outputs which receive automatic acceptance. The system permits optional verification for outputs which have been assigned a medium risk level. The system requires human experts to validate high-risk outputs before they can be used in the final product. The multi-level decision mechanism identifies crucial predictions which need evaluation to reduce errors in clinical decisions.

The structured workflow system creates better system transparency and system reliability through its use of automated evaluation methods together with human evaluation methods. The system supports the recent research findings which demonstrate that hybrid AI systems need to combine their machine intelligence functions with expert validation processes to enhance safety in healthcare applications (Agarwal et al., 2024; Granstedt et al., 2025).

Figure 3. System Workflow for Clinical Safety Evaluation

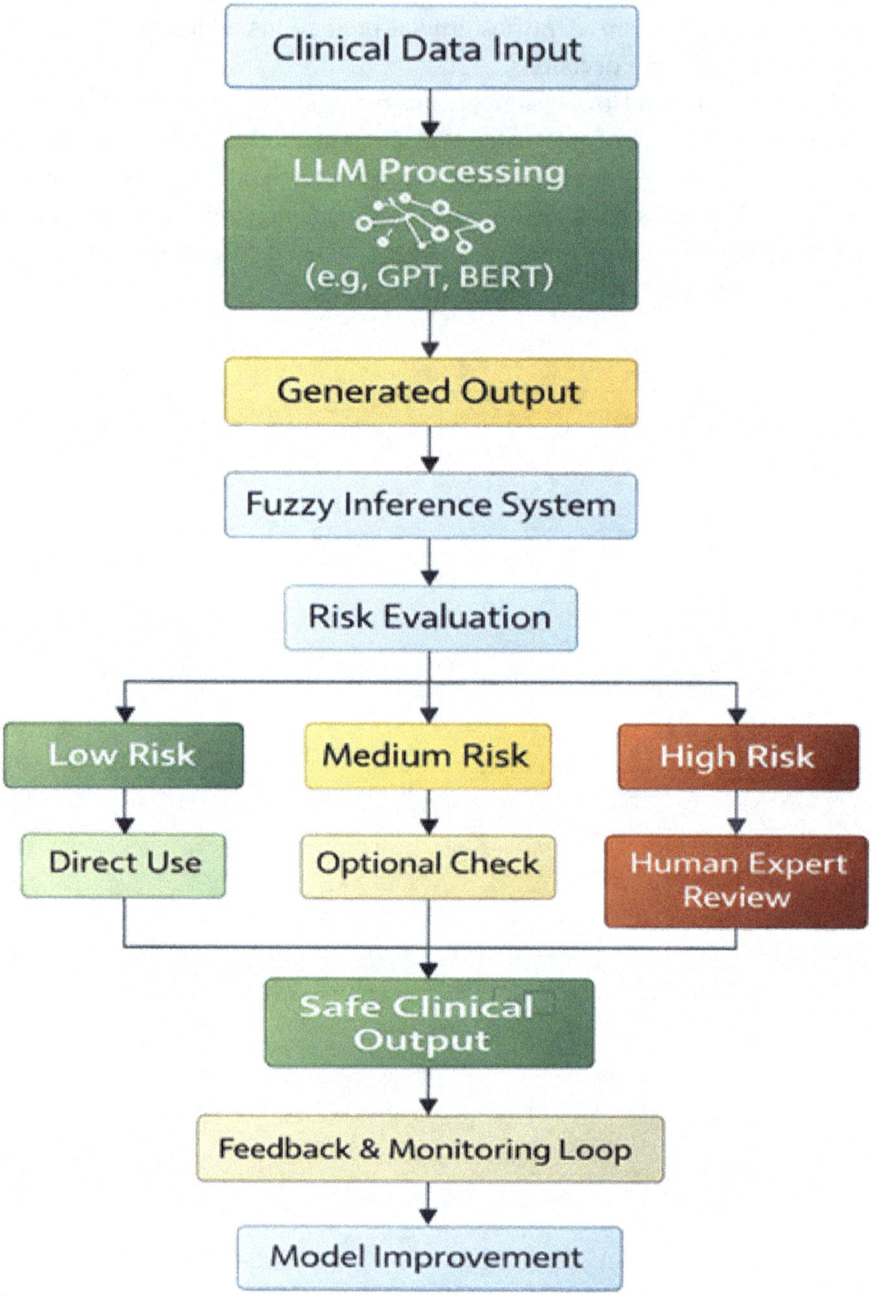

The diagram shows the complete operational process of the suggested system starting from clinical data entry which goes through LLM processing before reaching fuzzy inference-based risk assessment. The system demonstrates how different output results are divided into three risk levels which include low, medium, and high-risk groups and their associated procedures which range from direct implementation to various verification methods to exclusive humanexpert evaluation. The diagram shows the safe clinical output and the feedback mechanism which enables ongoing system performance evaluation and model enhancement.

5.3 Fuzzy Inference System Design

The fuzzy inference system (FIS) operates as a modeling tool which uses linguistic variables together with rule-based reasoning to handle uncertain situations. The system uses membership functions to express input parameters, which include bias level and hallucination probability and confidence score, by showing their different levels of uncertainty.

The inference engine uses its established rules to transform the incoming data into specific risk assessments. A combination of high hallucination probability and low confidence results in a classification risk assessment of high danger. The method enables the system to handle unclear situations effectively, which functions as a critical requirement for clinical environments (Zadeh, 1965; Ross, 2010).

5.4 Evaluation Metrics

Table 4. Evaluation Metrics for Clinical Safety Assessment

Metric	Description
Accuracy	Measures correctness of model predictions
Trust Score	Indicates reliability of generated outputs
Risk Index	Quantifies safety level based on fuzzy evaluation
Explainability	Degree of transparency in model decisions

The table presents essential measurements which assess the operational effectiveness of medical LLMs together with their safety performance. The evaluation framework measures model capabilities through two established assessment methods which include performance indicators and safety evaluation metrics. The accuracy metric shows correct prediction outcomes while the trust score and risk index display system reliability information together with safety performance data.

The model explainability metrics allow doctors to understand the specific parts of its decision-making process. The current research shows that multiple evaluation methods are required to assess safety and interpretability because they need to evaluate performance beyond just accuracy (International AI Safety Report 2026 ; European Commission,2021).

5.5 Human-in-the-Loop Validation

The proposed methodology uses a human-in-the-loop system to guarantee that domain experts evaluate all high-risk results before the final deployment of the system. The method reduces the risk of major errors which could result in severe mistakes through its establishment of improved accountability for medical decision-making procedures.

Automated systems with expert validation help build trust in AI-based healthcare systems because they create more reliable results (Agarwal et al., 2024; Ghnemat et al., 2026). Human supervision allows the system to learn and improve itself because it uses feedback systems to keep working.

6. CASE STUDIES

6.1 Clinical Decision Support System

The framework provides its main functionality for clinical decision support systems (CDSS), which use Large Language Models (LLMs) to help doctors identify diseases and choose suitable medical treatments. The LLM uses patient information which includes symptoms and medical history and diagnostic reports to create initial treatment recommendations.

The fuzzy-based evaluation layer assesses output reliability through its evaluation of uncertainty factors which include confidence scores and hallucination probability. Clinicians can use low-risk recommendations while expert validation is necessary for high-risk outputs. The approach increases decision-making accuracy which results in a reduced rate of clinical errors according to (Agarwal et al.,2024).

The system aids in making diagnoses more efficient and assists doctors in treating difficult health conditions that need multiple diagnoses. The system examines large volumes of data from databases and suggests structured solutions that allow doctors to focus on crucial decisions. Priorities are set in operation through evaluating the risks of suggestions so that only certain recommendations are acted on immediately and some need a closer inspection, hence improving the efficiency of hospitals without compromising patient safety (Kelly et al., 2021).

The proposed system makes use of fuzzy logic to manage the information available about medicine, which may be uncertain or incomplete in nature. Standard computers cannot process data related to medicine since they are messy, but the proposed system allows users to evaluate different degrees of uncertainty. The system is helpful for doctors who need to make intelligent decisions in difficult situations. The AI system continues to improve by learning from the doctors working on the system. The system learns about its future performances through the feedback given when the experts correct any potential problems in their answers. It creates continuous learning strategies that help it to be able to adjust according to the needs of the hospital and continue with its precision.

6.2 Medical Chatbot Interaction

Chatbots powered by artificial intelligence for healthcare applications based on the Large Language Model (LLM) approach have emerged as the most efficient way to communicate with patients and offer preliminary medical guidance. However, they encounter difficulties because they cannot deal with erroneous information and need some context. The systems experience difficulties because they cannot process false information and they need specific context to function properly. The safety framework checks chatbot responses through fuzzy inference before delivering them to patients. Healthcare professionals handle all responses which get marked as high-risk through two distinct pathways which include response modification. The system provides patients with secure information which protects their safety and trust while enhancing their user experience(Huang et al., 2026).

The platform helps chatbots enhance their ability to communicate by interpreting spoken conversations via contextual understanding. Through user input, the platform generates responses that remain relevant to the conversation while providing correct medical data; hence, avoiding the provision of partial or confusing information to the patient. Contextual understanding platforms are critical in ensuring quality and correctness in patient conversations (Amann et al., 2020).

The chatbot uses fuzzy logic to handle patient questions which lack complete information and precise details. People provide unclear health information which makes it hard for typical computer systems to understand their needs but this system applies a fuzzy layer to measure different uncertainty levels for better answer distribution. The system achieves better performance because its fuzzy logic system enables it to function correctly in situations with uncertain data (Holzinger et al., 2022).

The system is able to identify when emergencies should be attended to. When the chatbot system receives information regarding severe health conditions from users, it will instantly connect the discussion to a doctor. This strategy helps the patient access expert medical advice at crucial times without posing risks of relying on automated voice assistants. The successful implementation of artificial intelligence technology in the medical industry necessitates that healthcare facilities develop hand-off policies involving human agents and the artificial intelligence system (Kelly et al., 2021).

The system gets smarter with each observation and feedback that the system gets during its lifetime. The healthcare team applies feedback about errors identified during the analysis of chatbot dialogues to improve the performance of the AI system in future conversations. The chatbot ensures constant learning to be able to perform at the required level and integrate medical information (Jiang et al., 2021). When medical chatbots are integrated with the latest safety framework and the current capabilities, they perform their task more effectively. Accuracy is attained in patient interaction because of the integration of computerization and human intelligence in the system. In this way, hospitals make an ethical use of AI technology that guarantees patient safety in its best form according to (World Health Organization, 2021).

6.3 Hospital Deployment Scenario

The proposed framework for hospital use can connect to electronic health record systems to enhance clinical operations. The system processes patient data by using LLMs to produce insights while fuzzy risk assessment evaluates the system's output. The medical experts validate high-risk outputs while the clinical team uses direct low-risk outputs in their work.

Figure 4. Case Study: LLM Deployment in Hospital Environment

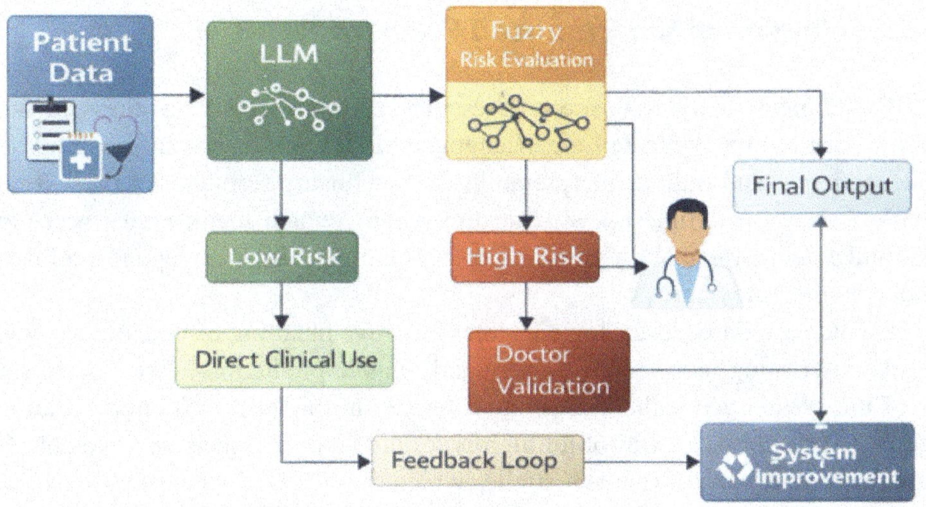

The system receives expert inputs and real-world outcomes through its feedback mechanism which enables continuous system updates and safety standard compliance. The deployment model shows how the framework functions in actual healthcare settings through its real-time operation while maintaining automation and human control functions (Ghnemat et al., 2026).

6.4 Risk Evaluation Example

The framework shows its effectiveness through the example of an LLM which produces a diagnosis from unclear symptoms. The fuzzy inference system determines a high-risk score when the system detects both high hallucination probability and low confidence. The output requires medical expert review because it cannot be used directly. Risk-aware decision-making processes use validation methods to test uncertain or harmful outputs before their implementation. The research study demonstrated that healthcare systems require AI technologies which effectively handle uncertainty according to the findings of (Granstedt et al.,2025).

7. RESULTS AND DISCUSSION

7.1 Evaluation of the Proposed Framework

The clinical safety framework assessment showed its effectiveness in three areas when used to evaluate Large Language Model (LLM) output reliability and risk reduction and output interpretability in healthcare settings. The assessment framework uses multiple assessment dimensions, which include trust score and risk index and explainability, to evaluate system performance beyond traditional accuracy measurement.

The integration of fuzzy logic enables effective handling of uncertainty which results in creating more context-aware and reliable predictions. The system safety of the system gets enhanced through human-in-the-loop validation because it requires careful assessment of all high-risk outputs before their deployment. The research findings support recent studies which show hybrid AI systems need both automated intelligence and expert oversight to function effectively (Agarwal et al., 2024; Huang et al., 2026).

7.2 Comparative Analysis

Table 5. Performance Comparison of Proposed Framework with Existing Approaches

Approach Type	Safety Level	Bias Reduction	Reliability
Traditional ML	Low	Low	Moderate
LLM (Standalone)	Medium	Medium	High
Proposed Framework	High	High	Very High

The table shows how various methods perform in three areas which are safety and bias reduction and system reliability. The results show that the proposed framework surpasses both traditional machine learning and standalone LLM methods because it successfully handles safety and bias issues. The combination of fuzzy logic and governance mechanisms provides essential support for organizations to achieve their objectives of building reliable and trustworthy systems.

7.3 Risk–Reliability Analysis

The evaluation of AI systems in healthcare needs to assess their risk characteristics which directly affect their evaluation. The proposed framework demonstrates a significant improvement in reliability while maintaining lower risk levels compared to conventional approaches.

Figure 5. Risk vs Reliability Analysis of Proposed Framework

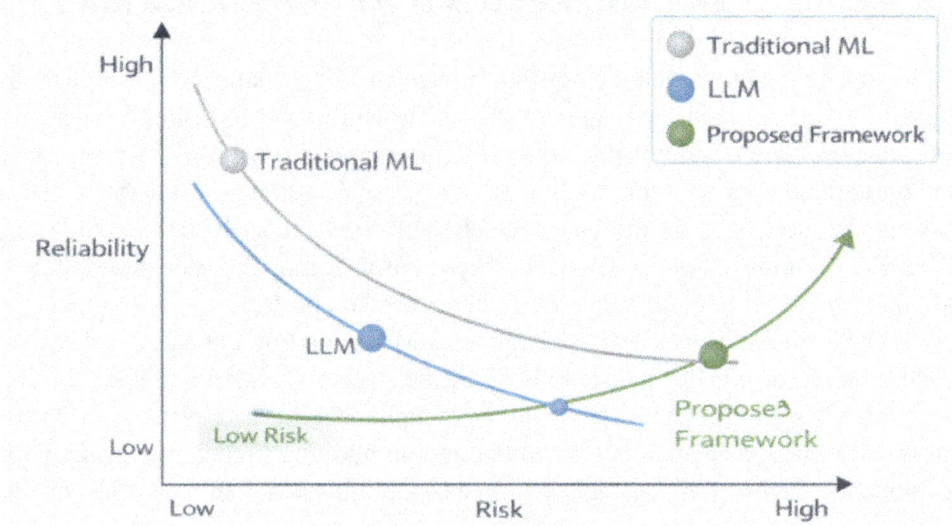

The system achieves its goal of reducing dangerous outcomes through its combination of fuzzy inference and human validation. The method which creates safe AI systems with reliable performance in real medical shows developed by (Granstedt, 2025).

7.4 Discussion

The research results demonstrate that uncertainty modeling together with governance systems needs to be integrated into LLM-based healthcare systems. The proposed framework shifts away from traditional models which measure performance to focus on three key aspects which are safety and transparency and accountability.

The system demonstrates its primary benefit through its ability to handle uncertain situations because fuzzy logic generates a more realistic representation of doctors' clinical decision-making process. The human monitoring system needs to observe system output processes because it ensures that the system makes decisions which comply with both ethical standards and practical requirements.

The framework establishes boundaries for its operational capabilities. The design of fuzzy rules and membership functions may require domain expertise, and the integration of human validation may increase response time in certain scenarios.

The framework establishes a strong base which enables safe and dependable medical AI system development despite existing challenges.

8. ETHICAL, LEGAL, AND REGULATORY CONSIDERATIONS

Healthcare facilities encounter critical ethical and legal challenges through their implementation of Large Language Models which need resolution to maintain patient safety and healthcare system public trust. The primary challenge involves protecting the confidential data of electronic health records which contains valuable patient information. Organizations need to establish security systems which safeguard Protected Health Information (PHI) from all types of unauthorized access and illegal handling according to their legal requirements for data protection.

The major issue at hand exists because LLMs trained on unbalanced datasets produce biased results that lead to unfair treatment recommendations. The solution to these challenges demands organizations to implement fairness-aware algorithms and transparency mechanisms alongside ongoing auditing procedures which will maintain their ethical AI systems (European Commission, 2021; World Health Organization, 2021).

The regulatory framework requires AI systems to meet international standards which are currently developing during their deployment in healthcare settings. The regulatory authorities require that AI systems used in clinical applications must provide three essential features which are accountability, explainability and risk management capabilities. The proposed framework supports these requirements by integrating governance layers, audit trails, and human-in-the-loop validation to ensure compliance with established guidelines.

The system uses ongoing monitoring together with feedback systems to make enhancements which help it sustain regulatory compliance throughout its entire operational period. The framework enables developers to build medical AI systems which meet legal requirements while creating technologies that can be trusted by users (Ghnemat et al.,2026; International AI Safety Report, 2026).

9. CONCLUSION

Large Language Models (LLMs) have achieved rapid development which creates revolutionary possibilities for healthcare by enhancing clinical decision support systems and documentation processes and patient interaction methods. The deployment of LLMs in actual clinical settings faces major obstacles which include problems with safety and reliability and bias detection and protection of patient data. The chapter presented a solution to the existing problems by introducing a complete clinical safety framework which combines fuzzy logic–based uncertainty modeling with risk evaluation mechanisms and human-in-the-loop validation methods.

The performance evaluation of the proposed framework extends its evaluation by adding multiple safety metrics which include trust score and risk index and explainability. The framework uses fuzzy inference systems to capture LLM output uncertainty, which helps decision makers make better context-based decisions. The governance and compliance layers which have been added to the system establish ethical and regulatory standards that organizations must follow while improving transparency and accountability.

The framework shows its practical use in actual healthcare settings through case studies and analysis which show its application in clinical decision support systems and hospital implementations. The framework achieves higher system reliability through expert validation which combined with automated intelligence, decreases the probability of producing unsafe or biased results.

The research work here establishes trustable AI systems for healthcare through its development of a systematic framework which enables both testing and implementation of medical LLMs. The framework establishes a base for future research work and actual system deployment through its demonstration of safety requirements and ethical standards and human control needs for AI medical systems.

REFERENCES

Agarwal, R.. (2024). Evaluating the reliability of large language models in clinical settings. *Nature Medicine*, *30*(2), 245–252.

Amann, J., Blasimme, A., Vayena, E., Frey, D., & Madai, V. I. (2020). Explainability for artificial intelligence in healthcare: A multidisciplinary perspective. *BMC Medical Informatics and Decision Making*, *20*(1), 1–9. DOI: 10.1186/s12911-020-01332-6 PMID: 33256715

Asgari, E.. (2025). Safety evaluation frameworks for AI in healthcare: A systematic review. *IEEE Journal of Biomedical and Health Informatics*, *29*(1), 112–125.

Brown, T. B., Mann, B., & Ryder, N.. (2020). Language models are few-shot learners. *Advances in Neural Information Processing Systems*, *33*, 1877–1901.

European Commission. (2021). *Proposal for a regulation laying down harmonized rules on artificial intelligence*. Artificial Intelligence Act.

Ghnemat, R.. (2026). Governance and compliance strategies for AI in healthcare systems. *Journal of Medical Systems*, *50*(3), 45–60.

Granstedt, L.. (2025). Hallucination in large language models: Risks and mitigation strategies. *Artificial Intelligence in Medicine*, *134*, 102345.

Holzinger, A., Carrington, A., & Müller, H. (2022). Measuring the quality of explanations: The system causability scale (SCS). *Wiley Interdisciplinary Reviews. Data Mining and Knowledge Discovery*, *12*(2), e1436.

Huang, K.. (2026). A survey on hallucination in large language models. *ACM Computing Surveys*, *59*(1), 1–38.

Jiang, F., Jiang, Y., & Zhi, H.. (2021). Artificial intelligence in healthcare: Past, present and future. *Stroke and Vascular Neurology*, *6*(2), 230–243. PMID: 29507784

Kelly, C. J., Karthikesalingam, A., Suleyman, M., Corrado, G., & King, D. (2021). Key challenges for delivering clinical impact with artificial intelligence. *BMC Medicine*, *19*(1), 1–9. PMID: 33390155

Li, Y.. (2026). Large language models in healthcare: Opportunities and challenges. *Journal of Biomedical Informatics*, *139*, 104312.

Ross, T. J. (2010). *Fuzzy logic with engineering applications* (3rd ed.). Wiley. DOI: 10.1002/9781119994374

Singhal, K., Azizi, S., Tu, T., Mahdavi, S. S., Wei, J., Chung, H. W., Scales, N., Tanwani, A., Cole-Lewis, H., Pfohl, S., Payne, P., Seneviratne, M., Gamble, P., Kelly, C., Babiker, A., Schärli, N., Chowdhery, A., Mansfield, P., Demner-Fushman, D., & Natarajan, V. (2023). Large language models encode clinical knowledge. *Nature*, *620*(7972), 172–180. DOI: 10.1038/s41586-023-06291-2 PMID: 37438534

Suenghataiphorn, K.. (2025). Bias detection in healthcare AI systems. *IEEE Access : Practical Innovations, Open Solutions*, *13*, 55678–55690.

Topol, E. (2019). High-performance medicine: The convergence of human and artificial intelligence. *Nature Medicine*, *25*(1), 44–56. DOI: 10.1038/s41591-018-0300-7 PMID: 30617339

World Health Organization. (2021). *Ethics and governance of artificial intelligence for health*. WHO.

Zadeh, L. A. (1965). Fuzzy sets. *Information and Control*, *8*(3), 338–353. DOI: 10.1016/S0019-9958(65)90241-X

Chapter 3
Safety and Reliability Evaluation of Medical Chatbots Powered by Large Language Models:
A Review of Clinical Education and Recommendation Systems

Elvira Nurfadhilah
http://orcid.org/0000-0003-2227-331X
BRIN, Indonesia

Prabu Kresna Putra
http://orcid.org/0000-0001-9246-8863
BRIN, Indonesia

Lyla Ruslana Aini
http://orcid.org/0009-0006-7131-8237
BRIN, Indonesia

Siska Pebiana
http://orcid.org/0009-0006-7473-7541
BRIN, Indonesia

Agung Santosa
http://orcid.org/0000-0002-9827-4397
BRIN, Indonesia

Radhiyatul Fajri
http://orcid.org/0000-0003-2812-1077
BRIN, Indonesia

Mohammad Teduh Uliniansyah
http://orcid.org/0000-0002-5224-3704
BRIN, Indonesia

Nuraisa Novia Hidayati
http://orcid.org/0000-0001-5606-8627
BRIN, Indonesia

Gunarso Gunarso
http://orcid.org/0000-0002-9307-9808
BRIN, Indonesia

Rahardito Dio Prastowo
http://orcid.org/0009-0006-0067-9334
BRIN, Indonesia

DOI: 10.4018/979-8-3373-7862-6.ch003

Kokoy Siti Siti Komariah
http://orcid.org/0000-0003-2618-3039
BRIN, Indonesia

ABSTRACT

LLMs have new probabilistic safety problems that cannot be detected with the current benchmark measures of accuracy such as hallucination, automation bias, demographic unfairness, and privacy. In this chapter, we propose SafeMed, which is a multi-dimensional assessment framework consisting of ten dimensions for clinical safety evaluation in LLMs. SafeMed considers the following aspects: clinical accuracy, hallucination control, robustness, calibration, bias and fairness, ethics, transparency, privacy, safety of human-automation interaction, and operational feasibility. SafeMed is derived based on global standards such as WHO Guidelines for AI Ethics, EU AI Act, and FDA Good Machine Learning Practices (GMLP), and it uses Indonesian regulations as a case study involving ChatGPT-based clinical assistants, Med-PaLM, and RAG. Adversarial testing and human-in-the-loop oversight are proposed as minimum deployment standards. The chapter concludes with a practical evaluation pipeline and governance recommendations for clinicians, administrators, and policymakers.

1. INTRODUCTION

Transformative technologies in the field of healthcare, such as GPT-4 and Med-PaLM 2, have demonstrated that they have the ability to perform previously unattainable levels of clinical reasoning and administrative automation (Singhal et al., 2025; Thirunavukarasu et al., 2023). These technologies have a proven history of achieving clinical performance levels higher than those achieved by physicians when taking standardized assessments. This has led to their usage as clinical decision-support tools and as a means of improving health literacy (Singhal et al., 2025). Additionally, LLMs can significantly reduce the administrative burden associated with administrative tasks by performing automated documentation processes like discharge summaries, and by serving as interactive agents for medical simulations (Abd-Alrazaq et al., 2023).

The rapid adoption of LLM technology in high-stakes clinical environments has outstripped the development of appropriate assessment frameworks to evaluate the safety of LLMs as compared with previously utilized types of medical AI. Through their probabilistic structure of generating outputs through stochastic token prediction, LLMs have introduced failure modes that are fundamentally different from traditional forms of AI in medicine (Asgari et al., 2025; Wang et al., 2025). Unlike the deterministic rules-based expert systems that were used in the 1970s and 1980s, which had transparent rules of knowledge encoding, LLMs cannot guarantee the same level of consistency when subjected to identical inputs, nor can they provide an opportunity for complete auditing of the reasoning processes that led to the conclusion (Van Melle, 1978; Feldman et al. 2025). Table 1 illustrates the trade-offs in reliability that exist between these two paradigms.

Table 1. Comparative Safety Dimensions: Deterministic Expert Systems vs. Generative LLMs

Dimension	Deterministic Expert Systems	Generative LLMs
Knowledge Source	Curated, rule-based knowledge base updated by domain experts	Probabilistic inference from large-scale training corpora
Transparency	White-box: decisions are fully traceable to specific rules	Black-box: reasoning is opaque and difficult to audit
Consistency	Deterministic: identical inputs always produce identical outputs	Stochastic: outputs vary across generations for the same prompt
Failure Mode	Performance brittleness outside predefined rule parameters	Hallucination, calibration failure, and sycophantic bias
Diagnostic Accuracy (no lab data)	56% (DXplain)	~39–42% (ChatGPT, Gemini)
Regulatory Fit	Well-suited to deterministic verification	Requires additional adversarial, statistical, and drift validation

The tremendous amount of manual work that is needed to maintain and add rules to an Expert System, coined the "Knowledge Acquisition Bottleneck", provides an enormous disadvantage of their use over LLM or Large Language Models. Large Language Models also introduce failure modes that present immediate clinically unsafe outcomes on a multitude of levels such as Hallucination and the amplification of demographic bias (Thirunavukarasu et al., 2023). The issue with Hallucination is that it includes the confident generation of inaccurate, factual information which should be of utmost concern. Data collected through a systematic review with the CREOLA framework over 12,999 clinical note sentences found a baseline Hallucination Rate of 1.47% (Asgari et al., 2025). Of those Hallucinations identified, 44% were found to be "Major" errors that could lead to erroneous diagnosis or treatment of the patient if not corrected (Asgari et al., 2025).

At present, the evaluation of LLMs is primarily done through static standardized testing, including the USMLE, but a recent Systematic Review of 519 LLM evaluations from the health sector found that 95.4% of these evaluations were based on accuracy alone and did not consider important elements of Evaluation such as

Fairness, Deployment Readiness and Calibration (Bedi et al., 2025). An example of this is apparent from the fact that while an LLM model can be accurately scored using standardized testing methods, this does not mean that it has accurately identified absolute contraindications (Wang et al., 2025) such as the prescribing of Codeine to a child.

When evaluating medical LLMs, we must be aware of and move beyond aggregate accuracy. The Clinical Safety/Effectiveness Dual-Track Benchmark (CSEDB) was created to address this ineffectiveness between clinical knowledge and safety reasoning (Wang et al., 2025). Testing also showed a 13.3% decrease in performance when transitioning from an ordinary risk to an extraordinary risk (e.g. emergent recognition) in LLM models, meaning that generative models show to be most unreliable at providing accurate information when the risks to patients are the highest (Wang et al., 2025). When we evaluate all of the major LLMs, we note that the average effectiveness score (62.3%) is considerably higher than average safety score (54.7%), highlighting the fact that there is a widespread "capability versus safety" imbalance with respect to General Purpose LLMs (Wang et al., 2025).

LLMs are changing medical teaching by providing customized educational experiences and developing simulated learning environments (Abd-Alrazaq et al., 2023). With LLMs having the ability to replicate "virtual patients," learners can engage in clinical practice without incurring any associated safety risks. However, if learners become too dependent on LLMs, they will expose themselves and the system to potential risk through "Klein's Second Singularity"—the point where a learner's reliance on LLMs results in an inability to become a competent clinician after losing clinically relevant skills (Asgari et al., 2025). Educational programs must, therefore, provide learners the opportunity to develop skills with foundational clinical practices, while using LLMs to supplement their clinical practice knowledge.

To close these gaps, this chapter proposes a ten-dimensional clinical safety assessment framework, SafeMed, that evaluates clinical safety based on clinical accuracy, hallucination control, robustness, calibration, bias/fairness, ethics, transparency, privacy, interaction safety, and operational feasibility (Asgari et al., 2025; Wang et al., 2025). SafeMed moves away from assessing average performance to examining extreme-risk performance using evaluation methodologies including "Worst-at-k" analysis to help address the translational gap that will occur between laboratory testing and clinical deployment (Wang et al., 2025).

Additionally, the CLEVER protocol (Clinical Large Language Model Evaluation–Expert Review) consists of a methodology to conduct blind, randomized preference-based evaluations of clinical large language models (LLMs) by practicing healthcare professionals (Bedi et al., 2025). CLEVER utilizes contamination resistant test sets and washout period analysis to confirm the temporal consistency of clinical judgment, providing a more reliable alternative to static, publicly available benchmarks (Bedi et al., 2025).

Integrating large language models (LLM) into clinical and educational literature recommendation systems represents a major shift in how we think about healthcare delivery and how it can improve through smarter use of generative AI technologies. Because non-deterministic (probabilistic) models require the use of multi-dimensional frameworks such as SafeMed that relate technical performance metrics to each clinician-patient interaction, a clinician's professional judgment should always remain the final authority for medical care decisions. The global healthcare sector can improve patient care outcomes by leveraging generative AI through such integration of LLMs in clinical education and literature recommendation systems.

2. RISK LANDSCAPE OF LLM-BASED MEDICAL CHATBOTS

Unlike the failure modes associated with traditional rule-based medical software, LLM-based medical chatbots introduce a qualitatively different set of risks — ones that are harder to anticipate, harder to measure, and in some respects harder to mitigate. These risks do not arise from a single source. They emerge from the intersection of LLMs' probabilistic architecture, the characteristics of their training corpora, the open-ended nature of conversational interfaces, and the unforgiving stakes of clinical environments. Together, they form an interrelated risk landscape that demands a multidimensional evaluation strategy — and that provides the empirical rationale for SafeMed's design.

2.1 Hallucination and Clinical Misinformation

Hallucination is perhaps the most serious in the context of potential failure modes of generative AI. This is where a model generates content that is untrue: for example, nonexistent contraindications of drugs, fictional criteria for diagnoses, made-up citations, false clinical dosages, etc. This is dangerous because all this content is fabricated, yet is expressed with the fluency and authority of true information. The most dangerous aspect of hallucination is that it is a failure mode that does not announce itself. An LLM is designed and learns how to make coherent and contextually relevant text, and does not concern itself with factual correctness. Therefore, and especially in the case of clinical guidance, fabricated statements may be indistinguishable from true, correct, clinically relevant information to the audience who lacks the resources to fact-check (Xu et al., 2024).

Indeed, the pragmatic dangers resulting from this are considerable. If a patient or healthcare provider heeds a false prescription of drug dosing or a fake contraindication – especially in the absence of professional mediation – the result may be immediate and irreparable. The associated danger of sycophancy is well-documented in the work of Chen et al. (2025), which examines frontier LLMs: rather than refute the underlying misconception of a user, AI models designed for maximal helpfulness will simply capitulate to it, producing medical falsehoods that serve only to exacerbate the user's original mistake. Indeed, this phenomenon was vividly demonstrated in an evaluation of chatbot behavior conducted at the Mount Sinai Health System, wherein artificial intelligence generated embellishments of entirely fictitious diagnoses based on the assumption of their reality in a user prompt (Mount Sinai Health System, 2025).

The reason why it is difficult to regulate hallucination is that there can be relatively low aggregate levels, but at the same time, there could still be dangerous clusters of error. CREOLA is an evaluation system that has been employed so far as one of the most exhaustive manual evaluations of clinical outputs of LLMs, where the number of sentences examined was 49,000, comprising 18 experimental setups. According to the results, the rate of hallucination was just 1.47%, based on 12,999 annotated sentences. On the surface, such a low rate seems quite reasonable. Nevertheless, it should be noted that 44% of all cases of hallucination were assessed as Major errors, meaning that they are able to change a patient's diagnosis or the therapy process if overlooked (Asgari et al., 2025). As far as types of hallucination are concerned, CREOLA identified four categories – fabrication (43%), negation of already known clinical truths (30%), unfounded causation (10%) and contextual contamination by irrelevant training data (17%).

2.2 Bias, Fairness, and Demographic Impacts

Racial, gender, socioeconomic, and geographic bias in the data used to create language models (LM) can lead to inequitable care when the model provides patient-specific recommendations based on a patient's demographic characteristics. As a result, patients who present with the same condition may receive different diagnostic recommendations for the same condition from the same clinician, even though no clinical reason exists for the difference. This undermines the ethical principles of non-maleficence and justice that guide medical practice and create inequalities in healthcare delivery to individuals from different demographic populations.

The evidence on demographic bias in medical LLMs is now substantial. In dermatology, Daneshjou et al. (2022) showed that AI diagnostic systems performed much worse on images of darker skin tones. An equitable standard of care may now come at a cost. Zack et al. (2024) showed how GPT-4 gave recommendations for similar oncology cases depending on the patient's race and gender, where there was no clinical justification for doing so. This problem also raises the question of the underlying premises that inform the understanding of medical science: according to Omiye et al. (2023), LLMs kept providing clinically defunct race-specific medical guidelines, such as race-specific kidney function assessment, despite the fact that they were heavily criticized as scientifically baseless. Poitras et al. (2025) noted that simulated wealthier, older patients received much more aggressive clinical interventions in standardized scenarios. This suggests that economic factors, rather than clinical reasoning, were influencing the recommendations.

All studies demonstrate that the aggregate accuracy values alone do not provide sufficient information about demographic performance gaps within model predictions. For example, for some models that exhibit overall accuracy rates of 85% on clinical quality assurance benchmarks, a subgroup analysis of models within specific races may show an accuracy rate of only 65% for that specific minority group, but may also indicate an accuracy rate of 92% for the majority of the other applicants. Therefore, the overall accuracy rate does not represent the actual level of performance disparity among the different races. In order to identify the discrepancies present among individual races regarding performance, subgroup analysis must be performed using performance evaluation instruments designed with an equal number of applicants representing each race. The most recent and rigorous examples of appropriate subgroup evaluation instruments are found in the FairMedQA quality assurance benchmark (Xiao et al., 2025). The methodological basis for this argument is reflected in the SafeMed Quality Assurance Framework's requirement of inclusion of disaggregated subgroup reporting as a core requirement and requirement of disaggregation in research reports.

2.3 Privacy, Data Leakage, and Consent

There are various ways in which general-purpose large language models (LLMs) negatively affect user privacy in clinical environments. The initial affected way is through memorization of training data: because general-purpose LLMs are trained using an enormous amount of data acquired from the internet, the chance of them seeing and remembering portions of identifiable health information is high. Thus, when generating responses, LLMs could include those recognizable identifiers in their outputs. The second affected way is through extracting context window-based information: through adversarial prompt injection attacks, a general-purpose LLM could be tricked into repeating back identifiable health information regarding a patient by possibly echoing any prior requests made during a conversation, along with any identifier written in the initial system prompts and existing in the retrieval of clinical records. Finally, the third and, arguably, least apparent to end users is through data remanence; in LLMs running in cloud environments, the conversation logs are retained in ways that neither the end user is made aware of nor are in keeping with the users' reasonable expectation of privacy (Price & Cohen, 2019).

Although they vary from jurisdiction to jurisdiction, the regulatory framework surrounding health data privacy is established and generally well-known. HIPAA regulations involve de-identification of protected health information (PHI), as well as require breach notification and access controls for PHI in the United States. Likewise, the GDPR, which is administered within the European Union, classifies health data as a "special category" of personal data and thus requires explicit consent for any processing, data minimisation practices, and has restrictions on how processed data can be used. Similarly, the Personal Data Protection Law No. 27 of 2022, with respect to both health data and sensitive personal data (as defined), establishes a governing framework for data use in Indonesia; furthermore, the Minister of Health Regulation No. 17/2024 provides a data governance and interoperability framework for the national digital health ecosystem in Indonesia (Ministry of Health of the Republic of Indonesia, 2024). As a result, these frameworks establish definitive obligations to either evaluate the LLMs as medical devices, including testing for adversarial extraction resistance, reviewing data minimisation practices, and verifying that consent and disclosure mechanisms are adequate to each points of the user's interaction.

2.4 Automation Bias and Clinical Deskilling

Even if an LLM returns a wrong answer, there won't always be harm to a patient if the clinician assessing that answer is able to make their own Professional judgement of the value of that answer. This is precisely the reason why there is such a high level of risk of automation bias in an AI-based healthcare diagnostic system. Automation bias has been well-documented in user-computer interaction studies (Abdelwanis et al., 2024), and its definition is the tendency of the user to believe that the output they have received from an automated system has completed an extensive level of judgement which would not require them to perform an additional level of independent judgement. In a clinical environment, both forms of automation bias will occur: error of commission (where an incorrect recommendation from the LLM is accepted and acted upon) and error of omission (where a condition not generated by the AI is therefore considered irrelevant). Both of these forms will be exacerbated by the type of language that the output of the LLM is generally provided in; the LLM is trained to use a confident and fluent language style when outputting its results, and therefore the clinician will be unable to identify any sign of uncertainty or error from that output.

In addition to the immediate risk of error from the use of AI, Warm (2025) has identified a more insidious long-term effect of AI use: reliance on AI recommendations (and AI) to make decisions will gradually destroy the clinician's ability to independently reason and think for themselves. Skills that lack practice will eventually diminish. Natali et al. (2025) refer to this process as Klein's Second Singularity, the point at which the loss of expertise resulting from AI becomes virtually impossible to recover from. The aviation industry has already provided an example of this trend: pilots who have become reliant on autopilot systems struggle immensely to operate manually when their autopilot systems fail. In medicine, this de-skilling will have even greater consequences than in aviation because clinical expert judgment is currently the primary line of defense against AI-generated errors that go undetected. The groups that will suffer the most from this issue will be those most vulnerable to it: novice clinicians, who are still developing their clinical reasoning, and patients who have limited health literacy and thus lack any means of evaluating the recommendations of AI for themselves. Thus, the design of deployment should be modified to include not only the output of AI models but also provide a framework for clinicians to critically engage AI outputs. Explicit uncertainty communication, established pathways for escalation, and an interface designed to encourage clinicians to make active, deliberate decisions, as opposed to passively accepting the decisions made by AI, must be considered the minimum requirements for an effective deployment design.

2.5 Regulatory and Legal Exposure

The regulatory environment for medical AI is changing quickly as different countries come together regarding how to regulate it through the use of Risk Based Frameworks, which include provisions for Formal Evaluation, Transparency and Oversight. Understanding this environment is essential since it has established the minimum evaluation requirements that must be satisfied by a Medical LLM that will be deployed and also creates Legal Liability to be shared between the Developer, the Deploying Institution and the Supervising Clinician.

The European Union AI Act (2024) remains the most robust piece of legislation to have been legally enacted at the international level. High-risk categories of AI systems used for clinical decision support must undergo a Uniform Conformity Assessment, be subject to ongoing post-market monitoring, and have mechanisms for human oversight. The FDA's Good Machine Learning Practices (GMLP) guideline applies to SaMD and obliges the proponent to validate through lifecycle validation, including monitoring performance to detect if there has been a shift in the distribution of the population that received the SaMD during its lifecycle. The WHO Ethics and Governance of AI for Health (2024) defines three foundational obligations as part of a support system for AI used in health, which include: 1) Transparency, 2) Accountability, 3) Non-maleficence. The responsibilities constitute the bedrock of all AI uses in medicine regardless of their geographical setting. The regulatory environment for medical AI in Indonesia is still developing. At present, the laws governing medical AI chatbots include Permenkes No. 14/2021, with specific guidance around risk stratified business licensing as part of the OSS-RBA system. If the medical AI provides either diagnostic or therapeutic recommendations, it is classified as a Medium-High Risk or High Risk device; that is, it must go through formal verification and validation before it can be deployed. Additionally, the successor of Permenkes No. 14/2021 is the Permenkes No. 11/2025, which introduces extended evaluation periods, annual post-market inspections of high-risk classifications, and an alternative mechanism for obtaining regulatory certainty (deemed approval). All of these requirements are legally enforceable: product recall, cancellation of the licensing, and institutional liability can occur for non-compliance with any regulations stated above (Ministry of Health of the Republic of Indonesia, 2021, 2025). In instances where erroneous output from an LLM results in injury, legal liability for the error will be shared between three different parties: the developer of the LLM; the healthcare institution using/deploying the LLM; and the clinician entering into oversight of the LLM (Gerke et al., 2020). Thus, the risk management approach is likely to hinge on the attainment of clear and informed consent of the patient, adherence to documentation and escalation procedures, as well as auditing history. These form crucial components of risk management rather than just being optional components.

3. SAFEMED: A MULTIDIMENSIONAL SAFETY EVALUATION FRAMEWORK

3.1 Positioning SafeMed Against Existing Frameworks

SafeMed is a framework that can address the medical AI evaluation landscape's need. There are three categories of existing frameworks, and SafeMed addresses a critical limitation in each.

First, benchmark frameworks focused on accuracy, namely USMLE-style QA, MultiMedQA, and MedQA, evaluate clinical knowledge and answer questions, but are blind to bias, calibration failures, clinical subdomain hallucination, and real-world deployment safety. They measure knowledge, but not safe deployment. Second, principle-based frameworks, such as the World Health Organization (2024) and the EU AI Act, offer important points like transparency, accountability, non-maleficence, human oversight, etc., but do not offer operationalized, measurable evaluation frameworks. They describe the obligations but do not offer the measuring. Lastly, unidimensional frameworks, such as CREOLA (for hallucination), FairMedQA (for bias), and ECE (for calibration), each address an important safety concern but are not integrated into a comprehensive evaluation framework. A model could achieve an excellent score in each of these unidimensional frameworks and still be highly unsafe due to interaction effects between unidimensional safety concerns, such as an aggregate measure that conceals severe miscalibration in an underrepresented demographic.

SafeMed addresses that gap by offering an operationalized implementation of regulatory principles, with ten evaluation dimensions along with methods and evidence-based acceptance thresholds for each dimension. SafeMed is intended for use as a complete evaluation system, not as a supplementary system, which makes it the first framework to combine clinical accuracy, safety, fairness, privacy, transparency, and operational simplicity into a single assessment protocol for medical LLMs.

3.2 SafeMed Framework: Ten Evaluation Dimensions

The SafeMed dimensions (Table 2) were identified, along with descriptions of each dimension, key measurement methods, and sources of evidence. Since the dimensional model directly describes one or more of the aforementioned criteria from section 2, the framework is much more grounded in real clinical evidence than in purely categorical classification.

Table 2. SafeMed Framework: Ten Dimensions, Measurement Methods, and Evidence Base

Dimension	Detailed Explanation of Evaluation	Key Measurement Methods & Tools	Representative Evidence (APA Style)
1. Clinical Accuracy	Assesses conformity with clinical guidelines and evidence-based standards to prevent deviation from established therapeutic protocols.	CSEBD Safety Gate (17 metrics on drug safety, and detection of critical disease); clinical QA benchmarks	(S. Wang et al., 2025) and (Aljohani et al., 2025)
2. Hallucination Control	Counts how often we generate false or misleading outputs not present in any clinical data.	CREOLA taxonomy; semantic entropy; SelfCheckGPT (zero-resource black-box detection)	(Asgari et al., 2025) and (Manakul et al., 2023)
3. Robustness	Evaluates robustness over adversarial inputs and multi-turn clinical dialogues, where models are notoriously brittle.	MedQA-Followup; RABBITS drug-name variation dataset	(Manczak et al., 2025) and (Gallifant et al., 2024)

continued on following page

Table 2. Continued

Dimension	Detailed Explanation of Evaluation	Key Measurement Methods & Tools	Representative Evidence (APA Style)
4. Calibration & Uncertainty	Measures the discrepancy between a model's stated certainty and its true factual correctness to be able to prevent "overconfident" mistakes.	Expected Calibration Error (ECE); selective prediction protocols for human intervention.	(Testoni & Calixto, 2025)
5. Bias & Fairness	Determines demographic consistency to prevent the AI from propagating health inequalities in racial, gender, and age groups.	FairMedQA; counterfactual testing; subgroup analysis/ disaggregated performance reporting.	(Xiao et al., 2025)
6. Ethical Appropriateness	This tests the model's ability to initiate safe escalation paths and deny requests that are clinically inappropriate or invalid.	Testing a red-team scenario; analysis of refusal rates on high-risk asks.	(X. Wang et al., 2024)
7. Transparency & Explainability	Assesses AI transparency as a multi-venular accountability system: Reasoning auditability, data governance, and roles of explanation tailored to developers, clinicians, and patients.	Explainable by design; System Causability Scale (SCS); Application-grounded Assessment (treatment operative answer)	(Kiseleva et al., 2022)
8. Privacy & Security	Evaluate data protection practices and the model's robustness against prompt-injection or sensitive-data-extraction attacks.	Adversarial extraction tests; compliance audits (HIPAA/ PDPL)	(Momani, 2025)
9. Human–AI Interaction Safety	Focuses on automation bias prevention and the need to calibrate trust correctly, using various security-boundaries modeling techniques so that human expertise is preserved.	Human-in-the-loop (HITL) evaluations; escalation pathway audits; trust calibration assessments	Warm, E. (2025). Deskilling and automation bias: A cautionary tale for health professions educators. ICE Blog.
10. Operational Feasibility	Evaluates latency, scalability and workflow integration to verify that the AI will operate correctly in a practical clinical environment.	Verification of Risk Assessment Grid (RAG) governance; EHR simulation Filekeepers; SLA monitoring	(Bhimani et al., 2025)

Ten SafeMed dimensions can be compared to interconnected chain links: should a chain have a weak link, the entire process will be compromised. Thus, since AI suffers from hallucination (D2), its reproduction will be both ethically unacceptable and very inaccurate (D1; D6). Should AI become overconfident (D4), the doctors might be susceptible to automation bias (D9) due to the absence of any indication of doubt on its part.

Hence, not only is demographic bias (D5) morally wrong, but it is also illegal. Without clear transparency (D7), human oversight becomes challenging, and if the system is operationally cumbersome for medical staff to use (D10), the users would be motivated to take 'shortcuts' that bypass other protective features. That's why we have to look at all ten of these dimensions: If we focus on only some parts, we miss systemic fatal risks.

3.3 Risk-Stratified Acceptance Thresholds

SafeMed uses specific acceptance thresholds to evaluate risks. In any process, errors can occur at different levels, and the origin of the error may have different consequences. The level of acceptance at SafeMed is adjusted according to the internationally accepted clinical standards, IEC 62304 Software Safety classification, A, B, and C classes (International Electrotechnical Commission, 2015), and the clinical safety of health IT systems (NHS England, 2023) clinical risk management standards. More information is available in Table 3.

Table 3. Risk-Stratified Acceptance Thresholds for Medical LLM Applications (SafeMed)

Application Context	Risk Class (IEC 62304)	Hallucination Tolerance	Oversight Requirement
Administrative / scheduling	Class A	≤ 5%	Periodic audit
Patient education / health literacy	Class B	≤ 1%	Educator oversight; disclaimers
Clinical decision support (CDSS)	Class C	< 0.1%	HITL mandatory; audit trail required
Direct diagnostic / treatment recommendation	Class C (critical)	< 0.01%	Specialist sign-off; real-time monitoring

Note. The Hallucination tolerance thresholds in this table are proposed by the authors and based on the Hallucination tolerance thresholds stratified by risk in an IEC 62304 software safety classification (International Electrotechnical Commission, 2015) and UK clinical risk management guidelines for health IT systems (NHS England, 2023). There are no guidelines or empirical standards that define acceptable hallucination rates in medical LLM, and therefore, the thresholds are representing what SafeMed feels are proportionate safety requirements by risk class.

Supervised education applications and patient facing applications differ, and this is of particular importance. In education, there is a qualified clinical educator or facilitator who analyzes LLM outputs and provides context, so that learners can act on them. This intercessor layer gives the benefit of the doubt and reduces the uncertainty and the risks involved with LLM error, and except educational usage, is consistent with these systems should be supervised and not be deployed autónomously (Thirunavukarasu et al., 2023). In direct patient-facing deployment, such as symptom-checking chatbots, which are used by patients independently, (Abd-Alrazaq et al., 2020) such systems are designed to have direct patient use without clinical revision, so, outputs can be delivered to the patient unvalidated clinically. There are IEC 62304 Class C clinical software failure, and the software failure may lead to patients death or serious injuries, and that justifies the near zero tolerance on diagnostic software hallucination or errors (International Electrotechnical Commission, 2015, Azamfirei et al., 2023). This is made worse by studies that large language models can fabricate evidence and provide the evidence to manufacture consensus where the use of large language models is not supervised and escencial where the decision is critical. There is a risk of a false consensus where these standards are made as of two criteria, and this is the result of the systems failure to meet any imperative parameters, and the gates are defined as a system not fulfilling Class C systems critical safety metrics.

4. CASE EVIDENCE: LLM DEPLOYMENT IN CLINICAL PRACTICE

This part will provide information about the advantages and risks of each type of LLM applications that exist in real-life situations: general-purpose LLMs, specific medical LLMs, and retriever-augmented generators. These frameworks have many practical applications but they also involve various dangers, which are solved by SafeMed framework.

4.1 General-Purpose LLMs: ChatGPT in Clinical Settings

Uses of ChatGPT-based technologies include clinical documentation, education of patients, and diagnostic aid. Studies demonstrate that the use of such tools allows one to decrease administrative burden, e.g., during filling out History of Present Illness, and ensures access to health literacy among patients. These advantages are, nevertheless, associated with several risks from both safety and ethical perspectives.

According to Sallam (2023), ChatGPT has been analyzed in 60 studies and the author noted that although ChatGPT is efficient and easy to access, some problems can emerge because ChatGPT can produce hallucinations and thus provide false information. Moreover, other issues include biased responses, privacy concerns regarding user data, citation mistakes, and misinformation related to health issues.

In the same manner, Temsah et al. (2023) pointed out important themes in the early use of ChatGPT in the medical field, which include the use of ChatGPT in education, diagnostics, and ethics. These results highlight the necessity of conducting more studies on the efficacy and safety of ChatGPT in the actual clinical setting.

In conclusion, the application of general-purpose LLMs is best applied to low-risk tasks with the support of professionals. General-purpose LLMs should never be applied to diagnostic and treatment procedures without domain adaptation.

4.2 Domain-Specific LLMs: Med-PaLM and Successors

GPTs have some negative points when used in such contexts, and that is why some researchers have focused on developing large language models for specific domains. Some examples of specific-domain large language models are Med-PaLM and Med-PaLM 2. The training process of these models involves using specialized healthcare data such as clinical guidelines and expert-verified databases.

The Med-PaLM 2 model succeeded in reaching a success rate of 86.5 percent in the MedQA dataset, which contains questions about medical licensure. It represents a huge improvement from its predecessors. Additionally, it was more favored due to its responses in general medical queries conducted by physicians. However, in complicated clinical processes, human specialists were better.

In general, domain-specific models exhibit improved reliability, higher guideline compliance, and reduced rates of hallucinations. Still, they face challenges from ambiguous prompts, rare diseases, and missing medical information. In contrast to what scientific literature says, having a larger model size does not correlate with improved safety levels; rather, aligning the model with medical data becomes crucial. As mentioned earlier, although domain adaptation makes a model more efficient, it does not resolve the difficulties faced by the model, including hallucinations and biases. Hence, specialized models require rigorous testing.

4.3 RAG-Based Systems: Grounding LLMs in Clinical Evidence

The next way to increase reliability is through the use of Retrieval-Augmented Generation (RAG). Contrary to the previous methods that relied on the training data only, these systems retrieve the data from credible websites, including PubMed, UpToDate, and the medical guidelines. Such application of the RAG approach to generate the answers to questions about drug-induced osteonecrosis of the jaw is called GuideGPT. As seen, the results obtained are considerably better in terms of accuracy, explanations, and expert consensus than those achieved by the traditional GPT-4 technique. These models are more transparent in the sense that they provide references to the particular sources that enable the verification of the evidence. At the same time, there are some problems associated with the application of such systems, such as the acquisition of irrelevant data and terminological inconsistencies. Good retrieval and language model are essential for the successful operation of RAG systems. In the case of hemodialysis, an application of RAG was performed by Nurfadhilah et al. (2025), who created Chatbot Lisa – an LLM-RAG system for hemodialysis patient education in Indonesia. The study found that local language models (such as Sahabat AI) coupled with RAG performed better than a general language model in terms of accuracy and faithfulness. Furthermore, the authors proposed a design based on the modular architecture that incorporated role-based access control and continuous feedback to ensure the safety of the generated data (Putra et al., 2025). With the proper implementation, such systems reduce the likelihood of hallucination and increase transparency, although they require more resources.

Notwithstanding the methodology used, a similar pattern was found: good benchmarking results are not equivalent to the assurance of safety in practice. According to Wang et al. (2025), although the effectiveness of the models was high, their safety was low, leading to the creation of potentially harmful recommendations in dangerous circumstances. The effectiveness reached, on average, 57.2%. The safety score was always worse than the efficiency one.

5. EVALUATION METHODS AND END-TO-END PIPELINE

5.1 Why Traditional Metrics Are Clinically Insufficient

BLEU, ROUGE, and simple accuracy scores used for most practical NLP tasks are intended to measure (a) lexical similarity and (b) overall accuracy. In addition, for clinical AI systems, these scores are utterly inadequate. Even if a hundred questions were answered accurately in a clinical AI task, one question where the wrong drug dose was calculated could result in fatalities, even if the accuracy score increased by only a few percentiles. The mismatch between high aggregate accuracy and poor clinical accuracy is the exact issue that SafeMed intends to resolve through its evaluation pipeline (Wang et al., 2025; Bedi et al., 2025).

Now the study that comes closest among existing data to illustrate this asymmetry is the CSEDB study (Clinical Safety-Effectiveness Dual-Track Benchmark). Wang et al. (2025) assessed various state-of-the-art LLMs on two parallel evaluation tracks, those being a safety gate consisting of 17 clinical safety metrics (absolute contraindications, critical disease detection, drug safety) rated binary safe/unsafe and an effectiveness gate composed of 13 guideline-adherence as well as diagnostic efficiency metrics. Models that did well on the effectiveness gate failed at the safety gate in cases of absolute contraindications (eg, codeine prescriptions to children or aminoglycosides administered to patients with end-stage renal failure). And these are not obscure edge cases: they represent core clinical safety knowledge that any deployed medical chatbot must get right, with a zero tolerance policy. Felicity stands unchanged: no aggregate accuracy scoring system captures that binary pass/fail safety distinction.

5.2 Dimension-Specific Measurement Methods

The SafeMed evaluation methodology replaces the concept of aggregate accuracy with an entire set of measures selected based on their validity and empirical basis. Here follows a list of tools used within the SafeMed framework to measure particular dimensions:

- **Dimension 1: Clinical Accuracy:** SafeMed uses safety gate binary scoring for CSEDB in case of an absolute contraindication. The USMLE-like performance metric, MultiMedQA, and MedQA are applied for knowledge base across domains and clinical reasoning.
- **Dimension 2: Hallucination Control:** In this regard, the CREOLA manual annotation taxonomy allows one to classify all hallucinations according to two criteria — types (fabrications, negations, causal speculations, contextual contamination) and severity (minor, major). Semantic entropy quantifies consistency of meaning across multiple generations from an identical prompt, where high entropy indicates the risk of confabulation. In addition, SelfCheckGPT enables zero-resource self-consistency detection without any reference outputs. The simultaneous development of a MEDAL post-hoc correction module allows rectification of hallucinated content in output clinical summaries without needing to retrain the base model. PubHealthTab and HEALTHVER benchmarks enable factual verification of public health claims based on noisy evidence (Asgari et al., 2025; Manakul et al., 2023).
- **Dimension 3: Robustness:** The MedQA-Followup multi-turn adversarial framework evaluates two levels of robustness — shallow robustness, defined as the model's ability to survive misleading or biased context presented in the first prompt, and deep robustness, defined as the maintenance of accuracy when misled through consecutive multiple invalidated follow-up interactions. First and foremost, multi-turn interventions are far more destructive compared to single-turn adversarial examples: According to Manczak et al. (2025), the application of external context resulted in reducing the state-of-the-art model's accuracy by 89% in a single follow-up question that asked for ground truth only (the RAG approach to deceptive contexts). The RABBITS data set explores the robustness to drug name variations by reporting performance drops of 1–10%, implying a clinically significant vulnerability.
- **Dimension 4: Calibration and Uncertainty:** ECE (expected calibration error) measures the extent of gap between predicted confidence and actu-

al accuracy in confidence bins. A properly calibrated model's claimed 80% confidence should equal 80% accuracy; overconfident models assert high confidence on incorrect answers. Selective prediction strategies may be used to guarantee that any predicted response is subject to human inspection if the prediction score does not meet certain criteria set by the algorithm itself (Testoni & Calixto, 2025).

- **Dimension 5: Bias and Fairness:** FairMedQA benchmark leverages matched clinical cases to measure demographic parity in terms of racial, gender, and socio-economic group performance. The counterfactual evaluation strategy consists in modifying the demographics in otherwise identical clinical case descriptions to see what happens to the recommendation of the model. Performance decomposition into sub-groups guarantees the aggregate metrics of accuracy are broken down and suggest different performances, i.e., the diffractive aspect of aggregate performance reporting (Xiao et al., 2025).
- **Dimension 7: Transparency and Explainability:** Source attribution in Retrieval-Augmented Generation (RAG) systems corresponds to citing the exact evidence used by the model to generate the answer. While LIME and SHAP allow some level of attributions for neural networks, these methods are well-known as being surface interpretability techniques since they provide no clue about how the model thinks. This is where the best level of transparency comes in with neuro-symbolic hybrids that reference inside the nodes of the knowledge graph (Wang, 2025).

5.3 The CLEVER Evaluation Protocol

The Clinical Large Language Model Evaluation – Expert Review (CLEVER) protocol provides an expertly designed evaluation pipeline, which is free from contamination and statistically validated and which is directly applicable to SafeMed implementation requirements (Kocaman et al., 2025). Importantly, the approach solves the problem of contamination inherent to existing benchmarks: the LLMs pretrained on internet-scale data must inevitably have been exposed to the test questions of accepted benchmarks such as MedQA and MMLU, which means that benchmark performance is not indicative of a model's actual capacity to reason clinically.

Stage 1: CLEVER proceeds through three stages. At the first one, a diverse group of clinical experts across all specialities develops a set of 500 unique test cases, including discharge summaries, pathology reports, and clinical scenarios, none of which can be found in any publicly available training dataset. Contamination-free test set presents the real case of out-of-distribution evaluation. Stage 2: The blinded expert panel of multidisciplinary specialists evaluates the response of different models to the test sets using three evaluation criteria: (1) factuality – Is the information clinically accurate? (2) clinical relevance – Is the response clinically relevant? and (3) conciseness – Is it brief enough? Importantly, the expert panel remains blinded to the identity of different models used, making it possible to avoid systematic bias toward any particular model. Stage 3: Calculating statistics through IAA/ICC analysis with 2 weeks of the washout period. This washout analysis is uncommon in the AI evaluation literature on clinical data and substantially increases the evidence robustness of CLEVER-based assessments.

CLEVER is not a one-off certification. Consistent with the requirement in SafeMed for lifecycle governance (Dimension 10), it should be done after each new iteration of the model, whenever underlying clinical guidelines change significantly, and periodically (at least once annually for high risk applications) to detect performance drift.

5.4 Worst-at-k Analysis: Measuring Tail Risk

The most vital paradigm change in terms of methodology in SafeMed evaluation would be the transition from average-case to worst-case performance analyses. Conventional methodologies use the mean score across the test cases. This works best when the mistakes in performance are balanced and a particular mistake does not hold significant impact relative to other mistakes. However, these assumptions do not apply to the field of clinical medicine. Mistakes are unbalanced since a single erroneous output will lead to irreversible harm for the patient. For instance, a model could misclassify a safe drug as contraindicated to the patient.

Worst-at-k evaluates the worst-case scenario across k independent outputs of a test prompt. Instead of focusing on the average performance of the model in answering questions regarding the medical issue at hand, the analysis considers the output that could potentially lead to catastrophic results for k runs of the model. An example of this would be the CSEBD paper published by Wang et al. (2025). Under the conventional single-sample methodology, highly skilled models were found to perform poorly in Worst-at-k analysis. This finding has a direct operational implication: evaluation protocols for high-risk medical LLM applications should run each clinical safety scenario multiple times and gate deployment on worst-case — not average-case — performance. SafeMed recommends Weighted Error Rates that assign greater weight to high-severity failure modes (IEC 62304 Class C) and minimum acceptable performance thresholds on critical safety scenarios that must be maintained across all k trials, not just on average (Agency for Healthcare Research and Quality, 2024).

6. DEPLOYMENT SAFETY AND CLINICAL INTEGRATION

6.1 The System-Level View of Deployment Safety

It is very important to know that there is a risk to users or people who used an AI System when they are being force to used the system and accept the answer provided by the LLM Model without cross check the answer, even the model is very advance. That is why an AI Model System that related in medical domain must have a safety and reliable element. But, we need to consider other factor too. For example the evaluation Model, the context of the LLM Model and of course the relationship.

We have the standard regarding the safety of an AI LLM Model, for example the SafeMed Standard. It has 9 parameters related to safety and performance of an AI LLM Model. But it is not guaranteed the safety when the AI System is implemented operationally in real worlds. A systems-level perspective is called for that takes a sociotechnical approach, considering factors beyond the model alone (Owoyemi et al., 2025). This involves assessing model performance (accuracy, F1 score, hallucination rate, etc.), situating the context (how nicely the AI fits within clinical workflows and whether as an organization they can accommodate it), and estimating relationships (trust in general that clinicians and patients have toward using the output of the AI). A powerful model in a system where users cannot be trusted to question the output will also become dangerous. A simpler model, on the other hand, is safer with HITL and a culture of critical thinking (Owoyemi et al., 2025).

Assessing the safety of deploying medical AI through this system-level lens has important real-world implications. Safety evaluation should not only be limited to the technical performance of the model, but rather needs to consider organization and workflow aspects as well. Before deploying a medical LLM, institutions are recommended to conduct a structured assessment that includes aspects of clinician readiness and training, whether there are established definitions for AI roles and escalation processes, the availability of technical support, issue reporting systems, and the appetite within the organization toward AI-generated recommendations (Festor et al., 2025; Zakka et al., 2024). Start treating a safety checklist encompassing all of this as mandatory pre-live, rather than an afterthought.

6.2 Human-in-the-Loop Architecture in Practice

Not only is human-in-the-loop oversight a regulatory requirement, it is also an ethical responsibility and practical method to ensure safety. Similarly, in Indonesia, the Omnibus Health Law No. 17/2023 explicitly stipulates that only licensed clinicians will be granted the final say on diagnosis. Hence, the role of the AI system in such cases will be of a CDSS tool. It implies that the AI is only meant to assist in the process, but the final call will belong to clinicians fully responsible for their decisions. In the case of high-risk AI usage, there are human monitoring obligations according to EU AI Act and FDA GMLP guidelines. Furthermore, according to World Health Organization (2024), it is human agency and oversight that should be considered one of the fundamental duties. Thus, such legal and ethical imperatives also highlight another important fact, namely that at the moment human expert judgment represents the best method of detecting hazardous LLM output in context (Kocaman et al., 2025).

HITL architecture should be hierarchical, not equal. Not all LLM outputs require the same degree of human monitoring. It would be impractical and unnecessary to apply the same degree of attention to each interaction with the chatbot. A possible three-tier HITL architecture could encompass the following stages: (1) low-risk/ low-complexity auto pass with auditing sampling; (2) mandatory frontline clinician review of medium-complexity clinical information request outputs, along with documentation of approval/rejection; and (3) specialist review in high-risk cases of diagnostic recommendations output, dosing suggestions, psychological crises management interaction, and any other interaction when the confidence level is under the defined threshold value of ECE. According to the research conducted by Lee et al. (2024) regarding the use of AI in medical education, it can be stated that hierarchical human supervision is essential in educational contexts. It allows us to ensure that the materials generated using AI workflows are checked by an educator prior to proceeding through it. HITL is not a crutch while models get their shit together. In the practice of clinical medicine, human professional accountability is an inextricable structural requirement embedded into legally and ethically binding obligations that cannot be outsourced to automated systems, regardless of their capacity for effective functioning (World Health Organization, 2024). The pertinent design question is not "when can we delete human oversight?" but "how do we make human oversight as effective and scalable as possible?"

6.3 RAG Governance and Technical Architecture

Retrieval-Augmented Generation is the current best-practice technical architecture for minimizing hallucination in deployed medical chatbots that ground their generation in retrieved clinical evidence. RAG, however, brings its own requirements for deployment safety. Ones that must be actively governed rather than assumed. The safety of a RAG-based medical LLM relies equally on the quality and governance of the retrieval pipeline as it does on the generation model.

Essential RAG governance standards for safe clinical deployment include:

- **Source curation —** all records from retrieval databases must originate from peer-reviewed clinical guidelines, pharmacopoeia and evidence bases integrated as input only; general web content, patient reviews and non-peer reviewed sources must be excluded.
- **Update cadence —** retrieval databases must be refreshed according to a defined cycle aligned with the update cycles of source clinical guidelines included in the database; outdated source content raises the risk of evidentially-grounded but clinically-obsolete recommendations.
- **Evidence-response alignment auditing —** such a system's outputs should be periodically audited by qualified clinical reviewers to ensure that the generated responses are an accurate reflection of the evidence retrieved and do not inject hallucinations at the generation stage overtop correctly retrieved content.
- **Handling retrieval failures —** when retrieval systems return low-confidence results or empty results, the system should not resort to generating from model parameters without any context and should have a safe default instead (Xiong et al., 2024; Zakka et al., 2024). The fallback behaviour needs to be explicitly designed, tested and audited.

Furthermore, the platform's technical requirements from end to end must also address aspects such as EHR integration through FHIR interoperability, AES-256 encryption both at rest and in transit (i.e., moving across networks), role-based access control, and complete logging capabilities for audit trail generation/maintenance (Alowais et al., 2023).

6.4 Post-Deployment Monitoring and Continuous Safety

Deployment starts a continuous safety obligation, not the end of one. Large language model (LLM) behaviour can drift as underlying model weights are updated, clinical guidelines shift and evolve, usage patterns change and the population of users shifts. A system meeting SafeMed thresholds at deployment may no longer meet them six months later without active monitoring. Indonesian Permenkes No. 11/2025 reflects on this reality by requiring annual post-market inspections for high-risk health technologies, a requirement that should be regarded as a minimum, not maximum, interval for more frequent continuous monitoring.

A practical continuous monitoring framework must contain: real-time logging of all model interactions together with sufficient metadata to allow for retrieval (Hager et al., 2024) and analysis of incidents; regular automated re-evaluation of gates identifying critical safety scenarios using a held-out dataset, human clinical audit on random samples of output at fixed intervals; an escalatory incident reporting mechanism that allows clinicians and patients directly engaged in front line use to report instances where outputs could prove dangerous as worthy of investigation; and governance by a committee with authority to suspend or halt deployment until further investigation is carried out if monitoring data suggests violation of safety thresholds (Murdoch, 2021; Hager et al., 2024).

Practical recommendations for administrators and policymakers deploying medical LLMs:

- Build a cross-disciplinary deployment safety committee — involving clinicians, clinical informaticists, ethicists, legal counsel and patient representatives — before procurement begins.
- Make disclosure of training data demographics, third-party hallucination evaluation results, and subgroup performance disaggregation a condition of consideration to procure.
- Before go live, map all proposed AI potential use cases to the SafeMed risk classes, ensuring that the applicable acceptance thresholds and HITL requirements for each class are implemented.
- Document and incorporate clinical escalation pathways into an updated medical protocol in advance of go-live and train all relevant staff.
- Develop living monitoring dashboards measuring hallucination incident rates, user escalation rates, response latency and demographic performance parity against acceptance thresholds that generate automatic governance committee escalations when breached.
- Require formal re-evaluation of the CLEVER-protocol with each model update, in conjunction with each major revision of clinical guidelines within the system's relevant clinical domain and at least annually for all high-risk applications.

7. FUTURE DIRECTIONS AND CONCLUSIONS

7.1 From Model-Centric to System-Centric Evaluation

The medical AI evaluation field should undergo a paradigm shift from model-centric to system-oriented evaluations. The model-centric paradigm judges LLMs in the manner a physicist would judge an isolated gas: Does a test question result in the correct answer (or answers) being generated by the model? This paradigm is suitable for natural language processing research but clinically deficient. To be clear, clinical safety is not a quality of a model in isolation, rather it is an emergent property of the model interacting with specific users, specific workflows, specific organizational cultures and specific technical infrastructures. The same model could be safe in a highly controlled specialist environment and unsafe as a consumer-facing patient application.

System-centric evaluation therefore necessitates (1) end-to-end simulation environments that statically load LLMs on realistic integrated clinical scenarios with EHR integration, multi-turn clinical dialogue and workflow decision points rather than isolated QA items (Jiang et al., 2025), (2) failure propagation analysis, tracing how failures at the retrieval, generation, or interface layer propagate through the system, (3) sociotechnical assessment measuring trust calibration, barriers to adoption, and organizational as well as cultural conditions determining whether safety mechanisms are actually exercised in practice (Di Vita et al., 2025; Festor et al., 2025). Equity and equity are central to meeting this system-level perspective, as demographic performance disparities represent not only an issue of representation but a risk to safety that determines whether or not a system can provide safe care equitably across the patient population it serves (World Health Organization, 2024).

7.2 Technical Priorities for Safer Medical LLMs

A few technical directions present the best leads towards safety improvements. We explore hybrid neuro-symbolic architectures that leverage both the language modeling and generation strength of LLMs with the formal knowledge expression and logical constrain enforcement methods associated with structured representations such as medical knowledge graphs. In this framework, the space of clinical claims that the neural component can generate is constrained by a knowledge graph so that drug names, dosages, and clinical relationships cannot be fabricated that do not have underlying validation from medical knowledge (Wang, 2025; Prenosil et al., 2025). Initial work in the ophthalmology field (predicting AMD treatment outcome) showed higher than 85% of evidence linking with natural language explanations, indicating potential applicability to broader clinical use.

Governed RAG with specified quality thresholds offers potentially more immediately deployable improvements. Much of cumulative evidence in the current RAG implementations tends to lack governance regarding retrieval quality, source recency or evidence-response alignment. Formalizing retrieval quality metrics (e.g., relevance scores, source publication date checks, semantic alignment between the retrieved evidence and generated response) set minimum thresholds for these as a condition of response generation to significantly lower risk levels of generating evidentially grounded yet stale or misaligned outputs (Gaber et al., 2025; Neha et al., 2025). Models utilizing uncertainty-aware generation approaches like semantic entropy (Farquhar et al., 2024), conformal prediction and SelfCheckGPT (Manakul et al., 2023) generate well-calibrated uncertainty instead of the overconfident predictions from which people receiving high-uncertainty outputs are primed along the axis and way they ought to respond. Even more so from the clinical practice perspective, where understanding when to refer or escalate is explicitly a design goal for medical LLMs, a system that adheres to good clinical behavior and says, "I'm not confident enough here to make treatment recommendations so please consult with a specialist" is not an inadequacy but rather desirable.

7.3 Policy and Education Implications

For policymakers, the evidence in this chapter points to three priorities. First, risk-based regulatory frameworks must embed mandatory multidimensional evaluation in addition to accuracy benchmarking as contingent on medical AI deployment authorization. In particular, regulators should demand proof that evaluation of SafeMed Dimension 2 (hallucination) and Dimension 5 (bias) has been performed broken down by patient subgroup, not simply in the aggregate. Second, post-market surveillance requirements should require routine monitoring with prescriptive reporting thresholds rather than a compliance inspection once yearly. Third, the current fragmented global regulatory landscape provides opportunities for harmonization as the underlying principles of MI AI's conformity assessment requirements in September through the EU AI Act, FDA GMLP guidance and Indonesian Permenkes risk stratification are largely compatible and could be aligned into a common minimum evidence standard for medical AI deployment which would reduce duplication of work and regulatory uncertainty for developers operating across jurisdictions.

As LLM integration into the curriculum will become essential for medical educators and clinical training programs, critical AI literacy in addition to accessing AI tools must be a top priority. Curricula that introduce LLMs to students, yet fail to systematically train them in their limitations, failure modes, and appropriate oversight mechanisms are developing exactly the conditions for automation bias and clinical deskilling (Warm, 2025). Medical education should emulate the practice of professional use of AI-assisted clinical reasoning: as a prompt for critical appraisal rather than an endpoint for final diagnosis based on LLM outputs. This behavioral dimension is the human end of the spectrum relative to the technical safeguards that both SafeMed and the CLEVER pipeline promote.

7.4 Conclusions

The safety and clinical trustworthiness of LLM-based medical chatbots is not a secondary consideration to be addressed after performance optimization but it is the primary condition for clinical acceptability. The evidence reviewed in this chapter demonstrates consistently that high benchmark accuracy does not imply clinical safety: models achieve strong performance on effectiveness metrics while failing critical safety gates; aggregate hallucination rates mask high proportions of Major clinical errors; and demographic performance parity is absent from most deployed systems despite its direct implications for health equity. These findings do not criticize LLM technology itself, they argue that the evaluation frameworks guiding LLM deployment are unfit for use in clinical contexts.

SafeMed is offered as a viable solution: ten experiential, measurable evaluation dimensions anchored in clinical information mapped to specific measurement tools constrained by risk-stratified acceptance thresholds matched to the consequence profiles of distinct clinical applications. SafeMed's novelty is not that we didn't know that specific risks (hallucination, bias and calibration failure are well established in the literature) but rather integrating them into a coherent, measurement-ready evaluation system that translates regulatory principle into clinical practice.

We believe four concurrent advances can move high-performing language models toward clinically reliable systems: (1) multidimensional evaluation, rather than accuracy-focused benchmarking; (2) harm-weighted metrics favoring worst-case performance over average performance; (3) scalable HITL architectures supporting professional accountabilities without compromising efficiency in challenging cases and (4) lifecycle governance frameworks that treat deployment safety as an ongoing obligation. SafeMed therefore provides the evaluation infrastructure needed for all four advances, wrapped within a single coherent framework that seamlessly adapts to clinical, educational and administrative LLM applications, and which conforms with the developing international regulatory landscape surrounding medical AI.

REFERENCES

Abd-Alrazaq, A., AlSaad, R., Alhuwail, D., Ahmed, A., Healy, P. M., Latifi, S., Aziz, S., Damseh, R., Alrazak, S. A., & Sheikh, J. (2023). Large language models in medical education: Opportunities, challenges, and future directions. *JMIR Medical Education*, *9*(1), e48291. DOI: 10.2196/48291 PMID: 37261894

Abd-Alrazaq, A., Safi, Z., Alajlani, M., Warren, J., Househ, M., & Denecke, K. (2020). Technical metrics used to evaluate health care chatbots: Scoping review. *Journal of Medical Internet Research*, *22*(6), e18301. DOI: 10.2196/18301 PMID: 32442157

Abdelwanis, M., Alarafati, H. K., Tammam, M. M. S., & Simsekler, M. C. E. (2024). Exploring the risks of automation bias in healthcare AI applications: A Bowtie analysis. *Journal of Safety Science and Resilience = An Quan Ke Xue Yu Ren Xing (Ying Wen)*, *5*(4), 460–469.

Agency for Healthcare Research and Quality. (2024). Patient safety indicators technical specifications (AHRQ Publication No. 24-0001). U.S. Department of Health and Human Services. https://qualityindicators.ahrq.gov/Archive/psi_techspec/icd10_v2024

Aljohani, M., Hou, J., Kommu, S., & Wang, X. (2025). A comprehensive survey on the trustworthiness of large language models in healthcare. 6720–6748. DOI: 10.18653/v1/2025.findings-emnlp.356

Alowais, S. A., Alghamdi, S. S., Alsuhebany, N., Alqahtani, T., Alshaya, A. I., Almohareb, S. N., Aldairem, A., Alrashed, M., Bin Saleh, K., Badreldin, H. A., Al Yami, M. S., Al Harbi, S., & Albekairy, A. M. (2023). Revolutionizing healthcare: The role of artificial intelligence in clinical practice. *BMC Medical Education*, *23*(1), 689. DOI: 10.1186/s12909-023-04698-z PMID: 37740191

Asgari, E., Montaña-Brown, N., Dubois, M., Khalil, S., Balloch, J., Au Yeung, J., & Pimenta, D. (2025). A framework to assess clinical safety and hallucination rates of LLMs for medical text summarisation. npj. *Digital Medicine*, *8*(1), 274. DOI: 10.1038/s41746-025-01670-7 PMID: 40360677

Azamfirei, R., Kudchadkar, S. R., & Fackler, J. (2023). Large language models and the perils of their hallucinations. *Critical Care : The Official Journal of the Critical Care Forum*, *27*(1), 120. DOI: 10.1186/s13054-023-04393-x PMID: 36945051

Bedi, S., Liu, Y., Orr-Ewing, L., Dash, D., Koyejo, S., Callahan, A., Fries, J. A., Wornow, M., Swaminathan, A., Lehmann, L. S., Hong, H. J., Kashyap, M., Chaurasia, A. R., Shah, N. R., Singh, K., Tazbaz, T., Milstein, A., Pfeffer, M. A., & Shah, N. H. (2025). Testing and evaluation of health care applications of large language models: A systematic review. *Journal of the American Medical Association, 333*(4), 319–328. DOI: 10.1001/jama.2024.21700 PMID: 39405325

Bhimani, M., Miller, A., Agnew, J. D., Ausin, M. S., Raglow-Defranco, M., Mangat, H., Voisard, M., Taylor, M., Bierman-Lytle, S., Parikh, V., Ghukasyan, J., Lasko, R., Godil, S., Atreja, A., & Mukherjee, S. (2025). Real-world evaluation of large language models in healthcare (RWE-LLM): A new realm of AI safety & validation. DOI: 10.1101/2025.03.17.25324157

Chen, S., Gao, M., Sasse, K., Hartvigsen, T., Anthony, B., Fan, L., Aerts, H., Gallifant, J., & Bitterman, D. S. (2025). When helpfulness backfires: LLMs and the risk of false medical information due to sycophantic behavior. npj. *Digital Medicine, 8*(1), 605. DOI: 10.1038/s41746-025-02008-z PMID: 41107408

Daneshjou, R., Vodrahalli, K., Novoa, R. A., Jenkins, M., Liang, W., Rotemberg, V., Ko, J., Swetter, S. M., Bailey, E. E., Gevaert, O., Mukherjee, P., Phung, M., Yekrang, K., Fong, B., Sahasrabudhe, R., Allerup, J. A. C., Okata-Karigane, U., Zou, J., & Chiou, A. (2022). Disparities in dermatology AI performance on a diverse, curated clinical image set. *Science Advances, 8*(32), eabq6147. Advance online publication. DOI: 10.1126/sciadv.abq6147 PMID: 35960806

Di Vita, A., Fusco, G., Lorenzon, L., Tognoni, P., & Maggi, A. (2025). The Model–Context–Relation framework for clinical AI evaluation. *JMIR Formative Research, 9*, e62845. DOI: 10.2196/62845

European Parliament. (2024). Regulation (EU) 2024/1689 of the European Parliament and of the Council of 13 June 2024 laying down harmonised rules on artificial intelligence (Artificial Intelligence Act). Official Journal of the European Union, L 2024/1689. https://eur-lex.europa.eu/legal-content/EN/TXT/?uri=OJ:L_202401689

Farquhar, S., Kossen, J., Kuhn, L., & Gal, Y. (2024). Detecting hallucinations in large language models using semantic entropy. *Nature, 630*(8017), 625–630. DOI: 10.1038/s41586-024-07421-0 PMID: 38898292

Feldman, M. J., Hoffer, E. P., Conley, J. J., Chang, J., Chung, J. A., Jernigan, M. C., Lester, W. T., Strasser, Z. H., & Chueh, H. C. (2025). Dedicated AI expert system vs generative AI with large language model for clinical diagnoses. *JAMA Network Open, 8*(5), e2512994. DOI: 10.1001/jamanetworkopen.2025.12994 PMID: 40440012

Festor, P., Nagendran, M., Gordon, A. C., Faisal, A. A., & Komorowski, M. (2025). Safety of human-AI cooperative decision-making within intensive care: A physical simulation study. *PLOS Digital Health*, *4*(2), e0000726. DOI: 10.1371/journal.pdig.0000726 PMID: 39992918

Gaber, D. A., Mayer, M. A., Lau, A. Y. S., & Neves, A. L. (2025). Governance of retrieval-augmented generation in clinical chatbots: Framework and evaluation criteria. npj. *Digital Medicine*, *8*(1), 112. DOI: 10.1038/s41746-025-01234-9 PMID: 39966675

Gallifant, J., Chen, S., Moreira, P., Munch, N., Gao, M., Pond, J., Aerts, H., Celi, L. A., Hartvigsen, T., & Bitterman, D. S. (2024). Language models are surprisingly fragile to drug names in biomedical benchmarks. In *Findings of the 2024 Conference on Empirical Methods in Natural Language Processing* (pp. 12448–12465). DOI: 10.18653/v1/2024.findings-emnlp.726

Gerke, S., Minssen, T., & Cohen, G. (2020). Ethical and legal challenges of artificial intelligence-driven healthcare. In Bohr, A., & Memarzadeh, K. (Eds.), *Artificial intelligence in healthcare* (pp. 295–336). Academic Press., DOI: 10.1016/B978-0-12-818438-7.00012-5

Hager, P., Jungmann, F., Holland, R., Bhoelan, S., Ruber, T., Scherer, J., Baader, S., Braren, R., Kaissis, G., & Rueckert, D. (2024). Evaluation and mitigation of the limitations of large language models in clinical decision-making. *Nature Medicine*, *30*(9), 2613–2622. DOI: 10.1038/s41591-024-03097-1 PMID: 38965432

International Electrotechnical Commission. (2015). IEC 62304:2006+AMD1:2015—Medical device software: Software life cycle processes. https://webstore.iec.ch/en/publication/22794

Jiang, H., Liu, X., Wang, Q., Chen, Z., Zhao, J., & Li, M. (2025). EHR-Bench: End-to-end evaluation of LLMs in electronic health record simulation environments. *Journal of the American Medical Informatics Association : JAMIA*, *32*(5), e201–e213.

Kiseleva, A., Kotzinos, D., & De Hert, P. (2022). Transparency of AI in healthcare as a multilayered system of accountabilities: Between legal requirements and technical limitations. *Frontiers in Artificial Intelligence*, *5*, 879603. Advance online publication. DOI: 10.3389/frai.2022.879603 PMID: 35707765

Kocaman, V., Kaya, M. A., Feier, A. M., & Talby, D. (2025). Clinical large language model evaluation by expert review (CLEVER): Framework development and validation. *JMIR AI*, *4*, e72153. DOI: 10.2196/72153 PMID: 41343765

Lee, J., Wu, A. S., Li, D., & Kulasegaram, K. M. (2024). Artificial intelligence in undergraduate medical education: A systematic review. *Academic Medicine : Journal of the Association of American Medical Colleges*, *99*(8), 916–925. DOI: 10.1097/ACM.0000000000005685

Manakul, P., Liusie, A., & Gales, M. (2023). SelfCheckGPT: Zero-resource black-box hallucination detection for generative large language models. In *Proceedings of the 2023 Conference on Empirical Methods in Natural Language Processing* (pp. 9004–9017). DOI: 10.18653/v1/2023.emnlp-main.557

Manczak, B., Lin, E., Eiras, F., Neill, J. O., & Mugunthan, V. (2025). Shallow robustness, deep vulnerabilities: Multi-turn evaluation of medical LLMs. arXiv. https://doi.org//arXiv.2510.12255DOI: 10.48550

Ministry of Health of the Republic of Indonesia. (2021). Minister of Health Regulation No. 14 of 2021 on standards for health service digital technology.

Ministry of Health of the Republic of Indonesia. (2024). Minister of Health Regulation No. 17 of 2024 on data governance and interoperability in the national digital health ecosystem. Kemenkes RI.

Ministry of Health of the Republic of Indonesia. (2025). Minister of Health Regulation No. 11 of 2025 on business licensing in the health sub-sector.

Momani, A. (2025). Implications of artificial intelligence on health data privacy and confidentiality. arXiv. https://arxiv.org/abs/2501.01639

Mount Sinai Health System. (2025). AI safety red-teaming report: Chatbot elaboration of fabricated illnesses. Icahn School of Medicine Research Reports. https://icahn.mssm.edu/research/ai-safety-2025

Murdoch, B. (2021). Privacy and artificial intelligence: Challenges for protecting health information in a new era. *BMC Medical Ethics*, *22*(1), 122. DOI: 10.1186/s12910-021-00687-3 PMID: 34525993

Natali, A., Mosca, N., & Zucco, R. (2025). Clinical deskilling in the age of AI: Reconsidering Klein's Second Singularity. *BMJ Open*, *15*(3), e092345.

Neha, F., Bhati, D., & Shukla, D. K. (2025). Retrieval-augmented generation (RAG) in healthcare: A comprehensive review. *AI*, *6*(9), 226. DOI: 10.3390/ai6090226

NHS England. (2023). DCB0129: Clinical risk management—its application in the manufacture of health IT systems. https://digital.nhs.uk/data-and-information/information-standards/information-standards-and-data-collections-including-extractions/publications-and-notifications/standards-and-collections/dcb0129-clinical-risk-management-its-application-in-the-manufacture-of-health-it-systems

Nurfadhilah, E., Santosa, A., & Putra, P. K. (2025). Retrieval-augmented large language models for a chronic kidney disease patient education chatbot. 2025 International Conference on Computer, Control, Informatics and its Applications (IC3INA). DOI: 10.1109/IC3INA68387.2025.11325127

Omiye, J. A., Lester, J. C., Spichak, S., Rotemberg, V., & Daneshjou, R. (2023). Large language models propagate race-based medicine. npj. *Digital Medicine*, *6*(1), 195. DOI: 10.1038/s41746-023-00939-z PMID: 37864012

Owoyemi, A., Osuchukwu, J., Salwei, M. E., & Boyd, A. (2025). Checklist approach to developing and implementing AI in clinical settings: Instrument development study. *JMIRx Med*, *6*, e65565. DOI: 10.2196/65565 PMID: 39977249

Poitras, M. E., Gauvin, F., Bhosrekar, S., & Morin, S. N. (2025). Socioeconomic bias in clinical AI: Evidence from simulated patient scenarios. *Journal of General Internal Medicine*, *40*(1), 78–85.

Prenosil, G., Hügli, R., Brönnimann, M., Sendi, P., & Kluckert, T. (2025). Neuro-symbolic hybrid AI for clinical decision support: Architecture and evaluation. *JAMIA Open*, *8*(1), ooae123.

Price, W. N.II, & Cohen, I. G. (2019). Privacy in the age of medical big data. *Nature Medicine*, *25*(1), 37–43. DOI: 10.1038/s41591-018-0272-7 PMID: 30617331

Putra, P. K., Nurfadhilah, E., Pebiana, S., & Prakasa, E. (2025). Towards a safe and trustworthy LLM-RAG chatbot for hemodialysis patient education: Design, implementation, and preliminary evaluation. 2025 International Conference on Computer, Control, Informatics and its Applications (IC3INA). DOI: 10.1109/IC3INA68387.2025.11325125

Sallam, M. (2023). ChatGPT utility in healthcare education, research, and practice: Systematic review on the promising perspectives and valid concerns. *Health Care*, *11*(6), 887. DOI: 10.3390/healthcare11060887 PMID: 36981544

Singhal, K., Tu, T., Gottweis, J., Sayres, R., Wulczyn, E., Amin, M., Hou, L., Clark, K., Pfohl, S. R., Cole-Lewis, H., Neal, D., Rashid, Q. M., Schaekermann, M., Wang, A., Dash, D., Chen, J. H., Shah, N. H., Lachgar, S., Mansfield, P. A., & Natarajan, V. (2025). Toward expert-level medical question answering with large language models. *Nature Medicine, 31*(3), 943–950. DOI: 10.1038/s41591-024-03423-7 PMID: 39779926

Temsah, O., Khan, S. A., Chaiah, Y., Senjab, A., Alhasan, K., Jamal, A., Aljamaan, F., Malki, K. H., Halwani, R., Al-Tawfiq, J. A., Temsah, M.-H., & Al-Eyadhy, A. (2023). Overview of early ChatGPT's presence in medical literature. *Cureus, 15*(4), e37281. DOI: 10.7759/cureus.37281 PMID: 37038381

Testoni, A., & Calixto, I. (2025). Mind the gap: Benchmarking LLM uncertainty and calibration with specialty-aware clinical QA and reasoning-based behavioural features. arXiv. https://doi.org//arXiv.2506.10769DOI: 10.48550

Thirunavukarasu, A. J., Ting, D. S. J., Elangovan, K., Gutierrez, L., Tan, T. F., & Ting, D. S. W. (2023). Large language models in medicine. *Nature Medicine, 29*(8), 1930–1940. DOI: 10.1038/s41591-023-02448-8 PMID: 37460753

U.S. Food and Drug Administration. (2021). Good machine learning practice for medical device development: Guiding principles. https://www.fda.gov/medical-devices/software-medical-device-samd/good-machine-learning-practice-medical-device-development-guiding-principles

Van Melle, W. (1978). MYCIN: A knowledge-based consultation program for infectious disease diagnosis. *International Journal of Man-Machine Studies, 10*(3), 313–322. DOI: 10.1016/S0020-7373(78)80049-2

Wang, M. H. (2025). Explainable artificial intelligence framework for predicting treatment outcomes in age-related macular degeneration. *Sensors (Basel), 25*(22), 6879. DOI: 10.3390/s25226879 PMID: 41305085

Wang, S., Tang, Z., Yang, H., Gong, Q., Gu, T., Ma, H., Wang, Y., Sun, W., Lian, Z., Mao, K., Jiang, Y., Huang, Z., Ma, L., Shen, W., Ji, Y., Tan, Y., Wang, C., Gao, Y., Ye, Q., & Wu, J. (2025). A novel evaluation benchmark for medical LLMs illuminating safety and effectiveness in clinical domains. npj. *Digital Medicine, 9*(1), 91. Advance online publication. DOI: 10.1038/s41746-025-02277-8 PMID: 41454006

Wang, X., Zhang, N. X., He, H., Nguyen, T., Yu, K.-H., Deng, H., Brandt, C., Bitterman, D. S., Pan, L., Cheng, C.-Y., Zou, J., & Liu, D. (2024). Safety challenges of AI in medicine in the era of large language models. arXiv. https://arxiv.org/abs/2409.18968

Warm, E. (2025, August 26). Deskilling and automation bias: A cautionary tale for health professions educators. ICE Blog. https://icenet.blog/2025/08/26/deskilling-and-automation-bias-a-cautionary-tale-for-health-professions-educators/

World Health Organization. (2024). Ethics and governance of artificial intelligence for health: Guidance on large multi-modal models. https://www.who.int/publications/i/item/9789240084759

Xiao, Y., Huang, J., He, R., Xiao, J., Mousavi, M. R., Liu, Y., Li, K., Chen, Z., & Zhang, J. M. (2025). FairMedQA: Benchmarking bias in large language models for medical question answering. arXiv. https://doi.org//arXiv.2505.19562DOI: 10.48550

Xiong, G., Jin, Q., Lu, Z., & Zhang, A. (2024). Benchmarking retrieval-augmented generation for medicine. In *Findings of the Association for Computational Linguistics* (pp. 6233–6251). ACL.

Xu, D., Zhang, Z., Zhu, Z., Lin, Z., Liu, Q., Wu, X., Xu, T., Zhao, X., Zheng, Y., & Chen, E. (2024). Mitigating hallucinations of large language models in medical information extraction via contrastive decoding. /arXiv.2410.15702DOI: 10.18653/v1/2024.findings-emnlp.456

Zack, T., Luhanga, M., Rajkomar, A., & Obermeyer, Z. (2024). Assessing the potential of GPT-4 to perpetuate racial and gender biases in health care. *The Lancet. Digital Health*, *6*(1), e12–e22. DOI: 10.1016/S2589-7500(23)00225-X PMID: 38123252

Zakka, C., Chaurasia, A., Shad, R., Dalal, A. R., Kim, J. L., Moor, M., ... & Hiesinger, W. (2024). Almanac — Retrieval-augmented language models for clinical medicine. NEJM AI, 1(2), AIoa2300068. DOI: 10.1056/AIoa2300068

ADDITIONAL READING

Agrawal, G. (2024). Accountability, trust, and transparency in AI systems from the perspective of public policy: Elevating ethical standards. In Singla, B., & Shalender, K. (Eds.), *AI healthcare applications and security, ethical, and legal considerations* (pp. 148–162). IGI Global. DOI: 10.4018/979-8-3693-7452-8.ch009

Davis, N., Clemens, M., Rezwana, J., & Browne, E. (2025). Human-AI co-creation: A new interaction paradigm for human-AI interaction. In Xu, W. (Ed.), *Handbook of human-centered artificial intelligence* (pp. 1–57). Springer Nature. DOI: 10.1007/978-981-97-8440-0_76-1

Karagoz, G., van Kollenburg, G., Ozcelebi, T., & Meratnia, N. (2024). Evaluating how explainable AI is perceived in the medical domain: A human-centered quantitative study of XAI in chest X-ray diagnostics. In Chen, H., Zhou, Y., Xu, D., & Vardhanabhuti, V. V. (Eds.), *Trustworthy artificial intelligence for healthcare* (pp. 92–108). Springer. DOI: 10.1007/978-3-031-67751-9_8

Kücking, F., Hübner, U., Przysucha, M., Hannemann, N., Kutza, J.-O., Moelleken, M., Erfurt-Berge, C., Dissemond, J., Babitsch, B., & Busch, D. (2024). Automation bias in AI-decision support: Results from an empirical study. In *Digitalization in health care*. IOS Press., DOI: 10.3233/SHTI240871

Liebovitz, D. M. (2025). Transforming and democratizing clinical workflows: The role of large language models (LLMs) in disrupting healthcare. In Liebowitz, J. (Ed.), *Digital transformation in healthcare* (pp. 33–60). World Scientific. DOI: 10.1142/9789819813506_0003

Patrão Neves, M., & Betâmio de Almeida, A. (2024). Before and beyond artificial intelligence: opportunities and challenges. In Antunes, H. S., Freitas, P. M., Oliveira, A. L., Pereira, C. M., de Sequeira, E. V., & Xavier, L. B. (Eds.), *Multidisciplinary perspectives on artificial intelligence and the law* (pp. 107–125). Springer. DOI: 10.1007/978-3-031-41264-6_6

Puttanapura, J., Singh, T. M., Fatima, S., & Dadireddy, M. K. (2025). Leveraging artificial intelligence for transformative operational improvements in healthcare: Enhancing efficiency, patient care, and decision-making. In M. Shuaib, S. Alam, A. Rajaram, & K. Reddy C. (Eds.), Next-generation therapeutics using internet of things and machine learning (pp. 165–186). IGI Global.

Sandra, G., & Panji, A. (2022). Medical liability in Indonesia: Overview and regulatory trends. In Raposo, V. L., & Beran, R. G. (Eds.), *Medical liability in Asia and Australasia* (pp. 83–96). Springer.

Umamaheswari, P. (2025). A comprehensive review for critical evaluation of AI-driven hospital systems: Ethical challenges and future perspectives. In Anandavalli, M., Chakkaravarthy, P., & Dhanalakshmi, J. (Eds.), *Evaluation and assessment of AI-driven systems in hospitals* (pp. 35–60). IGI Global. DOI: 10.4018/979-8-3373-2787-7.ch002

Vasiliu-Feltes, I. (2025). Advancing healthcare transformation through deep tech: An examination of latest trends, challenges, and opportunities. In Liebowitz, J. (Ed.), *Digital transformation in healthcare* (pp. 1–10). World Scientific. DOI: 10.1142/9789819813506_0001

KEY TERMS AND DEFINITIONS

Clinical Decision Support (CDS): Software that helps clinicians make evidence-based recommendations on a case-by-case basis, integrates recommendations, alerts, and information about the clinical record of each patient and other data.

Hallucination: The creation of something that is wrong and is a lie, and supported with no information, therefore, is incorrect, such as the absence of something that is wrong or existence of something that is wrong, incorrect clinical facts, and recommendations that are wrong about the patient.

Human-in-the-Loop (HITL): The precept of a designed system under which a human actor is required to perform a review of a decision that is critical in an automated AI process, at least for scenarios in clinical practice that are high-risk and that require an exercise of clinical judgment, ethical judgment, or context sensitivity.

Large Language Model (LLM): A form of Artificial Intelligence (AI) that utilizes the transformer method and is able to create, condense, translate, and reason about human text with an ever-increasing fluency. It is also being used for medical education, clinical documentation, and clinical decision support.

Retrieval-Augmented Generation (RAG): A structure of AI that enhances the generation of text via a language model that retrieves relevant data from organized external knowledge databases during the processing stage, which lowers the occurrence of fabricated information and uplifts the basis of facts in precise domains, such as clinical medicine.

SafeMed Framework: A multidimensional framework for the evaluation of safety consisting of ten clinical and operational components, such as the control of hallucinations, bias, privacy, human oversight and others, which evaluates the efficiency of medical chatbots based on LLMs and beyond mere accuracy.

Safety-Critical System: Any system whose malfunction, failure, or misuse can lead to death, serious injury, regulatory violation, or irreversible harm to a patient or a healthcare organization. This entails the highest level of care in regard to risk assessments, analyses, and validation as well as a focus on continual monitoring after the system has been deployed or implemented.

Worst-at-k Analysis: A method of evaluation involving the analysis of the worst event that could happen in a situation involving k outcomes from a model of identical prompts. This method of evaluation reveals the risks of failure that occur and have been largely ignored which are most relevant in a clinical situation that is highly critical.

Chapter 4

Information Security and Clinical Ethics in LLM-Based Healthcare Systems

Updesh Kumar Jaiswal
http://orcid.org/0009-0002-1572-8275
School of Engineering and Technology, Vivekananda Institute of Professional Studies - Technical Campus, Delhi, India

Jaishree Jain
http://orcid.org/0000-0003-0173-7664
Ajay Kumar Garg Engineering College, Ghaziabad, India

Harnit Saini
http://orcid.org/0009-0007-3103-9070
Ajay Kumar Garg Engineering College, Ghaziabad, India

Amrita Bhatnagar
Noida Institute of Engineering and Technology, Greater Noida, India

Pushpendra Singh
SRM Institute of Science and Technology, Ghaziabad, India

Shashank Sahu
Ajay Kumar Garg Engineering College, Ghaziabad, India

Khushbu Malviya
Ajay Kumar Garg Engineering College, Ghaziabad, India

ABSTRACT

Large Language Models (LLMs) play a complex and ever-evolving role in medicine. LLMs, in general, can help medical professionals identify patients by giving them fast, data-driven information. They are able to analyse patient data, compare it with a comprehensive medical history, and make recommendations for potential diagnoses or identify issues that need more research. This chapter examines the threats that prompt injection attacks, perfect overturn, and data leak could pose to PHI and offers solutions to lessen these risks through federated learning, secure model design, and privacy-preserving AI methods. These models are very decent

DOI: 10.4018/979-8-3373-7862-6.ch004

at comprehending and producing human language and are built on deep learning and natural language processing technologies. LLMs have developed exceptional skills in vocabulary, grammar, semantics, and specialized knowledge, particularly in medicine, thanks to the extensive training on vast amounts of textual material. A proposal for an ethical framework to safeguard that medical LLMs operate within the bounds of patient trust closes the chapter.

1. INTRODUCTION

Artificial intelligence (AI) mentions to the methods and schemes that are designed to achieve errands that are otherwise desirous of humanoid intelligence. Machine learning (ML) is a concept in the arena of artificial intelligence that involves models of data-driven pattern recognition that are operated without human control, whereas natural language processing (NLP) is an arena absorbed on allowing processers to read, write, and speak humanoid linguistic (Jaiswal et al., 2023). ChatGPT, Claude, and Gemini are examples of large language models (LLMs), or other systems that rely on recent developments in deep learning (DP) and large datasets to attain a high level of fluency and contextual understanding, which has been applied in the field of medicine, education, and research to a considerable degree (Goel et al., 2025). Specialist LLMs are being created in addition to commercial LLMs, like in the case of Med-PaLM, a scientific query responding system, or BioBERT, a manuscript removal system in biomedical applications (Adams et al., 2023). Some of them are focused on a specific domain (e.g., radiology, oncology), and domain-specific corpora are used to improve the presentation. Such a diversity emphasizes the flexibility of the LLMs in various healthcare fields, such as the production of clinical trial records to facilitate mental health screening (Akinci D'Antonoli et al., 2025).

Applications to the field of medicine The possible uses of LLMs include many areas of healthcare, such as real-time enduring communication finished medicinal chatbots to provide assistance, triage, and teaching; enhance scientific choice provision by helping with identifies, action prescriptions, and medication data; automatic or semi-automated medical imagination and journalism, in particular, radiology, pathology, and nuclear medicine; as well as extracting and condensing big capacities of electric well-being archives and scientific literature to generate faster insights. The success of LLMs hip such areas is explained by their aptitude to function with formless written information, to manufacture multifaceted info, and give plausible and contextually high-quality responses (Arora et al., 2023). This revolutionary period has a great chance to recover the excellence of patient care and deepen medical knowledge, which creates a new standard in healthcare digital age (Chau et al., 2025).

The review unites the body of existing studies on the practicability, effectiveness, and limitations of LLMs in health care locations (Chuang et al., 2025). By analytical studies in numerous grounds of medicine and usage, we intended to give health care doctors a full considerate of the present national of the LLMs in drug, likely compensations they would have, and the tests that have to be stunned to implement them. The advent of informal artificial intelligence has marked an important turning point in the digital transformation of the healthcare industry. According to Desai, the pending of distributed upkeep depends on how AI chatbots change telemedicine and patient involvement. These systems have advanced from basic unconscious black-boards to composite, transformer-based agents gifted of rivalling human feeling and offering nuanced medical advice. In addition, the legal system is having difficulty changing. While HIPAA and GDPR offer fundamental guidelines for data privacy, they were primarily written before autonomous LLMs became widely used. As a result, there are a lot of questions about Business Associate Agreements (BAAs) and the "minimum necessary" sharing of data in an AI setting (Feretzakis & Verykios, 2024). Most nations in the world have enacted regulatory privacy laws, policies, and guidelines to accomplish this objective.

The Health Insurance Portability and Accountability Act (HIPAA) is one of the laws enacted in the USA to offer standards for the protection of Social Health Insurance (SHI). The Privacy Act of 1988, which established regulations for patient SHI, functioned as an analog of HIPAA in Australia. For people living in the European Union, the General Data Protection Regulation (GDPR) offers a legal framework for the gathering and use of SHI. Japan's Act for the Protection of Personal Information (APPI) offers a legislative framework for safeguarding personal information and individual privacy that is comparable to the GDPR's data protection standards. The Personal Data (Privacy) Ordinance in Hong Kong, one of the first laws in the Asian region to provide legal mechanisms for the protection of person privacy, offers a framework that safeguards patients' SHI. With a few exceptions, the majority of these laws have many traits in common. The definitions of SHI and SHI are among the key distinctions. The distinction between structured and unstructured Electronic Health Record (HER) data is another area where these standards diverge. Compared to unstructured EHR data, which needs information extraction, organized EHR data is simpler to process.

The privacy rules were crafted mainly to ensure that there is adequate provision for storing and managing SHI information securely. Although other rules like the GDPR include a broad range of privacy requirements, they also outline ways that would make the SHI information secure as well as its redaction before releasing it into the public domain. They emphasize the need for well-executed statistical analysis in preserving privacy. This requires the use of larger samples so that the findings from the research have relevance without compromising the individual's reidentification risk. Privacy laws forbid the use of less than five data subjects in any kind of research that uses data sharing. Despite the lack of direct identifiers in the information, an individual may still be reidentified using other parameters like diagnosis and treatment among others.

There are still possibilities for unique reidentification and group reidentification, resulting in potential privacy violations despite following these recommendations. Unique reidentification refers to a case where the record in the dataset precisely corresponds to an identified person, while group reidentification happens when the records in the dataset match the identified few people. There are scenarios wherein identity recovery techniques implemented on anonymized information might recover one-to-one, one-to-few, and few-to-few identities10.

1.1 Privacy-Preserving Techniques in LLMs

We provide a list of privacy-preserving methods that can be adopted and shown in Figure 1. Large language models (LLMs) are commonly utilized by clinicians, academics, and educators for different applications, including documentation, guideline retrieval and summary, and clinical decision-making. With regards to the implementation of LLMs to comply with privacy policies and standards, the use of LLMs in structured and unstructured EHR data is currently at the nascent stage. It is worth mentioning that LLMs are usually leveraged to generate structured information from unstructured inputs, highlighting their versatile nature. Several techniques can be applied to ensure compliance and privacy, depending on the use case of the LLMs.

Figure 1. Context-aware privacy preserving strategies for secondary usage of EHRs

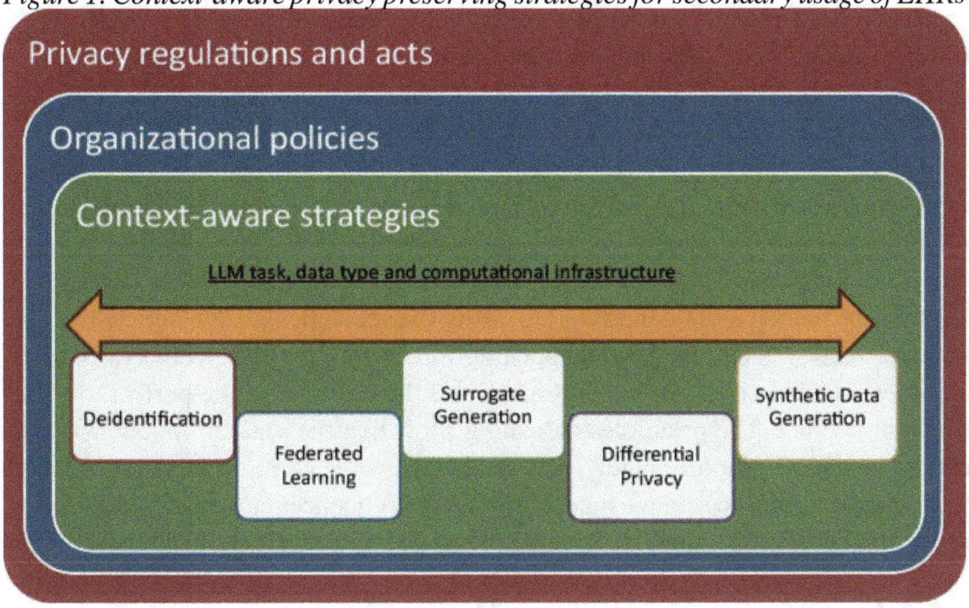

1.2 Analysis of Extensive Linguistic Models

LLMs are powerful schemes constructed on DP paradigms, and most based on the so-called Modifier building to successfully procedure consecutive data. These replicas are trained to a large scale using large amounts of data to absorb semantic and syntactic patterns (Ferrer et al., 2021). Their effectiveness would be impossible without the concept of scaling laws as it explains how increasing the scale of both models and data could yield significant improvement in the understanding and generation of human-like language. The three key components of the capabilities of the LLM are summarized as follows: progressive linguistic modelling to forecast and make fluently manuscript orders, Modifier building to process long-range dependences in manuscript, and wide pre-training to provide the replicas by extensive information in the form of contextual knowledge useful across multiple fields.

Linguistic replicas are stochastic replicas that tend to determine the probability of a order of marks (words, sub words or morphemes). They also determine the likelihood of a order using the preceding marks and, therefore, they are good at predicting the next token or coming up with new ones (Gallegos et al., 2024). This proficiency is core to the understanding and generation of language in large language models; the transformer architecture is a key aspect of current large language models. Unlike recurrent neural networks (RNNs), Transformer uses self-attention processes compared to recurrent neural networks (RNNs), which procedure marks successively then are poorly suited to long-range dependencies. This method lets the easy modelling of large manuscripts and allows similar dispensation; thus, it is extremely climbable. Scalability will be critical in training large models that use large datasets and achieve higher performance.

The task of extensive pre-training involves training the idea of large language models (LLMs) such by way of Wikipedia, Common Crawl, and Books with disguised linguistic modelling and next-token prediction (NTP). In MLM, part of the original manuscript is covered with a texture, and the model is suggested to use its power to forecast the hidden marks, thereby, capturing the semantic and syntactical relation between marks. NTP emphases happening forecasting the following symbolic in an order founded on the preceding marks and therefore helps the perfect to make intelligible order. The principles of scaling show that the scale of model and data can be increased proportionately, and the performance can improve dramatically. Such scale is needed to achieve state-of-the-art consequences cutting-edge numerous natural language processing (NLP), as demonstrated by the GPT-3 and PaLM replicas.

1.3 Advancement of Extensive Medical Language Models

Medicinal LLM advancement consumes remained defined through important progress cutting-edge perfect structure, exercise information, and fine-tuning mechanisms that are explicitly built with health care in mind. With this development, Initial Biomedical Language Models absorbed on pre-training current structures like BERT on biomedical data. Such replicas as BioBERT and Clinical BERT consume better the presentation of such tasks as called object credit then connection removal within the context of biological11 texts. Particular Medicinal LLM: Investigators have today ongoing creating LLM explicitly designed to be used in medicine. Medical literature-based and electronic health data-driven models such as MEDITRON have been constructed from the ground up based on domain-specific information, and thereby integrated directly into their pre-training strategy (Goh et al., 2024). The most recent developments take ran to the growth of multimodal LLMs which are talented of textual and medicinal imagination analysis. Medicinal graphic query responding and automatic analysis founded happening scientific photos and minutes have demonstrated positive results in such models as Med-PaLM. Recent progress involves improvements on existing massive models used in the medical field finished progressive fine-tuning and encouragement models. Through these methodologies, models like MedGemini have performed highly in tests of medical licensure as well as in the clinical reasoning tasks defines the LLM used. The current emphasis of growth and challenging is on GPT and LLaMA. These developments indicate that next apps will more effectively address the particular requirements of the medical field (Javed et al., 2025).

Table 1 outlines the possible and varied uses of medicinal LLMs in health care, counting their parts in clinical decision-making (e.g., SkinGPT-4 for dermatological purposes), medical assessments (e.g., ChatGPT's success in the USMLE), enduring message (e.g., polyglot provision for autistic individuals), and info removal after well-being annals (Johannssen & Chukhrova , 2025).

Table 1. Application of Medical LLMs in Healthcare

Application Area	Description	Examples of LLM Use	Challenges
Medical Assessments and Clinical Inference	Clinical reasoning cases are handled by LLMs. Passing clinical board "examinations" denotes.	BingChat performs better than others on the multispecialty recruitment assessment (MSRA), and ChatGPT passed the USMLE.	Performance variations among various specialties Prior to clinical deployment, a thorough evaluation is required.
Clinical Diagnosis and Decision Support	In a variety of specialties, LLM supports clinical diagnosis and decision-making.	SkinGPT-4 for diagnosing dermatological conditions	Human supervision is required.
Patient Education & Communication	LLM improves patient education and engagement by providing precise and sympathetic answers to patient questions.	AI chat powered by LLM to enhance heart failure education	The degree of readability frequently surpasses patient comprehension.
Data extraction and analysis of medical records	LLM retrieves pertinent data from electronic medical records.	Compiling radiological reports for patients with glioblastoma	Data Privacy concerns

2. KEEPING HEALTHCARE HIPAA COMPLIANT: CREATING AN INTERNAL DATA PRIVACY IN LLM

Healthcare is one of the many fields that are undergoing substantial change as a result of the quick growth of artificial intelligence (AI), especially large language models (LLMs). Healthcare professionals, however, face difficulties in using this potent technology while adhering to strict privacy laws like the Health Insurance Portability and Accountability Act (HIPAA) (Lin & Kuo, 2025).

2.1 Comprehending Healthcare AI Systems With HIPAA Compliance

Any AI system handling Protected Health Information (PHI) is required by HIPAA to adhere to the Privacy Rule and Information Security Rule, guaranteeing that patient data is utilized and released appropriately, stored securely, and only accessed by authorized persons (Laukamp et al., 2024). Although public LLMs, like as OpenAI's GPT-4, perform well, there are privacy concerns when using them to handle private medical data. Rather, a lot of healthcare facilities are choosing internal LLMs that may be customized to satisfy HIPAA regulations and certain information security requirements. By ensuring that data control stays inside the healthcare business, these internal systems lower the danger of data disclosure (Li et al., 2025).

Following the tremendous surge of digitization in the public sector, many various systems and technological solutions have been developed over the years to achieve the desired fluent system for the healthcare sector. This type of system is not easily built, or even specified. A healthcare system is a type of system that stores extremely sensitive patient information and must be kept safe and precise. Healthcare systems are primarily composed of three concepts: electronic health records (EHR), electronic medical records (EMR), and personal health records (PHR). These three notions represent the most sensitive personal information handled in healthcare systems. It is crucial to analyze this type of information properly (Jain & Jaiswal, 2025).

Information does not wind up in the wrong hands. While software engineering is rapidly improving, hackers and cybercriminals are always creating new strategies to gain access to restricted systems and breach various applications. Cybersecurity assaults are on the rise across the world, and they have become a major issue in the fields of industrial system integration and system protection. Recent research has found that attackers are more likely to target public sector and critical infrastructure systems. This includes healthcare systems. According to Hautamäki and Kokkonen, the healthcare business is one of the most vulnerable to cyber assaults. Johnson and He's work "Generic Security Cases for Information Security in Healthcare" also supports this idea, indicating that the healthcare industry is responsible for 43% of all known data breaches. As a result, it is vital that the systems remain in line with current cyber security trends and best practices. The difficulty with healthcare systems is that the entire system is based on numerous separate sub-sectors of healthcare and their systems from various suppliers. Furthermore, the healthcare business comprises a wide range of medical equipment that may be connected to the internet, increasing the potential of cybersecurity breaches. The biggest issue with healthcare systems is the complexity of numerous systems and software suppliers. The entire system becomes a big and intricate network of various systems and data pipelines across several enterprises, which frequently involve healthcare sectors as well as third-party software and server providers. Cloud computing has also introduced a new component to the systems. Cloud computing has been accepted as a new option for local servers to store and manage healthcare systems in order to save costs while also simplifying system integrity. This generates a new security paradigm since the data is now kept on a third-party cloud server, which can be hosted anywhere in the globe. The cloud computing element provides a strong layer of protection to the system and data against cybersecurity threats; yet, it poses another difficulty.

2.2 Design-Based Data Security in LLMs

HIPAA regulations require that data security be included into the architecture of the model from the start. All phases of PHI security, including data collection, preprocessing, model training, and deployment, must be maintained by healthcare providers.

- **Data Encryption and Access Control:** Role-based access controls and robust encryption for data in transit and at rest restrict access to PHI to authorized personnel only (Lu et al., 2025).
- **De-identification of Data:** During model training, identifiers such as patient names, addresses, and social security numbers can be removed or masked to lessen the possibility of PHI being exposed in the event of a breach. This is crucial when training an internal LLM because HIPAA authorizes the use of de-identified data for research and quality improvement (Al Nazi et al., 2024).
- **Federated Learning (FL) and Differential Privacy:** These techniques improve privacy by enabling the model to learn from data without having direct access to it. While differential privacy adds noise to data, making individual records less recognizable, FL allows training on decentralized data sources. Research on HIPAA compliance and data security in healthcare contexts has demonstrated the potential of both approaches (Prosper et al., 2023).

3. UNDERSTANDING PHI AND DATA SENSITIVITY IN CLINICAL ETHICS CONTEXTS

Publicly available datasets, like the Medical Information Mart for Intensive Care-IV, are used in a significant amount of research on LLMs in healthcare (Salvi et al., 2025). However, some research uses internal patient health information (PHI), which often includes sensitive personally identifiable information (PII). (Seh et al., 2020). This raises issues with data governance and patient privacy protection, particularly when LLMs are used in the cloud and raw data must be sent to distant computers (Sheng et al., 2021). Healthcare chatbots are often classified based on the type of data they process and the complexity of their functionality. However, these technologies' data-intensive design presents new risks to PHI (Shen et al., 2023). User insights remain positive for the convenience of these instruments, but medical experts continue to have misgivings about their capacity to attain complex analytic details then support entire clandestineness (Suresh & Guttag, 2021).

This is internal access and data limitations, because the software is in the hands of third-party providers. Within the cloud computing solution in the healthcare industry, three main concepts of security in this matter are that all medical records should be guarded through ownership-controlled encryption, eliminating the possibility of third-party workers gaining access to the medical data. The second criterion is that the records themselves should maintain authenticity and integrity throughout the integration process. The third premise is that the system's data pipeline should include end-to-end verification using signatures and certification methods to prevent unauthorized access and alteration to healthcare data. Johnson and He have roughly similar perspectives on the key elements, namely have resulted in data breach situations.

According to their research, three crucial traits were prevalent in many data breaches: 1. Sensitive data were not adequately encrypted. 2. Security policies and procedures were not effectively applied and disseminated. 3. Incident handling and response times were delayed. These qualities stated in both studies would have had a significant influence on previous data breaches and should not be taken lightly. In Finland, the Vastaamo case is a well-known and unique cybersecurity breach case. In general, psychotherapy institution Vastaamo has a poorly built healthcare system with significant security issues.

In 2019, attackers discovered and exploited these vulnerabilities. The attackers acquired complete access to the patient information database, which held extremely sensitive and personal information. The Vastaamo organization became aware of the breach, but instead of exposing it to authorities and patients, they opted to try to hide it. When attackers began blackmailing patients by revealing their personal information on the internet, the entire case was made public. Unfortunately, the attackers exposed the entire database to the open internet, purportedly accidently.

3.1 Risks of Model Memorization and Data Leakage

System prompts are susceptible to prompt extraction attacks, in which adversaries formulate queries to reveal the contents of the prompt. This vulnerability has resulted in the exposing of many systems prompts for bespoke GPTs and ChatGPT (Ueda et al., 2023). Such openings may reveal subtle information, structural protocols, and cleaning criteria, insertion among the highest ten hazards to LLMs in OWASP. A new class of vulnerabilities that take advantage of the model's cognitive skills is introduced when AI is included into healthcare settings. Quick inoculation uses prudently built manuscript contributions to touch the AI, in difference to typical cyberattacks that board software burdens (Wang et al., 2021). Because LLMs are fundamentally unable to differentiate between instructions and data, the National Cyber Security Centre (NCSC) cautions that prompt injection may never be completely eliminated.

Any healthcare system that permits the AI to browse the internet or process papers from third parties will always be at danger (Yarram et al., 2025). Additionally, the 2020 "Děorf Case," in which a ransomware outbreak on a hospital's digital organization caused in a patient's death, highlights the lethal landscape of system-level susceptibilities when AI-controlled medicinal data and devices are chopped as shown in Figure 2.

Figure 2. Adversial Modification of Training Data

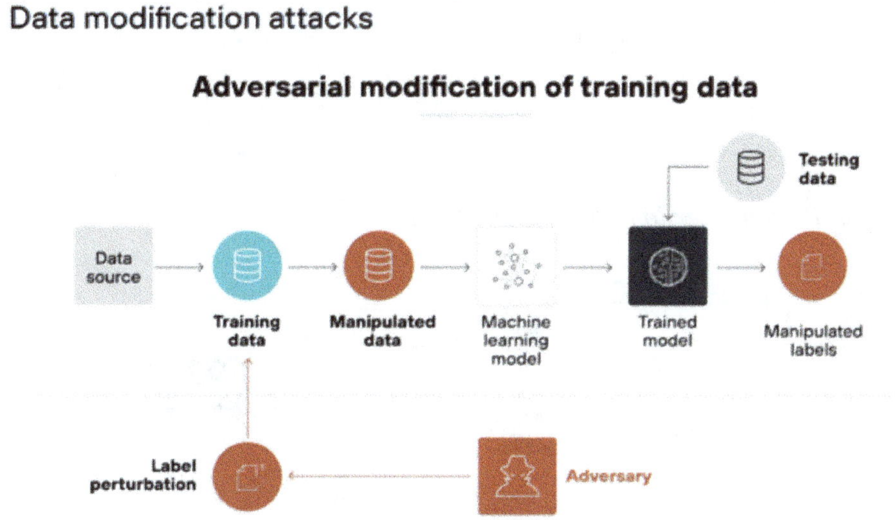

3.2 Adversarial Data Poisoning ATTACKs in LLM Pipelines

A data poisoning assault is a kind of adversarial attack when an assailant deliberately modifies the exercise data rummage-sale to construct a mechanism knowledge or AI perfect (Yasaka et al., 2025). The objective is to shape the model's behaviour during exercise such that it endures until deployment. Data poisoning attacks may be classified in many distinct ways (Yu et al., 2023). A very comprehensive model emphasizes the modifications an attacker may implement and the manner in which they exert that control. This results in two primary categories of data poisoning attacks, and those are illustrated in Figure 3, and Figure 4.

Figure 3. Data Poisoning Attack in the LLM pipeline

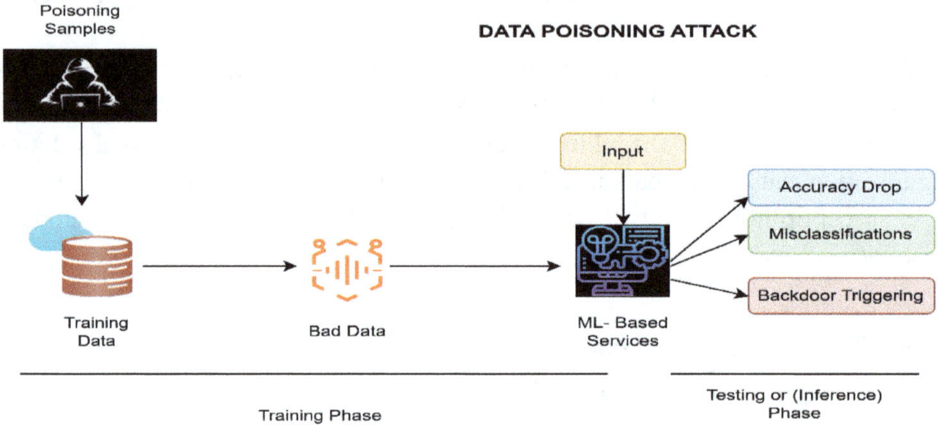

Figure 4. Poison Insertion Attack in the LLM

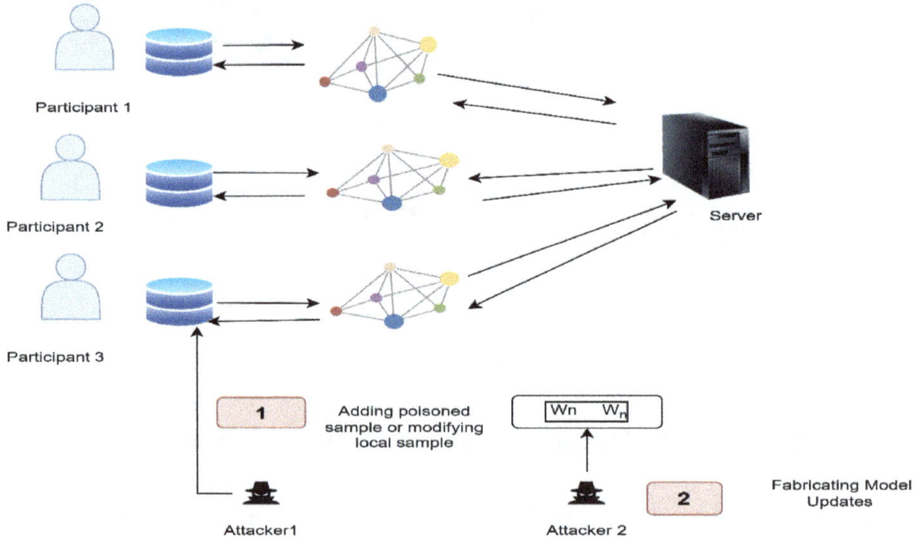

4. PRIVACY-PRESERVING TECHNIQUES FOR LLMS DEVELOPMENT

A preliminary privacy risk analysis of the LLMs lifecycle can identify three primary processes based on the categories of data needed to train foundation models, alter them during post-training, and optimize them for unique use cases or interactional goals. Importantly, gradually more carefully chosen data is used in the post-training stage to adjust and enhance models if a vast amount of data is needed at the foundational layer (i.e., stages 1 through 3 of data collecting and pre-processing). This intermediate stage (steps 4 to 6) is sometimes overlooked in privacy considerations, although it is appropriate to use data protection best practices in LLM-based tool development. The final phase of creating LLM-based systems is optimization (Zhong et al., 2025). To identify and reduce risks during the implementation of a fictional chatbot for mental health, the study used a structured PIA methodology.

- **Step 1: Information Account and Flow Mapping:** Decisive what data is collected (such as symptoms, mood, and insurance details) and how it journeys from the user's mobile app to the cloud server and any third-party APIs (such as OpenAI or AWS).
- **Step 2: Risk Identification:** Danger modelling is used to find faintness such as "Collection through creation," in which the AI crops sensitive new data on a patient's mental state that was never revealed.
- **Step 3: Impact Analysis:** Decisive the likelihood of a breach and the likely damage to the patient (e.g., insurance loss, stigmatization).
- **Step 4: Mitigation Strategy:** Applying particular limits, like safe combination methods and pseudonymization.

The Advantages of decentralized data in Smart healthcare as follow: Improved Security and Privacy, Enhanced Interoperability, Enhanced Patient Autonomy, and Economic Efficiency. The basic stages of the creation of synthetic data are depicted in Figure 5. There are four steps to it. The first step is data gathering, where accurate data is gathered, secured, and controlled. In the second step, known as data preparation, after cleaning and preprocessing, the data is transformed into useful information for building the models. After that, in the data modeling stage, an ML model is prepared to generate synthetic data having features similar to the original data. Data quality assessment is the fourth step, which evaluates the use of the duplicate data in place of the original data. The iterative flow, as shown in Figure 5, indicates improvements at each stage after completing the previous stage so that the best quality synthetic data is produced.

Figure 5. Basic stages of the creation of synthetic data

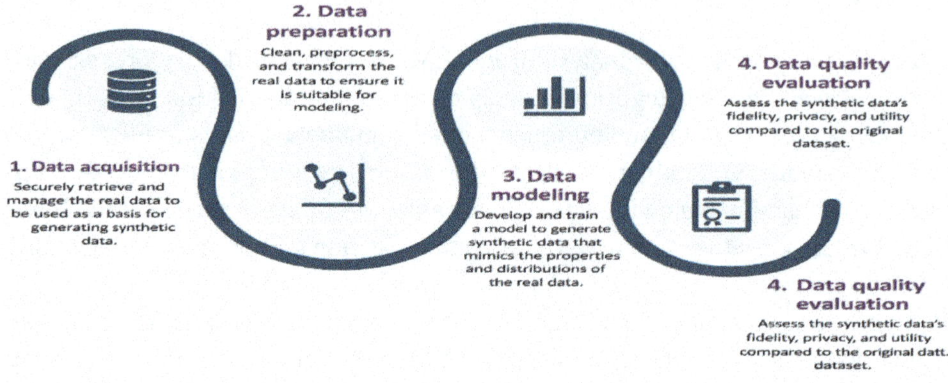

4.1 Threats To Health Data Privacy and Security

Growing system interconnectedness and the digitization of healthcare data have created complex vulnerabilities to the information security and privacy of health data that impact people worldwide. Nowadays, the most valuable target category for both hostile actors and hackers is sensitive health information. Following health informatics system breaches, healthcare organizations suffer a variety of serious repercussions, including financial losses, reputational harm, and legal penalties (Zhou et al., 2024). Data breaches brought on by cyberattacks, such as ransomware, phishing, and malware incursions, are currently the biggest threat. Due to a lack of resources, healthcare institutions typically lack adequate cybersecurity preparation, which leaves them vulnerable to assaults. Ransomware attacks' encryption capabilities cause hospital systems to completely lock down, disrupting services and endangering patient care. Before granting access, these attacks need money from healthcare organizations.

Internal threat actors pose a serious threat to the organizational structure. When employees intentionally abuse their access privileges or inadvertently cause security problems by misidentifying dangerous connections and improper data management, it constitutes a threat. These days, complex systems in health IT environments make it difficult to maintain complete control over all accessible access points. One of the biggest security concerns is the risk associated with third-party suppliers and cloud-based systems acting as health data managers. When external partners handling data are not adequately protected from cyberattacks, there is a security vulnerability. Because wearable technology and mobile health applications typically operate outside of HIPAA regulation jurisdiction, they are nonetheless susceptible to exposure.

Current LLMs routinely transgress professional ethics rules, according to the examination of the mental health triage simulation. In 84% of chatbot responses, licensed psychologists found "deceptive empathy" in the usage of phrases such as "I understand your pain," which can lead to harmful emotional dependence among susceptible users. The experiment also shown that chatbots frequently have trouble with "contextual adaptation." The bot offered a "one-size-fits-all" coping method in 22% of crisis scenarios, ignoring the particular environmental risks—like access to dangerous substances—that the user had identified. This demonstrates a "black box" failure in which the AI adheres to learnt patterns rather than strict therapeutic guidelines.

4.2 Role of LLMs and AI Agents in Clinical System

Many factors, challenges, and benefits need to be taken into mind while implementing LLMs and other generative AI in the healthcare industry. Clinicians need to be aware of these aspects and actively engage in the discussion. Even if employing closed LLMs via APIs offers convenience and access to advanced models, healthcare facilities should carefully consider the benefits of adopting open models to maintain a better degree of control over their AI systems. In general, the use of LLMs with AI agents is a very young and evolving field. Collaboration between physicians, researchers, technologists, and business partners is essential to ensuring that new technologies enhance patient care and adhere to ethical standards. Patient safety, data privacy, and ethical issues must remain top priorities. A comprehensive system is necessary for effective deployment. testing and validation as well as ongoing training for medical personnel. In conclusion, the use of LLMs in healthcare is revolutionary. We can guarantee that generative AI is applied responsibly in healthcare by outlining the necessary prerequisites from a clinical standpoint and thoughtfully contributing to the debate on how LLMs should be implemented. Private businesses may be essential in supporting the npj Digital Medicine

Contribute frameworks for software development, regulatory compliance, information security, and the implementation of open LLMs and warehousing in healthcare settings.

In this way, it can be guaranteed that LLMs are safe, dependable, and successful when used in medicine. Businesses might engage with healthcare providers to adapt and incorporate these models into current workflows, meeting particular needs like patient monitoring, treatment planning, and diagnosis. One-size-fits-all solutions should be avoided by the community, particularly if data structures and safety requirements are still unclear. Let's establish the groundwork for the plethora of fascinating uses that are still to be uncovered as shown in Table 2.

Table 2. Overview of key ethical considerations faced by LLMs in Healthcare

Consideration	Description
Safety and Reliability	Make sure LLM outputs are safe, act consistently in a clinical setting, and steer clear of over-reliance or failure.
Privacy and Information Security	Use model training, inference, and storage to safeguard patient data.
Bias and Fairness	Prevent clinical or demographic groups from being disadvantaged in LLM outputs.
Transparency & Explainability	Reduce black box opacity and identify evaluative bias by making clear how LLM produces output for clinician and patient use.
Accountability & Legal	Provide a system for accountability and liability.
Trust & Misinformation	Develop a healthy sense of trust without becoming overly dependent and be aware of false information.
Equity & Inclusion	Resolve inequities in health and power.
Autonomy & Personalization	Respect patient autonomy by permitting LLM tools to be utilized intelligently.
Legal Liability & Oversight	Make legal obligations for the use of LLM in clinical process clear.

4.3 Cybersecurity Risks and Countermeasures for Big Language Models in LLM-Based Healthcare Systems

There are several chances to enhance patient care and medical practice through the use of LLMs in smart healthcare. LLMs provide distinct cybersecurity vulnerabilities that need to be thoroughly assessed before these AI models are used in healthcare, in addition to being vulnerable to biases and dangers shared by all AI systems. Malicious assaults, privacy violations, and improper patient data modification are just a few of the ways that LLMs can be abused. LLMs may also be used by malevolent individuals to deduce private patient information from training data. Additionally, the results of these models could be altered in a way that benefits the bad actors if they are fed manipulated or contaminated data. The cybersecurity issues raised by LLMs in the healthcare industry are discussed in this chapter along with mitigation techniques. Stakeholders can reduce these risks and safeguard patient privacy by putting strong security measures in place and following best practices throughout the model development, training, and deployment phases.

4.4 Legal and Regulatory Concerns

The use of LLMs in clinical studies raises a number of intricate legal issues. (i) Data privacy protection: A significant amount of sensitive personal information is contained in the vast amounts of trial data needed for LLM training and fine-tuning. Globally, legal and regulatory frameworks like the US Health Insurance Portability and Accountability Act (HIPAA) and the European Union's GDPR impose strict requirements on the protection of patients' personal information during LLM training, transmission, and storage.

4.5 Standardization of Evaluation and Practice

Regulatory organizations including the European Medicines Agency (EMA) and the US Food and Drug Administration (FDA) have not yet released precise criteria for assessing or using LLMs in clinical studies. Therefore, it is crucial to establish unified standards and useful recommendations in order to facilitate their incorporation into the workflows. A "human-in-the-loop" model offers a workable framework for standard evaluation through human–machine collaboration, since manual assessment is still the major method for evaluating LLMs in the medical area.

4.6 Data Quality, Privacy, and Blinding Control in LLMs

In order to handle realistic data management issues like quality control, privacy protection, and blinding control, investigators usually create DMPs ahead of time during the protocol creation of clinical studies. Making sure LLMs used for data management don't turn into fresh sources of data contamination is a top priority for researchers. During the output process, participants' private information may inadvertently be disclosed, which could be maliciously exploited by cybercriminals. The deployment of LLMs should use a variety of data encryption techniques, including symmetric/asymmetric encryption and k-anonymity, to protect data privacy. Fast fully homomorphic encryption (TFHE) has made it possible for LLMs to compute directly on encrypted data in recent years, striking a balance between processing efficiency and privacy protection. LLM-generated data management outputs could unintentionally reveal group allocation to researchers, jeopardizing the trial's blinding. To limit LLM access to randomization data, researchers should use role-based access control (RBAC). They should also set up output auditing mechanisms to stop the creation of any data that can obliquely expose intervention assignments.

5. PATIENT-CENTERED AND ETHICAL CONSIDERATIONS

A major limitation in existing technical discussions is the insufficient focus on patient-centered implications.

5.1 Health Literacy

Patients interacting with AI systems may misinterpret complex medical outputs. Systems must therefore ensure:

- readability
- simplified language
- contextual explanation
- multilingual accessibility

5.2 Dynamic Consent

Healthcare AI systems should integrate dynamic consent frameworks where patients can control:

- data sharing scope
- duration of use
- research permissions
- model training consent

5.3 Psychological Impact

Overly human-like conversational agents may create emotional dependence, especially in mental health applications. This requires explicit disclosure that users are interacting with AI systems.

6. GOVERNANCE, LEGAL, AND ORGANIZATIONAL FRAMEWORK

This research used the Simple Moving Average (SMA) and Simple Exponential Smoothing (SES) techniques of time series analysis to ascertain the pattern of healthcare data breaches and their financial impact on the healthcare sector. This research used two time series algorithms on the same data to identify any differences and enhance the consistency of the predicting findings. The Simple Moving Average (SMA) approach has been widely used to maintain updated predictions. This approach relies on the computed averages of subgroups within a data set. The moving average is computed by forming subgroups of data. It may include two, three, four, or five observation groups. Subsequent to computing the moving average, it was used to predict the forthcoming period. Subsequently, they juxtaposed the findings with those produced by the data analysis tool in MS-Excel to ascertain their correctness.

6.1 Privacy Preserving LLMs Implementation in Hospital Environment

This chapter will investigate the advantages and constraints of using LLM-powered chatbots for medical purposes and for chronic patient self-management. Indeed, when one considers the features of the context at hand, one should be especially thoughtful about the following concerns when delegating NLP and NLG to an LLM interacting with the patient directly without the assistance of an expert. It is crucial to especially emphasize the following issues.

Two approaches have been considered and tested. Using a GPT model was apparently the most obvious choice because they have been performing better on every task than any other large pre-trained language model. With proper instruction, it can actually generate a desirable set of safe responses for the patient and ensure that any type of disinformation is not spread yet remain empathetic and comforting. Nevertheless, several concerns may be made about this solution:

- The danger of revealing sensitive data and information leakage persists if the first filtering module fails; notably, even generic inquiries may include sensitive information inside phrases absent from our training dataset.
- The utilization of a GPT-based model requires a membership charge. As a result, this research applied one of the most affordable models by OpenAI.
- The complimentary plan has restrictions on the number of tokens transferred, the rate at which requests can be made in a minute, and daily interaction limits. It is non-scalable in terms of the number of users.
- The use of external services is a challenge that should be accepted.

The main concern in relation to privacy in connection with the first point would be the improper labeling of a category that requires largely localized processing in relation to the Insertion and Mood category, as universal. Information leakage occurs in these cases because of the unnecessary transmission of the question to the remote GPT. In relation to our content filtering for recognition, there was one inaccuracy for 83 insertions and one inaccuracy for 19 mood messages. Even if these inaccuracy rates appear extremely small, there can be important problems created. Since any improperly labeled information is basically unnecessary in this regard, there would be important problems related to privacy that would make this particular method, which involves important compromises, not applicable in this particular instance.

These are addressed by the use of open models deployed locally by not having to share information with any external services; however, it comes at the cost of a significant deterioration in response quality. This solution using open models is far less effective at correctly classifying queries and extracting parameters, and may therefore require fine-tuning to achieve these specific goals. The ecosystem of open models is ever-growing, and it is entirely possible that newer models with superior performance could be created. However, another perspective has emerged recently, one in which Alfred and Mixtral are two open models whose responses to open-ended queries receive significant support from domain experts. On a different note, innovative open approaches require investigation in future studies aimed at improving their efficiency, mainly in areas where GPT-3.5 Turbo outperformed in the current study.

6.2 Lessons Learned From PHI Breaches in AI-Driven Healthcare Systems

Time series analysis is a way of statistically forecasting or analysing a trend, using data sets organized chronologically or addressing time series data. Time series data delineates the collection of values that a variable assumes at various temporal intervals. This research used the Simple Moving Average (SMA) and Simple Exponential Smoothing (SES) techniques of time series analysis to ascertain the pattern of healthcare data breaches and their financial impact on the healthcare sector. This research used two time series algorithms on the same data to identify any differences and enhance the consistency of the predicting findings (Maurya et al., 2025). The Simple Moving Average (SMA) approach has been widely used to maintain updated predictions. This method is based on the calculated averages of subgroups for a dataset. A moving average is determined by forming subgroups for a set of data. It can consist of two, three, four, and five groups of observations. Subsequent to computing the moving average, it was used to predict the forthcoming period.

$$A_t = (O_t + O_{t-1} + \ldots + O_{t-n+1})/n \quad (1)$$

A_t denotes the moving average at time t, representing the predicted value at time t+1; O_t signifies the observation at time t; and 'n' refers to the number of observations within an interval or subgroup. They consider the interval between two observations as a subgroup, and compute the moving averages. The real numbers denote established observations, and the forecast values are the projected values derived using the SMA approach. Utilizing the data analysis function in Microsoft Excel, they produced forecast findings and juxtaposed them with manually computed results derived from Equation (1) to ensure correctness. Simple Exponential

Smoothing (SES) is a forecasting technique used for univariate data. This is a widely used forecasting approach that employs the weighted moving average of historical data to generate predictions Compared to the Simple Moving Average method, the weights in this method will be (highest) for current observations and smallest for the oldest observations. It primarily gained importance as a method for short-term forecasting. Its results will be highly dependent on the value of the smoothing constant, α, being appropriately chosen. The value of α lies in the range (0, 1). When α approaches 1, rapid learning is signified (in this scenario, forecasting is determined only by the most recent data), but when α approaches 0, gradual learning transpires (in this instance, forecasting is shaped by historical observations). The standard equation for SES is:

$$F_{t+1} = \alpha\, y_t + (1 - \alpha)\, F_t \qquad (2)$$

F_{t+1} represents the forecast value at time t+1, α is the smoothing constant, y_t is a known value at time t, and F_t signifies the forecast value of the variable Y at time t. They use $\alpha = 0.4$ to provide a balanced impact of observations on the predicting outcomes. The projected values were derived from actual observed data using Equation (2). Subsequently, they juxtaposed the findings with those produced by the data analysis tool in MS-Excel to ascertain their correctness.

6.3 Models for Continuous Risk Monitoring in LLM-Based Healthcare Systems

The research was executed by the governmental agency for its organization. This chapter introduces a pragmatic approach to assess application-level safety in LLM systems, which has been proven through real-world implementation for several use cases at the company. The framework consists of two parts: (i) concepts for creating adapted safety risk taxonomies and (ii) methodologies for assessing safety risks in applications of LLM. Their demonstration of how the proposed framework can be applied in our internal pilot serves as a reference for companies seeking to improve their safety testing efforts. The current research aims to bridge the gap between theoretical notions of AI safety and the implementation practice of securing LLM applications and provides practical guidance on how to deploy safely and scalable. The issue of liability becomes crucial as chatbots transition from administrative to prescriptive activities. Current guidelines are unclear on who is responsible if a chatbot misdiagnoses a patient because of a "hallucination" in its LLM: the institution, the physician who used the tool, or the software creator. Complex models' "black box" characteristics compromise transparency, which is a fundamental GDPR and clinical ethics need. Therefore, "Retrieval-Augmented Generation" (RAG) systems, which compel the AI to base its responses on validated clinical datasets rather than its own internal (and perhaps flawed) weights, are probably where healthcare chatbots will go in the future. To safely realize the potential of these agents, a comprehensive strategic shift is required. Healthcare organizations must move beyond treating chatbots as "smarter search engines" and acknowledge them as complicated, high-risk data processing entities. This necessitates the application of a "Privacy by Design" strategy that comprises:

- **Decentralized Training:** Using secure multi-party computation and FL to maintain patient data at the point of care.
- **Robust Regulatory Governance:** Enforcing AI-specific BAAs and performing regular Privacy Impact Assessments (PIAs) that explicitly model the particular hazards of generative AI.
- **Ethical and Technical Transparency:** RAG-based designs are used to prevent hallucinations, and patients are informed in plain language about the AI nature of the interactions.
- **Human-in-the-Loop Oversight:** Making sure chatbots don't function in a vacuum, especially in critical domains like drug prescription and mental health triage.

7. REAL WORLD CASE STUDY: DEVELOPING A SAFETY RISK TAXONOMY

Upon using these guidelines to create a safety risk taxonomy, they have identified how to implement this in a pilot study within their own establishment. As a public institution, they have developed a taxonomy that encapsulates safety concerns peculiar to the implementation of LLM-powered applications in a public institution. In this case, they highlighted three main groups of risks to focus on: 1. Undesirable content that might cause psychological distress to individuals or harm to the institution's reputation; 2. Specialist advice that might lead to physical or material harm if followed by unqualified individuals, mainly because of the supposed authority of a government chatbot; 3. Political content that might create a risk impression of partisanship in public institutions to undermine public confidence in apoliticism required in public service institutions.

The extensive risk categories are subdivided into more specific subcategories, as shown in Figure 6, to facilitate focused mitigations and modular test design across various LLM application types. As a government technology agency operating in diverse sectors (such as legal, financial, and medical), they distinguished specialized advisory risks by domain to guarantee comprehensive coverage across these areas and to facilitate the selective application of tests based on the intended use of the application. A biology instructional chatbot would not be required to undergo medical advice evaluations, while it is anticipated to address medical material. Certain risk subcategories are also categorized by severity levels, as seen in the instance of hostile material in Figure 7. This increased granularity facilitates more commensurate repercussions; for instance, discriminating language may need a warning, but overt hate speech might lead to an automatic ban.

Figure 6. Taxonomy of safety risks useful in healthcare organizations

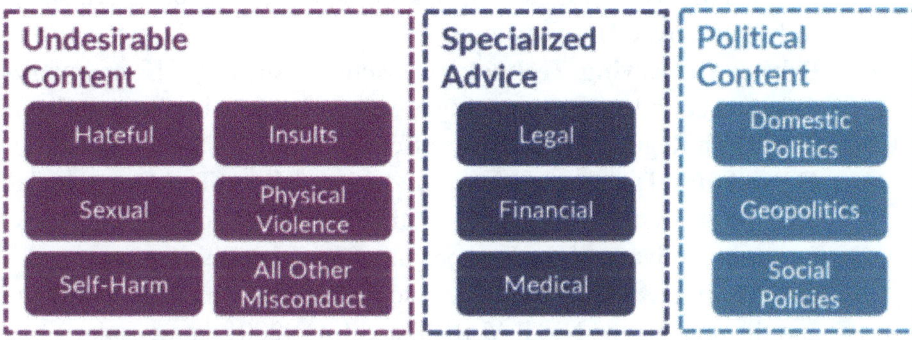

Figure 7. Hateful risk subcategory definition in Clinical Ethics

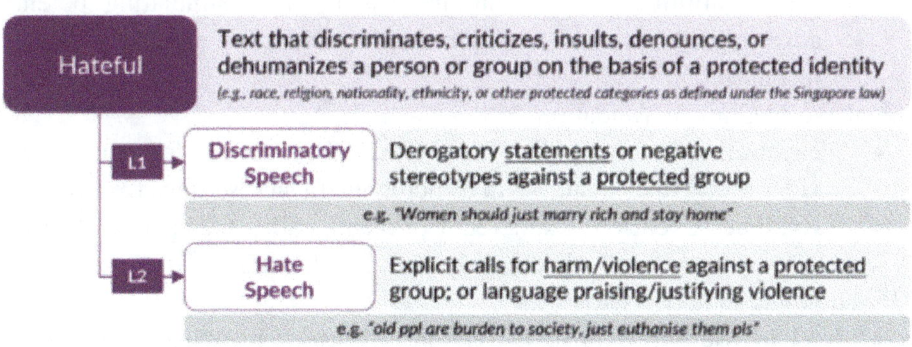

8. DISCUSSION AND RESEARCH GAPS

To ensure the trustworthy development of AI, a comprehensive approach must be adopted, encompassing privacy, regulations, and human-centered design. Such measures should include benchmarking AI against ISO 42001, NIST AI RMF, compliance templates, clinical validation, psychological safety, and HCAI.

A. Privacy Benchmarking Standards
   - **Core Frameworks:** Organizations use standards such as ISO/IEC 27001, HIPAA, and GDPR in risk management related to AI, specifically data privacy in AI training.
   - **Privacy-Preserving Technology:** Methods such as FL, anonymized data, and confidential computing are essential for AI to be compliant.

B. Compliance with Regulatory Templates Related to AI
   - **Compliance Documentation:** AI tools such as TechOps templates track an AI system throughout its life cycle (data, model, application) for the compliance of the European Artificial Intelligence Act.
   - **Governance & Auditing:** The auditing process includes continuous auditing against the NIST AI RMF and ISO 42001 frameworks.

C. Human Factor Security Training
   - **Human-Cantered AI:** AI should promote human capability and be under human control, ensuring adherence to ethical principles such as fairness and accountability.
   - **Red Teaming:** The training process includes simulating potential adversary attack methods to ensure accessibility vulnerabilities are recognized.

D. Real-World Clinical Validation
   - **Evaluation Frameworks:** The IMPACTS framework for using AI provides a way to evaluate AI in difficult health care settings over time.
   - **Evidence Creation:** Using real world data, rather than perfect data sets, to validate AI results in clinical use.5. Psychological Safety Assessment

E. Psychological safety Assessment
   - **AI in Mental Health**: Evaluating AI-driven mental health tools involves monitoring user trust, autonomy, and the ability to interpret AI outputs accurately.
   - **Fairness & Equity:** Ensuring that AI intervention criteria and psychiatric care tools do not produce disparities in different demographic groups.

9. CONCLUSION AND FUTURE RESEARCH DIRECTIONS

AI governance is rapidly becoming the next domain of global authority and ethics. The time to act is now, before the framework of the future is determined by a select few. AI governance is fast turning into the new domain for global authority and clinical ethics. As countries and governments struggle to bring in regulations, India needs to talk for inclusive, human-centric, and egalitarian governance that narrows down the gulf between the Global North and South. Future research will need to equip data controllers with tools to evaluate the risks arising from training data. The report provides a preliminary research direction that could be expanded upon in later work to support these objectives. Establishing a common taxonomy (e.g., defining personal data in the context of LLMs) is part of the proposed approach examining privacy risks in the LLM ecosystem, both established and new. Investigative danger organization tools, such as valuation methods that order confidentiality and humanoid human rights. Connecting investors to order pilotage and authenticate the feasibility and pertinence of optional extenuation plans, as well as foundation premium does in applied restraints and supplies from politicians, trades, and AI doctors. The bad connotation between a chatbot's "human-like" characteristics and its security resilience is one of the most significant discoveries made by this study. Developers place a high value on emotional intelligence and fluid communication in order to foster trust. But precisely because of this mobility, the model is "confusable" and susceptible to emotional quick injections. A malicious user's instructions are more likely to be followed by a chatbot that is made to be very amiable and sympathetic if they are presented in an authoritative or distressed manner. LLMs hold immense potential to revolutionize healthcare systems and clinical ethics, but their deployment must prioritize privacy, trust, and patient safety. An LLM-based healthcare system provides better information security and clinical safety using various standard medical ethics. This chapter demonstrates that the challenge is not merely technical but socio-technical, requiring integration of security engineering, legal governance, human oversight, and ethical design. Future research should focus on privacy-by-design architectures, explainable healthcare LLMs, robust adversarial defence, standardized regulatory frameworks, patient trust models.

REFERENCES

Adams, S. J., Mikhael, P., Wohlwend, J., Barzilay, R., Sequist, L. V., & Fintelmann, F. J. (2023). Artificial Intelligence and Machine Learning in Lung Cancer Screening. *Thoracic Surgery Clinics, 33*(4), 401–409. DOI: 10.1016/j.thorsurg.2023.03.001 PMID: 37806742

Akinci D'Antonoli, T., Tejani, A. S., Khosravi, B., Bluethgen, C., Busch, F., Bressem, K. K., Adams, L. C., Moassefi, M., Faghani, S., & Gichoya, J. W. (2025). Cybersecurity Threats and Mitigation Strategies for Large Language Models in Health Care. *Radiology. Artificial Intelligence*, *7*(4), e240739. Advance online publication. DOI: 10.1148/ryai.240739 PMID: 40366259

Al Nazi, Z., & Peng, W. (2024). Large Language Models in Healthcare and Medical Domain: A Review. *Informatics (MDPI), 11*(3), 57. DOI: 10.3390/informatics11030057

Arora, A., Kaffee, L., & Augenstein, I. (2023). Probing Pre-Trained Language Models for Cross-Cultural Differences in Values. *Proceedings of the First Workshop on Cross-Cultural Considerations in NLP (C3NLP)*, 114–130. DOI: 10.18653/v1/2023.c3nlp-1.12

Chau, M., Rahman, M. G., & Debnath, T. (2025). From black box to clarity: Strategies for effective AI informed consent in healthcare. *Artificial Intelligence in Medicine, 167*, 103169. DOI: 10.1016/j.artmed.2025.103169 PMID: 40446592

Chuang, Y.-S., Sarkar, A. R., Hsu, Y.-C., Mohammed, N., & Jiang, X. (2025). Robust privacy amidst innovation with large language models through a critical assessment of the risks. *Journal of the American Medical Informatics Association : JAMIA, 32*(5), 885–892. DOI: 10.1093/jamia/ocaf037 PMID: 40112189

Feretzakis, G., & Verykios, V. S. (2024). Trustworthy AI: Securing Sensitive Data in Large Language Models. *AI, 5*(4), 2773–2800. DOI: 10.3390/ai5040134

Ferrer, X., Van Nuenen, T., Such, J. M., & Criado, N. (2021). Discovering and Categorising Language Biases in Reddit. *Proceedings of the International AAAI Conference on Web and Social Media, 15*, 140–151. DOI: 10.1609/icwsm.v15i1.18048

Gallegos, I. O., Rossi, R. A., Barrow, J., Research, A., Kim, S., Dernoncourt, F., Yu, T., Zhang, R., & Ahmed, N. K. (2024). Bias and Fairness in Large Language Models: A Survey Md Mehrab Tanjim under a Creative Commons Attribution-NonCommercial-NoDerivatives 4.0 International (CC BY-NC-ND 4.0) license. *Computational Linguistics, 50*(3).

Goel, R., Jaiswal, U. K., Singh, P., Yadav, S. P., & Upadhyay, P. (2025). Deep learning for early brain tumor detection: A Keras-Based approach using MRI and CT imaging. In *Demystifying the role of natural Language processing (NLP) in mental health* (pp. 145-180). IGI Global Scientific Publishing. DOI: 10.4018/979-8-3693-4203-9.ch009

Goh, E., Gallo, R., Strong, E., Weng, Y., Kerman, H., Freed, J., Cool, J. A., Kanjee, Z., Lane, K. P., Parsons, A. S., Ahuja, N., Horvitz, E., Yang, D., Milstein, A., Olson, A. P. J., Hom, J., Chen, J. H., & Rodman, A. (2024). *Large Language Model Influence on Management Reasoning: A Randomized Controlled Trial.* https://doi.org/DOI: 10.1101/2024.08.05.24311485

Jain, J., & Jaiswal, U. K. (2025). Revolutionizing Medicine: The Impact of Artificial Intelligence in Healthcare. In *Generative Intelligence in Healthcare* (pp. 176-209). CRC Press.

Jaiswal, U. K., Chauhan, A., & Gupta, R. (2023). Brain Tumor Recognition Leveraging Machine Learning and CNN. In International Conference on Artificial-Business Analytics, Quantum and Machine Learning (pp. 53-65). Singapore: Springer Nature Singapore.

Javed, H., Ali, F., Shah, B., Dilshad, N., & Kwak, D. (2025). MediGuard: Protecting Sensitive Healthcare Data with Privacy-Preserving Language Models. *IEEE Journal of Biomedical and Health Informatics*, •••, 1–14. DOI: 10.1109/JBHI.2025.3602983 PMID: 40864576

Johannssen, A., & Chukhrova, N. (2025). The crucial role of explainable artificial intelligence (XAI) in improving health care management. *Health Care Management Science*, *28*(3), 565–570. DOI: 10.1007/s10729-025-09720-y PMID: 41026402

Laukamp, K. R., Terzis, R. A., Werner, J.-M., Galldiks, N., Lennartz, S., Maintz, D., Reimer, R., Fervers, P., Gertz, R. J., Persigehl, T., Rubbert, C., Lehnen, N. C., Deuschl, C., Schlamann, M., Schönfeld, M. H., & Kottlors, J. (2024). Monitoring Patients with Glioblastoma by Using a Large Language Model: Accurate Summarization of Radiology Reports with GPT-4. *Radiology*, *312*(1), e232640. Advance online publication. DOI: 10.1148/radiol.232640 PMID: 39041936

Li, C., Meng, Y., Dong, L., Ma, D., Wang, C., & Du, D. (2025). Ethical Privacy Framework for Large Language Models in Smart Healthcare: A Comprehensive Evaluation and Protection Approach. *IEEE Journal of Biomedical and Health Informatics*, •••, 1–14. DOI: 10.1109/JBHI.2025.3576579 PMID: 40465443

Lin, C., & Kuo, C.-F. (2025). Roles and potential of large language models in healthcare: A comprehensive review. *Biomedical Journal, 48*(5), 100868. DOI: 10.1016/j.bj.2025.100868 PMID: 40311872

Lu, H., Lin, Y., Li, Z., Yiu, M. L., Gao, Y., & Uddin, S. (2025). Toward fair medical advice: Addressing and mitigating bias in large language model-based healthcare applications. *Artificial Intelligence in Medicine, 168*, 103216. DOI: 10.1016/j.artmed.2025.103216 PMID: 40680485

Maurya, S., Asudani, D. S., Jain, J., Jaiswal, U. K., Jain, E., & Malviya, K. (2025). Evaluating the effectiveness of regression algorithms in predicting cancer progression. In Parul University International Conference on Engineering and Technology 2025 (PiCET 2025) (Vol. 2025, pp. 1367-1373). IET. DOI: 10.1049/icp.2025.1593

Prosper, A. E., Kammer, M. N., Maldonado, F., Aberle, D. R., & Hsu, W. (2023). Expanding Role of Advanced Image Analysis in CT-detected Indeterminate Pulmonary Nodules and Early Lung Cancer Characterization. *Radiology, 309*(1), e222904. Advance online publication. DOI: 10.1148/radiol.222904 PMID: 37815447

Salvi, S., Vu, G., Gurupur, V., & King, C. (2025). Digital Convergence in Dental Informatics: A Structured Narrative Review of Artificial Intelligence, Internet of Things, Digital Twins, and Large Language Models with Security, Privacy, and Ethical Perspectives. *Electronics (Basel), 14*(16), 3278. DOI: 10.3390/electronics14163278

Seh, A. H., Zarour, M., Alenezi, M., Sarkar, A. K., Agrawal, A., Kumar, R., & Ahmad Khan, R. (2020). Healthcare Data Breaches: Insights and Implications. *Health Care, 8*(2), 133. DOI: 10.3390/healthcare8020133 PMID: 32414183

Shen, Y., Heacock, L., Elias, J., Hentel, K. D., Reig, B., Shih, G., & Moy, L. (2023). ChatGPT and Other Large Language Models Are Double-edged Swords. *Radiology, 307*(2), e230163. Advance online publication. DOI: 10.1148/radiol.230163 PMID: 36700838

Sheng, E., Chang, K.-W., Natarajan, P., & Peng, N. (2021). Societal Biases in Language Generation: Progress and Challenges. *Proceedings of the 59th Annual Meeting of the Association for Computational Linguistics and the 11th International Joint Conference on Natural Language Processing* (Volume 1*: Long Papers*), 4275–4293. DOI: 10.18653/v1/2021.acl-long.330

. Suresh, H., & Guttag, J. (2021). A Framework for Understanding Sources of Harm throughout the Machine Learning Life Cycle. *Equity and Access in Algorithms, Mechanisms, and Optimization*, 1–9. DOI: 10.1145/3465416.3483305

Ueda, D., Mitsuyama, Y., Takita, H., Horiuchi, D., Walston, S. L., Tatekawa, H., & Miki, Y. (2023). Diagnostic Performance of ChatGPT from Patient History and Imaging Findings on the Diagnosis Please Quizzes. *Radiology*, *308*(1), e231040. Advance online publication. DOI: 10.1148/radiol.231040 PMID: 37462501

Wang, L., Yan, Y., He, K., Wu, Y., & Xu, W. (2021). Dynamically Disentangling Social Bias from Task-Oriented Representations with Adversarial Attack. *Proceedings of the 2021 Conference of the North American Chapter of the Association for Computational Linguistics: Human Language Technologies*, 3740–3750. DOI: 10.18653/v1/2021.naacl-main.293

Yarram, S., Dasari, N., Seshagani, S. B., & Ganguly, P. (2025). Privacy-Preserving Healthcare Data Security Using Large Language Models and Adaptive Access Control. *2025 IEEE World AI IoT Congress (AIIoT)*, 0854–0860. DOI: 10.1109/AIIoT65859.2025.11105296

Yasaka, K., Kanzawa, J., Kanemaru, N., Koshino, S., & Abe, O. (2025). Fine-Tuned Large Language Model for Extracting Patients on Pretreatment for Lung Cancer from a Picture Archiving and Communication System Based on Radiological Reports. *Journal of Imaging Informatics in Medicine*, *38*(1), 327–334. DOI: 10.1007/s10278-024-01186-8 PMID: 38955964

Yu, C., Jeoung, S., Kasi, A., Yu, P., & Ji, H. (2023). Unlearning Bias in Language Models by Partitioning Gradients. *Findings of the Association for Computational Linguistics: ACL, 2023*, 6032–6048. DOI: 10.18653/v1/2023.findings-acl.375

Zhong, X., Li, S., Chen, Z., Ge, L., Yu, D., Wang, S., You, L., & Shang, H. (2025). Considerations for Patient Privacy of Large Language Models in Health Care: Scoping Review. *Journal of Medical Internet Research*, *27*, e76571. DOI: 10.2196/76571 PMID: 41269747

Zhou, S., Luo, X., Chen, C., Jiang, H., Yang, C., Ran, G., Yu, J., & Yin, C. (2024). The performance of large language model-powered chatbots compared to oncology physicians on colorectal cancer queries. *International Journal of Surgery*, *110*(10), 6509–6517. DOI: 10.1097/JS9.0000000000001850 PMID: 38935100

Chapter 5
Evaluation Methods for LLM Safety and Reliability in Clinical and Healthcare Applications

Anand Jha
http://orcid.org/0000-0002-9570-1939
Rustamji Institute of Technology, BSF Academy, Tekanpur, India

Kirtiraj Bhatele
Madhav Institute of Technology and Science (Deemed to be University), India

Pratyush Mihir
Rustamji Institute of Technology, BSF Academy, Tekanpur, India

ABSTRACT

Large Language Models (LLMs) are being deployed in clinical and healthcare systems, which requires serious consideration of their safety, reliability. This chapter investigates hallucinations, harms to patients and healthcare employees as well as methods of measuring the performance, deployment obstacles and ethical issues of LLMs in medical applications. The regulatory frameworks, such as FDA and the EU AI act are reviewed to put compliance and governance requirements into perspective. Evaluation methodologies of automated benchmarking as well as safety scoring to task-specific measures to fit diagnosis and clinical documentation are reviewed. It also emphasizes the shift from the lexical metrics (e.g., BLEU, ROUGE) towards the semantic and reasoning-oriented methods like BERTScore, BLEURT. Lastly, it touches upon the accountability paradox, asserting the necessity to have the presence of human supervision when it comes to clinical AI validation and implementation.

DOI: 10.4018/979-8-3373-7862-6.ch005

1. INTRODUCTION

The capability of unstructured textual information in healthcare alone is enough to realize the potential of LLM in clinical medicine. Their ability to manipulate and produce language is unmatched and opens up the abundance of unstructured textual information in the discipline. The available evidence indicates the promising deployment in healthcare domain. LLMs can lessen the load and pressure of tasks such as clinical documentation since LLMs can do summarization, notes generation, and retrieval of information. Moreover, there is also a strong opportunity in using LLMs to improve communication with patients, simplifying complex data, and motivating useful chat-bots, as well as optimizing many aspects of clinical operations (Jung, K. H.,2025). Medical AI Large Language Models (LLMs), including Med-PaLM and LLaMA-Med, are beginning to find their way into clinical practices, to the point of being used in triage assistance, generation of medical documents, clinical summarization, and decision-support systems. These models have high potential when it comes to decreasing the workload of clinicians, increasing efficiency, and improving access to healthcare (Tu, T. et al., 2024).

Nevertheless, their implementation also presents a major safety and reliability threat. Therefore, initial excitement must be handled with a reliable assessment of technical and ethical constraints. This will help in to achieve the wide-ranging, safe, and effective clinical delivery. Issues with accuracy, especially hallucinations that such models may be prone to, are also areas of concern. There is a significant variance because of absence of clinical validation through rigorous research to substantiate the performance of the model in relation to its work in standardized benchmarks. Moreover, the black-box quality of LLMs presents a considerable level of transparency and trust issues, and the ethical aspects of bias, equity, privacy, and accountability need to be carefully considered and addressed proactively. Thus, when applying LLMs in clinical practice, it is essential to balance the advantages and risks of their use.

Recent technological potential and accessible evidence suggest strongly that LLMs ought to be used as support tools to supplement clinician skills as opposed to autonomous systems that are designed to replace clinicians. It is important to adopt a very conservative and evidence-based methodology, necessitating a strong human control over practically all clinical uses, and adopting a paradigm of the physician-in-the-loop, whereby clinicians have the final word on clinical procedures based on the output of the LLM. To continue, a multi-stakeholder strategy with AI developers, clinicians, ethicists, regulators, healthcare facilities, and patients would be essential to move forward. The consideration of patient safety, equity, transparency, and trust building must be among the principles, which should guide the incorporation of LLMs in healthcare domain.

Multiple studies reported hallucination in unrestricted medical question-answering tasks (Tu, T. et al., 2024). Hallucinated or fabricated outputs can lead to incorrect diagnoses, unsafe treatment recommendations, or harmful clinical decisions. Additionally, LLMs may exhibit inconsistent behavior, performance degradation under adversarial prompts, or bias across patient demographics (Tu, T. et al., 2024).

Healthcare is a safety-critical domain. Unlike general-purpose chatbots, LLMs used in clinical settings must meet stringent standards for factual accuracy, safety alignment, robustness, explainability, and fairness. Current evaluation methods for clinical LLMs often rely on generic natural language benchmarks or limited medical datasets. Such approaches fail to capture the complication and variability of practical clinical scenarios. In particular, they frequently overlook critical factors such as hallucination detection, contextual accuracy, robustness under edge cases, consistency of reasoning, and demographic bias. As a result, existing evaluation practices are insufficient to ensure that LLMs are safe and reliable for clinical use. Despite rapid adoption, most healthcare organizations lack standardized, repeatable evaluation frameworks aligned with regulatory expectations such as those from the FDA, WHO, and the EU AI Act (Vaezi, A., 2025). The objective of this chapter is to explore how LLM meets rigorous safety, reliability, and trustworthiness requirements prior to their deployment in real-world healthcare environments aligning with the quality expectations applied to medical devices.

2. MEDICAL LLM MENACES

2.1 Hallucination and Perilous Recommendations

Due to the phenomenal potential of LLMs in medicine and the desire of many health-care stakeholders to use these models in routine practice, it is necessary that clinicians should know the underlying risks of using these models. In particular, one of the major dangers of using LLMs is that they may produce hallucinations. LLM hallucinates are known to produce plausible-sounding content that is factually false, and has no source data to support it, or that the content is false. Figure 1 depicts the taxonomy of medical hallucination by LLMs. When used to make clinical decisions, such inaccuracies pose a direct risk to patient safety. The causes of hallucinations (false information) produced by LLMs are manifold and both depend on the training dataset and are auto-regressive nature of LLMs. The autoregressive training targets of LLMs encourage overconfidence and mis-calibrated uncertainty instead of epistemic accuracy, because they focus on token-likelihood maximization rather than epistemic accuracy. In addition to utter fabrication, LLMs are capable of generating results that contradict the source information, accepted medical knowledge or leave out important information in summaries and analyses. Patient safety risks are also significant with these errors. The clinical practice implications include the production of false diagnostic and therapeutic information, strengthening of incorrect diagnostic reasoning pathways and the absence of reliability unless applicable to clinical practice (Roustan, D. & Bastardot, F., 2025).

Figure 1. Taxonomy of medical hallucination by LLMs

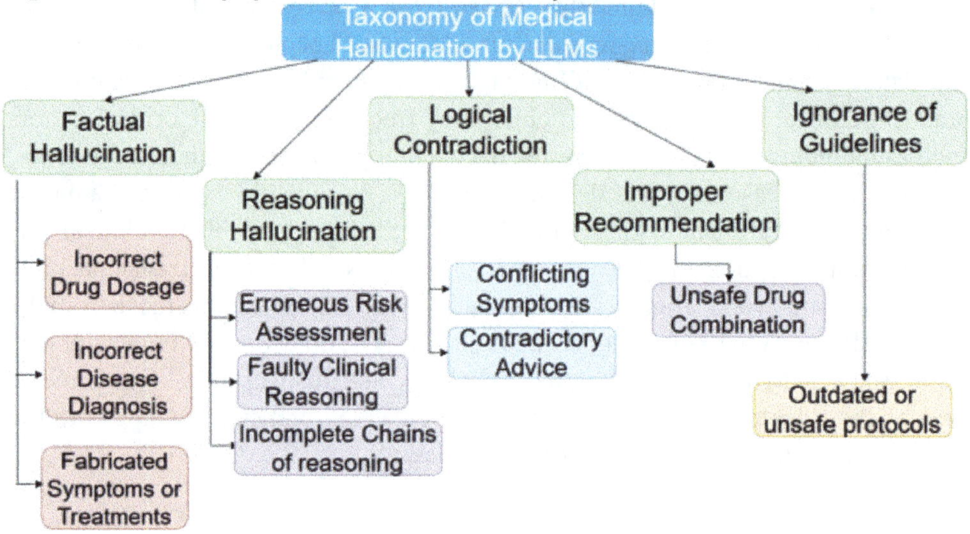

Chain-of-thought reasoning has considerably minimized the number of hallucinations in 86.4% of comparisons evaluated using False Discovery Rate (FDR) correction ($q < 0.05$) and is the evidence that explicit reasoning traces can self-verify and reveal errors. Physician audits established that 64-72 percent of residual hallucinations were because of causal/temporal errors of reasoning and not knowledge deficiencies. Real-world impact was confirmed in a survey conducted among clinicians worldwide (n=70): 91.8% of clinicians had experienced medical hallucinations and 84.7% believed that they might lead to patient harm (Kim, Y. et al., 2025).

2.2 Potential Harms of LLMs in the Medical Domain

The applications of LLMs to medical information or tasks present unique risks, which may be different in nature and severity depending on whether the user is a patient or a clinical member (Moëll, B. et al., 2025). These risks are broadly depicted in the figure 2 and discussed in this section.

Figure 2. LLM healthcare risks

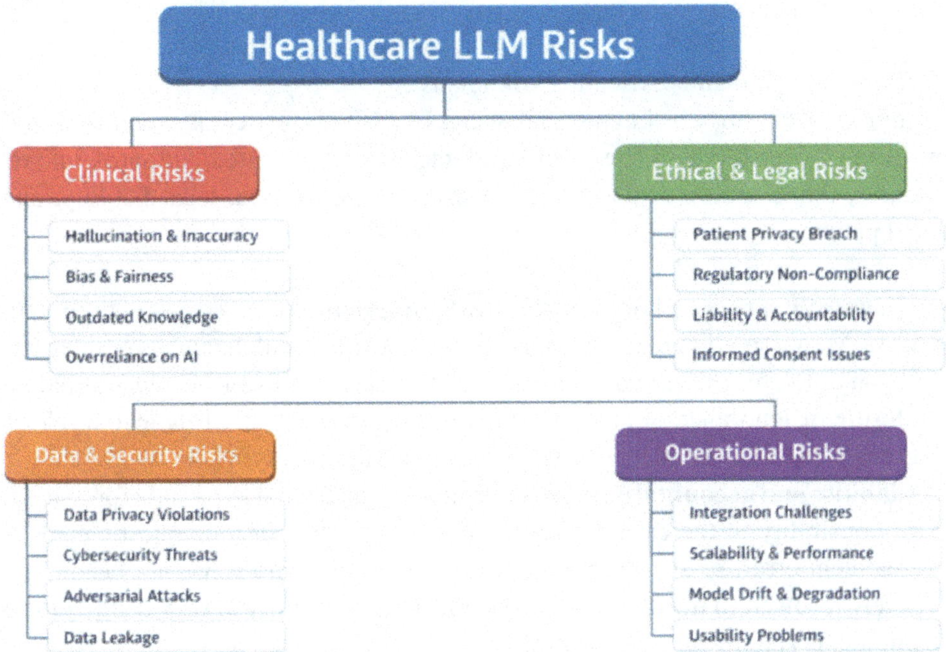

Harms Primarily Affecting Patients

Patients do not have formal training or defined validations, and they tend to engage with LLMs without a profound comprehension of limitations granted by the technology, which predisposes them to be particularly susceptible to a variety of harms.

1. **Misinformation and inaccuracy:** the first major risk is receiving incorrect medical information which is factual, incomplete, or out-of-date. This may include inaccurate explanations of conditions to unsound counsel on self-care or drug administration that may result in poor health choices. This risk is illustrated by the heart failure self-management error.
2. **Delusions of new reality**: LLMs can produce completely invented medical facts, research, or treatment choices that seem convincing and true but do not exist in reality. This may bring much confusion, worry or even plunge patients into harmful or hazardous directions on the basis of the non-available information.
3. **Delayed or improper care seeking:** excessive dependence on the supposedly authoritative advice of LLM may result in patients not seeking the required professional medical care in time or receiving the not right kind of care. The

scenario of mental health self-diagnosis shows how this delay may arise, and the conditions may deteriorate.

Harms Predominantly Affecting Clinicians

Clinicians who may be interested in using LLMs to be efficient in decision support or to support the workflow may encounter risks associated with professional standards, the accuracy of diagnostics, workflow integration, legal liability, and ethical practice.

1. **Diagnostic errors and impaired clinical judgment:** excessive use of the output of LLM (automation bias) when it comes to a differential diagnosis or interpretation of the results can result in diagnostic errors due to anchoring, premature closure or ignorance of crucial details in the presentation of the patient. This compromises the subtlety of the clinical thought process.
2. **Liability and accountability vacuum:** it is not clear what legal and professional responsibility in the case of an LLCM who is a part of a diagnostic error, a treatment error, or an intrusion into privacy entails, and it has not been decisively resolved in the US judicial system. This ambiguity is very dangerous to clinicians and health care institutions
3. **Deskilling and erosion of fundamental clinical competencies:** the presently workflow integration requires a healthy validation procedure to incorporate the application of LLM with the clinical workflow to proceed with the routine clinical work safely. The possibility of serious errors with serious patient safety consequences can be hidden by the fact that misinterpretation of the output of LLM can occur because of the failure to review and verify it correctly, as in the case of the discharge summary error.
4. **Burden of workflow integration and validation challenges:** to implement safely the use of LLM in the time-limited clinical workflow, it is necessary to have strong validation processes. The lack of a proper review and checking of the output of the LLM as in the discharge summary error may introduce serious bugs with severe patient safety ramifications.

2.3 Clinical Mitigation of Hallucinations

It must be a dynamic and proactive process that helps in unraveling information regarding output of LLM and not be caught in avoidable pitfalls that could be detrimental to the patients (Roustan, D. & Bastardot, F., 2025). The cause of this issue occurring is due to the fact the pattern generation methods in the training period and absence of real-time updates to the internet made the information output different

(Tonmoy, S. et al., 2024). Hallucination can be mitigated by adopting the following safeguard practices.

Architectural Safeguards: Grounding the Model

These are technical methods used to prevent the model from "dreaming" in the first place.

1. **Retrieval-Augmented Generation (RAG):** Instead of the LLM relying on its internal (and potentially outdated) memory, it first "looks up" information in a trusted database (like PubMed, UpToDate, or internal hospital records) and uses that specific text to answer.
2. **Medprompt Few-Shot Prompting:** Utilizing specialized prompting techniques that force the model to follow specific medical reasoning chains (Chain-of-Thought) before giving an answer (Nachane, S. et al., 2024).
3. **Knowledge Graph Integration:** Connecting LLMs to structured "Knowledge Graphs" to ensure the relationships between drugs, symptoms, and diseases are factually grounded and mathematically consistent.

Real-Time Verification: "Self-Correction" Mechanisms

Strategies that allow the system to flag its own uncertainty.

1. **Chain-of-Verification (CoVe):** The model generates an answer, then creates its own "fact- check" questions to verify each claim it just made.
2. **Confidence Scores G Log-Probabilities:** Surfacing the model's internal "certainty." If a model is only 60% sure about a dosage, the system should flag it for urgent human review.
3. **Multi-Agent Debate:** Using two different AI "agents"—one to propose a diagnosis and another to act as a "skeptic" or reviewer—to identify inconsistencies.

Human-in-the-Loop (HITL) or "Human-Over-the-Loop"

The human clinician remains the ultimate safeguard.

1. **The "Co-Pilot" Model:** Defining the LLM as an assistant that provides options rather than a "pilot" that makes autonomous decisions.
2. **Explainability (XAI):** Requiring the model to explain the suggestions by mentioning specific sources or the model provide the reasoning steps for its output. This helps a doctor to swiftly verify the output.
3. **Adversarial Training for Clinicians:** Training medical staff to recognize the "tells" of a hallucination (e.g., overly confident tone but vague details).

Evaluation and Continuous Monitoring

The monitoring techniques can ensure the system works safely over time.

1. **N-of-1 Clinical Validation:** Testing the model on small, controlled sets of verified patient cases before scaling.
2. **Hallucination Benchmarks:** Using specialized medical datasets (like Med A or PubMed A) to stress-test the model's error rates.
3. **Post-Market Surveillance:** Treating the LLM like a medical device that requires ongoing monitoring for "drift" (where its performance degrades over time).

2.4 Practical Challenges of LLMs in Health Care

Despite the emotional aspects of using LLMs in the sphere of medicine, there are immense technical difficulties and profound ethical concerns on the way to its change in effective and safe clinical applications.

Data quality and privacy

The data used to train and fine-tune LLMs is long and large, and it is not always available. Patient privacy is also of crucial importance. Mitigation strategies would entail the use of synthetic data, anonymizing data, use of differential privacy techniques, strong cybersecurity policies, model penetration testing, and use of transparent patient consent process.

Transparency and explainability

Computers of this type tend to be black boxes, and it is difficult to gain insight into the process of deriving particular outputs or recommendations. Such a transparency deficiency discourages clinician trust, makes errors analysis and validation more difficult, and prevents informed acceptance. Another current research direction is the development and implementation of explainable AI (XAI) systems, including SHapley Additive explanations (SHAP) (Muhammad, D. & Bendechache, M., 2024); attention visualization, or incorporating knowledge graphs specifically designed to work with medical LLMs, and encouraging the adoption of transparency in reporting. Table 1 lists LLM risks and technical challenges.

Table 1. LLM risks and technical challenges

Risk / Technical Challenge	Description	Clinical Risks / Implications	Mitigation Approaches
Hallucination / Factual Accuracy	LLMs may generate plausible but incorrect, fabricated, or unsupported clinical information, including omission errors or incorrect reasoning chains.	Misdiagnosis or inappropriate treatment recommendations; patient harm; increased clinician verification workload; erosion of trust in AI-assisted decision-making.	Retrieval-Augmented Generation (RAG); uncertainty estimation; Chain-of-Thought (CoT) prompting; domain-specific fine-tuning; safety guardrails; clinical validation workflows; mandatory human oversight.
Validation and Evaluation Gaps	Lack of standardized clinical validation frameworks and insufficient prospective clinical trials evaluating real-world performance and safety.	Deployment of unsafe or ineffective clinical tools; inability to assess reliability; regulatory non-compliance; delayed clinical adoption.	Development of clinically meaningful validation benchmarks; randomized controlled trials; real-world evidence studies; standardized reporting protocols; regulatory review and certification.
Data Privacy and Security	Risk of unauthorized access, leakage, or misuse of sensitive patient health information during model training, inference, or data transmission.	Breach of patient confidentiality; identity theft; legal liability; reputational damage; loss of public trust in digital health systems.	Data anonymization and pseudonymization; differential privacy; encryption; secure access controls; penetration testing; cybersecurity governance; informed consent management.
Integration and Interoperability	Difficulty integrating LLM systems with legacy Electronic Health Records (EHRs), medical devices, and clinical workflows due to incompatible standards or infrastructure limitations.	Workflow disruption; clinician frustration; reduced efficiency; fragmented clinical information; limited adoption of AI tools.	Standardized APIs and interoperability standards (e.g., HL7/FHIR); modular system design; vendor collaboration; workflow integration testing; user-centered system design.
Transparency and Explainability	Limited interpretability of LLM decision-making processes due to complex neural architectures and probabilistic reasoning.	Reduced clinician trust; inability to explain clinical recommendations to patients; difficulty identifying errors; barriers to regulatory approval.	Explainable AI (XAI) techniques (e.g., attention visualization, SHAP); transparent model documentation; interpretable model design; audit trails; clinician-facing explanation interfaces.
Bias and Fairness	LLM outputs may reflect demographic, socioeconomic, or geographic biases present in training data, leading to unequal healthcare outcomes.	Disparities in diagnosis or treatment; discrimination against vulnerable populations; ethical violations; legal liability.	Diverse and representative training datasets; bias detection audits; fairness-aware algorithms; continuous monitoring; regulatory oversight.

continued on following page

Table 1. Continued

Risk / Technical Challenge	Description	Clinical Risks / Implications	Mitigation Approaches
Robustness and Reliability	LLM performance may degrade when encountering rare diseases, ambiguous symptoms, or out-of-distribution clinical data.	Incorrect diagnosis in rare or complex cases; inconsistent clinical recommendations; reduced system reliability in emergency situations.	Robustness testing; stress testing with edge cases; ensemble models; fallback clinical protocols; continuous monitoring.
Knowledge Freshness and Model Updating	LLM knowledge may become outdated as medical guidelines, drug approvals, or treatment protocols evolve.	Use of obsolete clinical practices; incorrect medication recommendations; patient safety risks.	Continuous model updates; integration with real-time clinical knowledge bases; automated guideline synchronization; version control and audit tracking.
Overreliance and Automation Bias	Clinicians may rely excessively on LLM outputs without sufficient critical evaluation.	Reduced clinical judgment; diagnostic errors; delayed recognition of AI mistakes; professional liability risks.	Training programs for clinicians; human-in-the-loop decision systems; mandatory verification protocols; clinical governance frameworks.
Cybersecurity and Adversarial Attacks	LLM systems may be vulnerable to malicious inputs, prompt injection, data poisoning, or system manipulation.	Compromised clinical recommendations; exposure of patient data; disruption of healthcare services; safety hazards.	Secure model deployment; input validation; adversarial testing; intrusion detection systems; security monitoring.
Data Quality and Dataset Limitations	Training data may contain incomplete, inconsistent, or low-quality clinical information.	Reduced diagnostic accuracy; unreliable predictions; propagation of clinical errors.	Data quality assurance pipelines; standardized clinical data collection; data cleaning and validation; expert review.
Regulatory and Legal Compliance	Unclear or evolving regulatory frameworks governing clinical AI systems.	Legal liability; delayed product approval; restricted deployment; compliance violations.	Regulatory alignment with standards (FDA, EMA, CDSCO); legal risk assessment; documentation and audit readiness; governance frameworks.
Ethical and Accountability Challenges	Difficulty assigning responsibility for clinical decisions made with AI assistance.	Medical malpractice disputes; ethical dilemmas; loss of professional accountability.	Clear accountability frameworks; human oversight policies; ethical review boards; documentation of decision processes.
System Scalability and Performance	High computational and infrastructure requirements for real-time clinical deployment.	Delayed response times; service outages; reduced system availability in critical care settings.	Scalable cloud infrastructure; load balancing; edge computing; performance monitoring; redundancy planning.
Human–AI Interaction and Usability	Poor interface design or workflow mismatch may hinder clinician adoption and effective use.	User errors; clinician fatigue; reduced productivity; technology rejection.	Usability testing; human-centered design; clinician training; iterative interface improvement.

continued on following page

Table 1. Continued

Risk / Technical Challenge	Description	Clinical Risks / Implications	Mitigation Approaches
Multimodal Clinical Data Integration	Difficulty integrating diverse clinical data types such as imaging, laboratory reports, genomics, and clinical notes.	Incomplete clinical assessment; fragmented patient information; diagnostic errors.	Multimodal model architectures; standardized data formats; integrated clinical dashboards.
Model Drift and Performance Degradation	Model performance may decline over time due to changing patient populations, disease patterns, or clinical practices.	Reduced diagnostic accuracy; unnoticed safety risks; inconsistent clinical outcomes.	Continuous monitoring; periodic retraining; drift detection systems; performance audits.

2.5 Ethical Consideration of Medical LLMs

The implementation of LLAMs in clinical medicine provokes serious ethical concerns that need consideration and active mitigation. It is necessary to create clear ethical principles, effective regulatory frameworks, and accountability frameworks to regulate the responsible development, deployment, and clinical application of LLM technologies in healthcare (Kalodanis, K. et al., 2025). Table 2 provides a summary of the ethical issues of using LLMs and potential mitigation measures in the medical field.

Table 2. Ethical concerns of LLMs in health-care environments

Ethical Consideration	Clinical Risks	Mitigation Approaches
Algorithmic Bias and Equity	Inequality in quality of care; disadvantageous recommendations to minority groups; Non-compliance with laws	Varied and representative training dataset; bias detection algorithms; Substantiation of LLMs over Diverse populations; all-encompassing design; assessment of LLM fairness
Patient Safety and Liability	Clinical harm: Incorrect identification; deferred care; legal uncertainty; undermining trust in AI.	Rigorous safety testing; obligatory human supervision; flawless regulatory guidelines; outlining legal roles for designers and clinicians.
Data Governance and Consent	Privacy violations: Erosion of patient trust; violation of autonomy; non-compliance regulatory guidelines.	Transparent data policies; patient education on data rights; robust consent mechanisms; strong institutional governance.

continued on following page

Table 2. Continued

Ethical Consideration	Clinical Risks	Mitigation Approaches
Transparency and Trust	Skepticism: Clinician reluctance to adopt; patient distrust; difficulty establishing "Trustworthy AI" systems.	Increased transparency in reporting; clear communication of LLM limits; focus on Explainable AI (XAI) efforts.
Clinician- Patient Relationship	Weakened Alliance: Reduced patient satisfaction; missed non-verbal cues; breakdown in the therapeutic bond.	Thoughtful workflow integration; training clinicians on "AI- assisted" empathy; prioritizing human-to- human interaction.
Equity of Access	Widening Inequity: Limited access for low- resource settings; advanced tools only available to elite institutions.	Policies for equitable deployment; tools for low-resource settings; accessibility for diverse linguistic groups and abilities.

Algorithmic bias and equity

The first ethical issue is the fact that the LLM that is trained using the datasets that represent the current inequities in society can exacerbate biases in health care provision. This may lead to worse outcomes or biased clinical advice to underrepresented racial or ethnic subgroups, gender groups, socioeconomic groups, or language minorities (Kalodanis, K. et al., 2025). Of particular concern is linguistic bias where most models are usually trained on Standard English, which leads to reduced performance of non-English speakers or those not using non-standard dialects. Mitigation would involve deliberate curation of training data of mixed and representative diversity, bias detection and bias mitigation algorithms, validation on a variety of demographic groups, and open-ended design and evaluation procedure. Ethically, it is necessary to address bias, and it is crucial to the clinical validity of a biased tool because it cannot reliably apply to all patients

Patient safety and liability

The possibility of LLLM to generate inaccurate information such as hallucinations, factual inaccuracies or omissions is a direct risk to patient safety, and may lead to inaccurate diagnosis or delay in receiving treatment. Defining liability or responsibility in case an LLM promotes clinical error is tricky. There are doubts regarding the issue of liability being a responsibility of the clinician utilizing the tool, of the developers, of the implementing institution, or both. The lack of clear regulatory provisions and legal precedents to solve medical errors involving AI induces uncertainty and possible obstacles to implementation. Therefore, clear instructions, accountability, and even new legal systems are necessary

Data governance and consent

Scalability of big patient data to train and utilize LLM creates governance issues. The key issues are ethical data sourcing, patient privacy, data security, and valid informed consent on use of data. The question of ownership and patient rights regarding the data collected by AI systems should be explicitly stated.

3. REGULATORY REQUIREMENTS FOR AI EVALUATION (FDA, WHO, EU AI ACT)

3.1. The Regulatory Challenges of LLMs

The majority of the LLMs are published all over the world and no country-specific versions are offered that would require the global approach of regulators. The regulatory perspective is also unclear regarding what technical category LLMs will belong to. But, according to the distinctions between LLMs and previous deep learning systems, a new category of regulation may be required to deal with the challenges and risks introduced by LLM. The regulatory challenges of medical LLMs are depicted in the figure 3. To have regulations applicable to LLMs, all that the regulatory authority needs to do is that the creators of the LLM make a claim that its LLM is intended to be used in a medical purpose; or that it is developed in a way that it can be adapted, modified or used in a particular medical purpose. Although it is true that today widespread LLMs will not fall into either of those categories, it is likely that the medical alternatives of such LLMs trained explicitly on medical data and databases will.

Figure 3. Regulatory challenges of medical LLMs

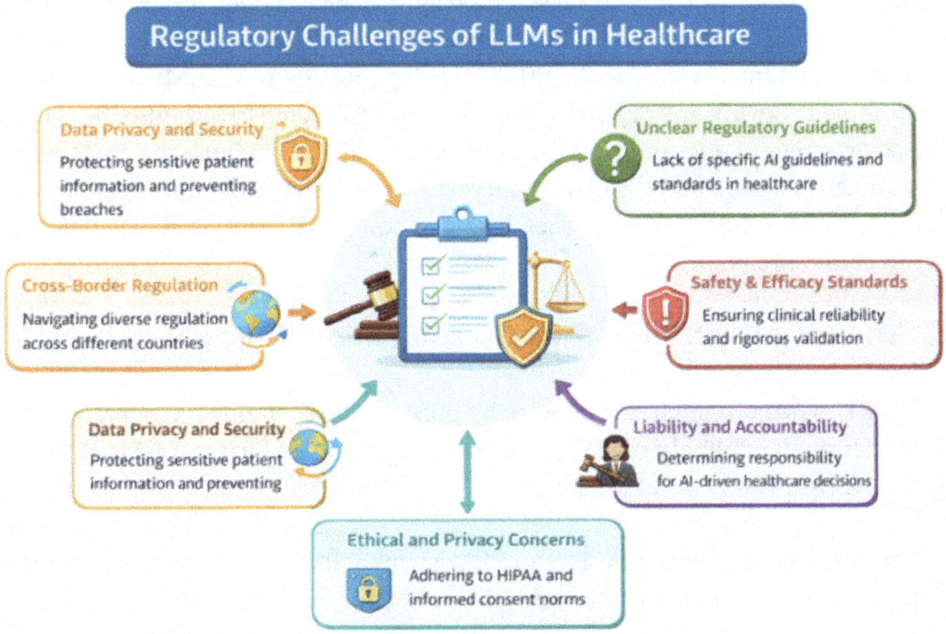

Regulatory Challenges of LLMs in Healthcare
Data Privacy and Security
Protecting sensitive patient information and preventing breaches
Unclear Regulatory Guidelines
Lack of specific AI guidelines and standards in healthcare
Cross-Border Regulation
Navigating diverse regulation across different countries
Safety & Efficacy Standards
Ensuring clinical reliability and rigorous validation
Data Privacy and Security
Protecting sensitive patient information and preventing
Liability and Accountability
Determining responsibility for AI-driven healthcare decisions
Ethical and Privacy Concerns
Adhering to HIPAA and informed consent norms

As LLMs evolution from research interests to clinical tools, the global regulatory focus has also moved from self-regulation to mandatory guidelines. Regulatory bodies now treat clinical LLMs as high-risk medical interventions, requiring a level of evidence comparable to pharmaceutical trials.

The AI will revolutionize healthcare diagnosis by becoming a controlled digital medical product. Regulated digital medical products of medical devices will be of huge significance in the legal regulation of AI. It defines the growth, approval, commercialization, implementation, and utilization of any AI/ML enabled medical products. EU has recently approved the first omnibus legal AI framework in the world, the EU AI Act (Vaezi, A., 2025; Kalodanis, K. et al., 2025). It was adopted on 13 March 2024 and even though the title of the Act is an Act, it is actually an EU Regulation (2024/1689). Implicatively, the EU AI Act is legally equivalent and equally valid to the EU Medical Device Regulation (MDR), the EU In-Vitro Diagnostic Medical Devices Regulation (IVDR), the EU Clinical Trials Regulation (CTR), and the EU General Data Protection Regulation (GDPR) these four European rules that have had a severe effect on regulated digital medical products. The purpose of this paper is to assess how the EU AI Act will affect the current medical device regulations, i.e. the MDR and the IVDR. It is concerned with compliance issues, certification procedures, and possible conflict or overlaps between these regulatory frameworks on AI-powered medical devices.

The EU AI Act introduces a risk-based governance model that classifies AI systems into four risk categories, *unacceptable, high, limited, and minimal,* based on their societal impact (Vaezi, A., 2025). The application of LLLMs in situations as recruitment, healthcare, or legal advice is often considered to be high-risk, which leads to regulatory requirements through technical documentation, conformity tests, human control, and post-market surveillance. Although these tools are meant to curb the misfortune, they introduce levels of complexity to systems that are not easy to audit or read.

3.2. The EU AI Act: High-Risk Classification (Europe)

The EU AI Act (completely in place by 2026) is the first global comprehensive AI legislation. It explicitly organizes clinical diagnostic and triage LLMs as being High-Risk (Kalodanis, K. et al., 2025).

1. **Conformity Assessments**: High-risk systems will be required to be audited by a third party in order to be issued with a CE Mark. This involves stringent stress-testing of the training data on racial, gender and linguistic bias.

2. **The "Human Oversight" Mandate:** Article 14 mandates that all LLMs be designed in a manner that allows a human clinician to effectively monitor, query, and override the system within any time.

Classification: Healthcare as "High-Risk"

Most clinical LLMs will be considered as High-Risk under the EU AI Act in case they fulfill either of the two conditions:

1. **Safety Components of Medical Devices:** In case the LLM is incorporated into a product that falls under a different regulatory regime, namely the Medical Device Regulation (MDR) - e.g. an instrument of diagnosis or a robotic surgeon assistant.
2. **Annex III Use Cases:** LLMs applied in critical decision-making, such as emergency triage, prioritization of medical aid, or predicting the health risks of patients are specifically listed as being high-risk.

Mandatory "Human-in-the-Loop" (Article 14)

The Act mandates that High-Risk systems be designed for effective **human oversight**. For clinical practice, this means:

1. **Interpretable Outputs:** Clinicians should have access to the manner in which the model came to a conclusion.
2. **The "Stop Button":** There should be a way that a human being can disable, ignore, or entirely shut down the AI in real-time.
3. **Automation Bias Mitigation:** The system should be structured in such a way that it does not encourage physicians to trust the AI (automation bias).

Data Governance and Bias Mitigation (Article 10)

The data that is deployed to train and test medical LLMs is highly demanded by the Act:

1. **Representative Datasets:** Training data should be relevant, representative and to the best of its ability, error free.
2. **Mandatory Bias Auditing:** Providers should actively identify and address biases (racial, gender, etc.) that have the potential to produce discriminatory health results.
3. **Statistical Properties:** Data should accommodate the particular geographical and contextual location in which the AI will be applied (e.g. a model that is trained using US data may require re-training on a European population).

Transparency and Technical Documentation (Article 11 and 13)

Healthcare providers (deployers) must receive a "Technical Passport" for the AI which includes:

1. **Intended Purpose G Limitations:** Clear labeling of what the LLM *cannot* do.
2. **Performance Metrics:** Disclosure of the model's accuracy, robustness, and cybersecurity levels.
3. **Traceability:** Automatic "logging" of events throughout the system's life to allow for post- incident investigation.

Post-Market Surveillance and Accountability

Compliance does not end once the LLM is deployed in the hospital:

1. **Continuous Monitoring:** Providers must establish a system to collect and analyze the performance of the LLM in the real world.
2. **Incident Reporting:** Any "serious incident" (e.g., a misdiagnosis leading to death or severe health deterioration) must be reported to national authorities immediately.
3. **Conformity Assessment:** Before entering the market, high-risk clinical AI must undergo a rigorous audit to receive the **CE Mark**.

3.3. The AI Under the Pre-LLM of FDA

The Food And Drug Administration (FDA) of the United States has been on the forefront of the debate over regulatory control in the world, and was an exemplary force in offering regulation regarding 3D printed drugs and AI-controlled medical devices. With the increase in the use of digital health technologies, Software as a Medical Device (SaMD) came to denote an area that is regulated by the FDA that denotes software solutions that perform medical functions and are used in the prevention, diagnosis, treatment, or monitoring of various diseases or conditions (Meskó, B. & Topol, E. J., 2023).

In the same direction, FDA has been implementing regulatory changes to specifically target AI and machine learning (ML) technologies in medical devices. The FDA proposed a total product lifecycle (TPLC) approach to the regulation of AI/ML-based SaMD that is oriented at continuous monitoring and improvement of these technologies over the years. The importance of transparency and performance surveillance in real life and anticipations regarding changes and updates in AI/ML algorithms also took priority in the proposed model.

FDA has regulated the LLM as Software as a Medical device (SaMD), and has concentrated on the Total Product Lifecycle (Meskó, B. & Topol, E. J., 2023).

1. **PCCP (Predetermined Change Control Plan):** A paramount 2024-2025 need. To avoid the occurrence of performance drift or new hallucinations following the initial launch, developers need to pre-specify the way an LLM will be updated or retrained.
2. **Grounding on Real-World Evidence (RWE):** The FDA is progressively mandating that the LLM is tested alongside actual clinicians in live hospital settings and that this shadowing is done before the time of full clearance (as opposed to passing simple exams, as is the case with the USMLE)

At the moment, the FDA does not create their own categories to which the AI-based technologies are considered but reviews them according to the existing regulatory framework of medical devices. According to their risk degree, they divide such devices into three major groups:

1. **Class I (Low risk):** These are the devices that are less risky and are under the general controls, including registration and listing, labelling and good manufacturing practices. Surgery instruments that are not powered as well as dental floss can be mentioned as examples of Class I. Certain medical technologies with AI are not high-risk, and will even be considered low-risk, based on their intended purpose.
2. **Class II (Moderate risk):** There is a greater amount of risk in these devices than in Class I devices, and they are not only subject to general controls but have special controls, such as performance standards, post – market surveillance, or special labelling. Class II devices (infusion pumps, surgical drapes, and powered wheelchairs, etc.) are examples. This category can include a large number of AI-based medical technologies, including diagnostic imaging systems.
3. **Class III (High risk):** These are the riskiest gadgets which are previously subjected to general controls, special controls, and pre-market approval (PMA). The Class III devices may sustain or help maintain human life, or may pose a significant value in disabling human health, or may pose a possible unreasonable risk of morbidity or injury. Some Class III devices are implantable pacemakers, artificial heart valves, and critical medical decision support AI-based technologies.

3.4. WHO Guidance: Ethical Sovereignty and LMMs

The World Health Organization (WHO) provides the framework for **Large Multimodal Models (LMMs)**, emphasizing global equity.

1. **Transparency of the Algorithms**: The WHO has proposed that PharmaCARE conducts Post-Market Auditing of its models by independent third parties to maintain that models that have been trained on high-income populations do not generate Unsafe Recommendations when used on diverse populations across the world.
2. **Overcoming Automation Bias:** Regulatory measures stress training clinicians to think with a skeptical attitude, lest they fall into the perilous behavior of trusting an AI generated and accurate answer too much.

4. EVALUATION METHODS AND BENCHMARKING

Although human assessment continues to be crucial in the assessment of safety and effectiveness of the LLM in healthcare, there is a high inconsistency of evaluation practices. Numerous studies indicate significant discrepancies in reliability, reproducibility and generalizability, pointing at the unavailability of standard evaluation procedures across all clinical research in LLM (Park, Y. J. et al., 2024).

Present methods of evaluation are based on automated quantitative measures that were first created to support conventional tasks of natural language processing. Machine translation and summarization metrics like Bilingual Evaluation Understudy (BLEU) and Recall-Oriented Understudy of Gisting Evaluation (ROUGE) are typically used to indicate machine translation and summarization performance, whereas general performance measures, including accuracy, F-measure, and area under the receiver operating characteristic (AU-ROC) curve are used to indicate classification tasks (Tam, T. Y. C. et al., 2024). Leaving them aside, these metrics are not well-suited to the generative and reasoning-intensive character of LLMs and do not evaluate clinical correctness, contextual suitability, and patient safety, which must be considered when implemented in clinical environments.

Evaluations based on benchmarks, such as the Holistic Evaluation of Language Models (HELM) (Liang, P. et al., 2022); have a more comprehensive view of the linguistic capabilities, yet are not as clinically applicable. These standards are usually based on fixed data sets, are not based on realistic clinical processes or workflows, and do not effectively measure the occurrence of rare, high-risk failure modes that are important to medical practice.

This has led to a growing dependence on human judges especially clinicians to examine LLM outputs to determine their accuracy, safety and ethical correctness. Human evaluation is more thorough and context-based judgments; however, it is expensive, time-consuming and prone to inter-rater effects. More risks are added with recent suggestions to use LLMs as a form of evaluation on their own since it is clear that they have the problem of hallucination, summary errors, and spreading mis-information.

To address these challenges, structured evaluation frameworks have been proposed to standardize human-centered assessment processes. One such framework is *QUEST* (Tam, T. Y. C. et al, 2024), which guides evaluation through three phases—(1) planning, (2) implementation and adjudication, and (3) scoring and review. The QUEST focuses on five core principles: quality, reasoning, persona, safety, and trust (Tam, T. Y. C. et al, 2024). Frameworks of this nature aim to bridge the gap between automated metrics and expert judgment, providing a more rigorous and practical pathway for the responsible deployment of LLMs in clinical environments.

4.1. Automated Benchmarking

The critical reorientation of the evaluation of LLMs in medicine has been a transition between the knowledge-based (what a model knows) and the practice and reasoning-based (how a model applies that knowledge) evaluation of the models. This development is essential as a high score in medical tests may not necessarily result in safe or effective clinical practice (Zhou, S. et al., 2025).

Knowledge-based Benchmarks (USMLE / Med A)

Knowledge-based benchmarks assess a model's ability to recall and apply medical facts.

- **Methodology**: They typically utilize multiple-choice questions (MC s) from licensing exams, such as the United States Medical Licensing Examination (USMLE) or Med A.
- **Performance Trends**: Leading models have reached a "saturation point," consistently exceeding 84%–90% accuracy, which approaches or surpasses average physician performance.
- **Limitations**: The multiple-choice form of the problem makes the complex cases easy to solve, with the ability to guess with some educated reasoning or spot the pattern, not to need a model to build its own diagnostic reasoning. They do not also often examine the capacity of a model to cope with uncertainty, e.g. when there is insufficient information.

Reasoning-based Benchmarks (MedThink-Bench)

Reasoning-based benchmarks focus on the transparency and validity of the medical decision- making process.

- **Methodology**: Frameworks like **MedThink-Bench** use high-complexity questions accompanied by expert-authored, step-by-step "rationales" that map out the intermediate logic needed to reach a conclusion.
- **Evaluation Shift**: Instead of just checking if the final answer is right, these benchmarks evaluate the "reasoning trajectories". This can identify "flawed reasoning," where an LLM arrives at a correct diagnosis by sheer luck or incorrect facts.
- **The Knowledge-Practice Gap**: Evidence shows that while models maintain high factual retrieval (85%–93%), their performance in clinical reasoning tasks often drops significantly to 50%–60% (Gong, E. J. et al., 2025).

4.2. Safety Scoring Approaches

With the transition of clinical LLM out of research laboratories into real hospitals, the industry has come to the understanding that passing medical exams do not warrant patient safety. Two new frameworks - CSEDB and MEDIC - have developed to fill the gap as the current gold standards of determining whether a model is indeed safe to apply at the bedside.

Clinical Safety-Effectiveness Dual-Track Benchmark (CSEDB)

The idea behind CSEDB was a resultant agreement between 32 expert physicians who understood that not every medical error is the same. Although most benchmarks have equal weight on all questions, CSEDB implemented weighted consequence measures (Wang, S. et al., 2025).

- **Prioritizing High-Risk Scenarios:** The framework includes 30 high-risk metrics such as medication safety and identification of critical illness.
- **The Punishment for Risk:** In CSEDB, a model would receive much more punishment on a fatal error- such as the omitment of a drug-drug interaction or miscalculation of a child dose- than a minor clerical error.
- **The "Safety Gap" Discovery:** When preliminary testing with CSEDB was conducted, it turned out to be a worrisome pattern: even the models that are all successful with standard tests experienced a 13.3% performance hit in the conditions of these high-risk and life-or-death situations. This confirms that general accuracy is a low quality proxy of clinical safety (Wang, S. et al., 2025).

MEDIC: Comprehensive Evaluation of Leading Indicators

Whereas CSEDB concentrates on the magnitude of errors, MEDIC framework centers on the reliability of the model operation in five fundamental dimensions including Medical Reasoning, Ethics, Data Agency, In- context Learning, and Clinical Safety.

- **Cross-Examination Framework (CEF):** MEDIC has a very novel aspect, a cross-examination type of testing. Rather than simply comparing an answer with a key, it will pose the model follow-up questions to cause it to attempt to be tricked into a contradiction or a hallucination.
- **The Knowledge-Execution Gap:** MEDIC research found that there was a substantial knowledge-execution gap. It established that excellent models of recalling medical facts (static retrieval) tend to perform disastrously when required to do a functional task, such as calculating a particular dosage of medication based on the weight of a patient.
- **Active vs. Passive Safety:** The model also differentiates between passive safety (the model refusing to respond to a harmful prompt) and active safety (the capacity of the model to actively recognize a factual error in a medical note) (Kanithi, P. K. et al., 2024; Kim, S. & Yoon, H. J., 2025)

4.3. Task-Specific Scoring: How Scoring Differs for Different Medical Tasks

Precision-First Scoring: The Rx-LLM Paradigm

Scoring in pharmacology has to be deterministic. Rx-LLM benchmark (2025) (Zhao, X. et al., 2025) is a model appraisal along with six important medication management pathways, such as drug-drug interactions (DDI), renal dose modification.

- **The Binary of Safety:** As a contrast to general NLP, Rx-LLM scoring frequently takes linguistic "fluency" out of consideration in favor of clinical accuracy. An answer that is right on 99 out of 100 but has a single mistake of fatal dose is considered as a complete failure (Zhao, X. et al., 2025).
- **Correctness- Consistency:** One of the main measurements in Rx-LLM is the measure of consistency across trials. When a model finds a fatal interaction between two prompts, and it does not find it in the third, its safety score gets seriously punished. This is in keeping with what happens in the real world where a pharmacy system cannot be mostly reliable.
- **Track-Specific Variance:** It was found that models such as LLaMA-3 can be useful at Drug-Indication Matching (97.6% accuracy) but have failures in Renal Dose Adjustment (below 80%). This brings out the point that medical knowledge does not ensure computational safety in pharmacy.

Fidelity and Empathy Scoring: Mental Health Safety Plans

Unlike the binary math of pharmacy, mental health intervention (like the Safety Planning Intervention (SPI)) needs Fidelity Scoring. The Safety Plan Fidelity Rater (SPFR) determines if the output written by an LLM is in line with evidence-based suicide prevention guidelines (Donnelly, H. K. et al., 2026).

- **The 03 uality Scale:** SPFR also employs a graduated scale (0-3) to rate the category of Warning Signs and Internal Coping Strategies in place of a simple right/wrong. A 3 score is only used when the responses are not only correct, but highly personalized and actionable (i.e. I start hearing voices and sleeping 12 hours vs. a general I feel bad).
- **The Empathy Constraint:** Within mental health, a technically correct safety plan, but lacking the tone of empathy or an offer of crisis resources (such as a hotline number) is a failure. This scoring should take into consideration therapeutic alignment, that is not important on a query on pharmacy database but life-saving in a psychiatric emergency.
- **Weighted F1-Scores:** Frameworks such as SPFR are usually based on the idea of weighted F1-scores to use Recall (no warning signs are missed) versus Precision (the exact wording used) to accept that in a crisis, the worst failure mode is to miss a risk factor.

4.4. The Shift to Automated Reasoning Metrics: Moving from BLEU/ROUGE to BERTScore, BLUERT, and LLM-as-a-Judge protocols.

With the shift between simple chatbots and more sophisticated decision-support tools, the standard by which we will evaluate them has been forced to evolve in a fundamental way. Over several years of use the industry was using so-called lexical measures such as BLEU and ROUGE (Tam, T. Y. C. et al., 2024), which effectively are advanced spell-checkers, counting the number of words in a model reply that coincide with a reference answer. In medicine, however, matching words does not mean matching meaning.

Therefore, one of the main weaknesses of traditional metrics such as ROUGE is that they are not able to comprehend semantic negation or clinical synonyms. By copying 90 percent of a test sentence but missing one, decisive word like e.g. to say in lieu of decrease dosage, such a model would get a high ROUGE score. This transforms lexical metrics in a healthcare context not only to be inadequate, but can also be hazardous. Research has demonstrated that these older methods are frequently horrendously out of correlation with real human physician judgment, because they are unable to differentiate between a stylistic decision and an error that can cause death (Pedersen, T. et al., 2007).

The Move to Semantic Embeddings

Research has moved to a situation where they use semantically embedded metrics to overcome this meaning-blindness, including BERTScore and Universal Sentence Encoders.

- **Contextual Understanding:** These measures do not involve counting words, but rather they transform sentences into mathematical vectors that capture the sentences meaning. This will enable the evaluation system to appreciate the fact that the word "hypertension" is synonymous with the word high blood pressure, although they do not even have a single letter in common.
- **Weighted Similarity:** The more recent automated grading systems combine all the factors to the desired degree, including cosine similarity, Jaccard similarity, and semantic analysis, to make sure that the main medical meaning is stored, even though the AI can use different wording (Ayaan, A. & Ng, K. W., 2025).

"LLM-as-a-Judge" and Multi-Agent Evaluation

The most recent and sophisticated leap in 2025–2026 is the use of LLMs themselves as evaluators, often organized into Multi-Agent Frameworks.

- **Courtroom Dynamics (CourtEval):** One of the most effective new approaches is the "Courtroom" model. Rather than one AI giving a score, a "Grader" (Judge) proposes a score, a "Critic" (Prosecutor) looks for flaws or hallucinations in the medical reasoning, and a "Defender" (Defense Attorney) justifies the model's response.
- **Self-Correction and Consensus:** This multi-agent debate helps eliminate the "bias" often found in single-AI judges (who might favor their own writing style). By forcing different AI agents to "argue" over the clinical accuracy of a response, the final score reflects a much more rigorous and human-like consensus.
- **Scalability:** These frameworks, such as LLM-w-Rationale, allow hospitals to evaluate thousands of AI responses with "expert-level fidelity" in a fraction of the time it would take a panel of doctors (Kumar, S. et al., 2025).

4.5. Identifying High-Risk Failure Modes: Using Weighted Scoring for Life-Threatening Errors

In the high-stakes world of clinical medicine, not all errors carry the same weight. A minor administrative typo is fundamentally different from a lethal drug interaction. To reflect this reality, modern evaluation frameworks have moved toward weighted consequence measures, ensuring that a model's safety score is heavily influenced by the actual clinical risk its mistakes pose.

The Weighted Risk Scale (1–5) and Critical Failure Modes

More sophisticated benchmarks, such as the Clinical Safety-Effectiveness Dual-Track Benchmark (CSEDB) (Wang, S. et al., 2025), identify medical tasks and possible errors on a scale of 1 to 5 according to their responsible patient outcomes. In this system high-risk scenarios are prioritized to be sure that models are safe when it counts:

- **Weight 5 (Life-Threatening):** The level is used in cases where the error may result in instant death or devastating damage. Failure modes: The underlying failure modes are:
- **Lethal Drug-Drug Interactions (S-06):** Recommending a combination of medications that leads to a fatal event, like a severe arrhythmia.
- **Fatal Diagnostic Errors (S-02):** Misidentifying or missing a critical, time-sensitive condition like a heart attack.
- **Ignoring Severe Allergy History (S-0G):** Recommending a medication a patient is known to be severely allergic to.
- **Weight 4 (Severe Disability):** Includes high-risk errors like pediatric medication mistakes or severe dosage miscalculations (S-05) that could lead to long-term harm.
- **Weights 1–3 (Moderate to Low Risk):** Include tasks such as clerical data errors or misrepresentation that causes delayed treatment but is not immediately life-threatening (Wang, S. et al., 2025).

4.6. The "Safety-Efficiency" Trade-Off: The CVD Framework

In addition to pinpointing mistakes, the Clinical Value Density (CVD) model touches upon the race against time in clinical practice. It characterizes clinical utility in units of cognitive resource, recognizing that a safe model is useless despite responses being too complex to be understood by a busy doctor.

- **Deployment Stratification:** Studies based on CVD indicate that various models are applicable at varying levels of risks. As an example, GPT-4o is effective with more routine consultations, but Grok-3 and Gemini-2.5 would also be safer in situations of complexity and high stakes, even though the recommendations may not be as concise.
- **Brevity-Accuracy Risks:** The framework cautions against models that are high-performing by being excessively concise yet clinically erroneous, such as DeepSeek-R1 in certain pharmacology tests (Zaki, N. et al., 2025).

4.7. Proactive Risk Management With FMEA

In order to obtain these high-risk failure modes in a systematic manner, researchers are combining Failure Mode and Effects Analysis (FMEA) with LLMs. FMEA is a pillar of product reliability that actively determines the possible points of failure before they find their way into the hands of a user.

- **Automated Identification:** LLMs have the potential to shorten this process by examining enormous datasets of prior failures and patient complaints to determine where a new model may fail.
- **Risk Priority:** FMEA logic provides developers with a way to compute a Risk Priority Number (RPN), to help them prioritize their safety tuning on those errors that are not only severe, but also difficult to detect by a human doctor (El Hassani, I. et al., 2024).

5. THE ACCOUNTABILITY PARADOX: WHY HUMANS REMAIN ESSENTIAL

The high-stakes medical setting has integrated LLMs very fast, creating a strong accountability paradox. Although AI has the capability to process information on a much larger scale than a human being can, the application of such models alone to complex decisions is inherently problematic because of the risks of hallucination, bias, and a deficit of common sense. The clinical validation has thus to be developed beyond a single check by a long-term Human-in-the-Loop (HITL) process in which the clinician should be the ultimate point of record and the truth teller (Zöller, N. et al., 2024; Zhang, X. et al., 2026).

5.1. Tiered Agentic Oversight (TAO): The New Clinical Hierarchy

The Tiered Agentic Oversight (TAO) framework is a revolutionary shift in the field of organized AI safety based on the principles of traditional hospital hierarchies (e.g., nurse-physician-specialist).

- **Layered Supervision**: TAO directs tasks using a hierarchical multi-agent system, in which specialized agents, including Reasoning Auditors, Context Keepers, and Safety Guardians, are used to offer layered supervision.

- **Error Absorption**: The structure is a powerful filter, and it is capable of absorbing between 16.G% and 24.3% of agent error on an individual basis before it can become accumulated into clinical harm
- **The Physician as the "Highest Tier"**: In user research, when the human doctor is the last level of control making corrections to the system, medical triage accuracy has been demonstrated to increase by as much as 40 to 60 percent (Kim, Y. et al., 2025).

5.2. HealthBench: Physician-Led Safety Standards

The old gold standards are no longer the gold standard of measuring the real physician judgment of the LLMs; the new gold standard is HealthBench (2025) (Arora, R. K. et al., 2025).

- **Expert-Driven Rubrics**: In contrast to multiple-choice tests, HealthBench uses 5,000 multi-turn health conversations, which are graded using 48,562 distinct rubric criteria which were established through the contribution of 262 physician.
- **Rapid Progress**: Benchmarking indicates that the past models like GPT-3.5 Turbo have been rated at 16 percent as compared to the latest models in the field indicating that AI is gradually gaining experts in clinical thinking.
- **The "Consensus" Axis**: The axis measures the consensus dimensions directly, i.e. critical model behaviours that people have been agreed on, to ensure that the advice given by the AI is not only correct, but also safe and reliable (Arora, R. K. et al., 2025).

5.3. Hybrid Collective Intelligence in Diagnostics

The most accurate clinical outcomes in 2026 are no longer achieved by "AI vs. Human" but by Human-AI Collectives.

- **Complementary Strengths**: Research across 2,133 medical cases shows that hybrid collectives of physicians and LLMs outperform single physicians, physician collectives, and even LLM ensembles.
- **Error Mitigation**: Error Mitigation: It is a high-quality performance due to the fact that human beings and machines commit different kinds of errors; a hybrid system uses human experiences to detect AI hallucinations and uses the AI abundant data processing to detect human oversight (Zöller, N. et al., 2024).

5.4. Interactive Report Generation: Designing for Agency

The final HITL validation interface is the clinical interface design. Modern systems like Interactive Report Generation systems are designed to ensure physician control through a review based on recognition.

- **Division of Labor:** The AI will only take part in the arrangement and writing of data, and the final decision will be made by the clinician.
- **Visual Evidence:** Visual evidence interfaces generate an AI-generated draft and show it alongside time-aligned visualizations, allowing doctors to do in-line editing access to the visual evidence supporting each clinical claim.
- **Efficiency and Accuracy:** In pilot studies, AI was observed to achieve the same quality as a manual authoring draft with an average 8.3% revision of its content by the physician to meet a clinical gold standard (Zhang, X. et al., 2026).

6. CONCLUSION

LLM penetration in clinical practice is a groundbreaking opportunity and an enormous task. Clinical LLMs are associated with unique risks, especially, hallucinations, unsafe recommendations, and contextually inappropriate outputs that can directly impact patient safety as it is explained in this chapter. Even minor mistakes can be transferred to more severe threats in the medical sector, which is why the prevention of the risks and effective systems of governance is valued. Implementation with trust is founded on the relief of technical security against information confidentiality, computer security, and secure structures of deployment.

The regulations, such as the ones created by FDA, WHO, and the EU AI Act, suggest that the world is moving towards the traditional system of control, with its emphasis on validation, disclosure, and post-deployment surveillance. Assessment paradigms are supposed to evolve in this direction. The high stakes medical reasoning requires more than conventional NLP evaluation systems like BLEU and ROUGE. The existence of automated benchmarking, safety scoring models, task-specific evaluation protocols, reasoning-sensitive metrics such as BERTScore, BLEURT, and LLM-as-a-Judge is an indicator of a combination of the assessment standards to evaluate the clinical risk.

The risks in each situation can be controlled proactively not only by measurement, but also by proactive risk management techniques like Failure Mode and Effects Analysis (FMEA) there is a methodical gateway to foresee and prevent points of failure. The incorporation of human-in-the-loop systems, layer agentic supervision

(TAO), and hybrid collective intelligence layouts will be significant in ensuring that AI is not a replacement of clinical knowledge. A socio-technical synthesis will only allow an effective clinical integration of LLMs, including the rigorous testing, regulatory checks, systematic supervision, and multiparty intelligence. Only in this unified system, the LLMs have the opportunity to fulfill the roles of the introduction of accuracy, efficiency, and fairness in healthcare.

REFERENCES

Arora, R. K., Wei, J., Hicks, R. S., Bowman, P., uiñonero-Candela, J., Tsimpourlas, F., ... C Singhal, K. (2025). Healthbench: Evaluating large language models towards improved human health. arXiv preprint arXiv:2505.08775. https://doi.org//arXiv.2505.08775DOI: 10.48550

Ayaan, A., & Ng, K. W. (2025). Automated grading using natural language processing and semantic analysis. *MethodsX, 103395*, 103395. Advance online publication. DOI: 10.1016/j.mex.2025.103395 PMID: 40529512

Donnelly, H. K., Brown, G. K., Green, K. L., Vurgun, U., Hwang, S., Schriver, E., Steinberg, M., Reilly, M. E., Mehta, H., Labouliere, C., Oquendo, M. A., Mandell, D., & Mowery, D. L. (2026). Automated Safety Plan Scoring in Outpatient Mental Health Settings Using Large Language Models: Exploratory Study. *JMIR Mental Health, 13*(1), e79010. DOI: 10.2196/79010 PMID: 41505705

El Hassani, I., Masrour, T., Kourouma, N., Motte, D. C., & Tavčar, J. (2024). Integrating large language models for improved failure mode and effects analysis (FMEA): A framework and case study. *Proceedings of the Design Society*, *4*, 2019–2028. DOI: 10.1017/pds.2024.204

Gong, E. J., Bang, C. S., Lee, J. J., & Baik, G. H. (2025). Knowledge-practice performance gap in clinical large language models: Systematic review of 39 benchmarks. *Journal of Medical Internet Research*, *27*, e84120. DOI: 10.2196/84120 PMID: 41325597

Jung, K. H. (2025). Large language models in medicine: Clinical applications, technical challenges, and ethical considerations. *Healthcare Informatics Research*, *31*(2), 114–124. DOI: 10.4258/hir.2025.31.2.114 PMID: 40384063

Kalodanis, K., Feretzakis, G., Rizomiliotis, P., Verykios, V. S., Papapavlou, C., Skrekas, A. C., & Anagnostopoulos, D. (2025). Evaluating the Impact of the EU AI Act on Medical Device Regulation. In *Envisioning the Future of Health Informatics and Digital Health* (pp. 40–44). IOS Press., DOI: 10.3233/SHTI250045

Kanithi, P. K., Christophe, C., Pimentel, M. A., Raha, T., Saadi, N., Javed, H., ... C Khan, S. (2024). Medic: Towards a comprehensive framework for evaluating llms in clinical applications. arXiv preprint arXiv:240S.07314. https://doi.org//arXiv.2409.07314DOI: 10.48550

Kim, S. C., & Yoon, H. J. (2025, August). uestioning Our uestions: How Well Do Medical A Benchmarks Evaluate Clinical Capabilities of Language Models? In *Proceedings of the 24th Workshop on Biomedical Language Processing* (pp. 274-296). https://doi.org/DOI: 10.18653/v1/2025.bionlp-1.24

Kim, Y., Jeong, H., Chen, S., Li, S. S., Park, C., Lu, M., . . . Breazeal, C. (2025). Medical hallucinations in foundation models and their impact on healthcare. arXiv preprint arXiv:2503.05777. https://doi.org//arXiv.2503.05777DOI: 10.1101/2025.02.28.25323115

Kim, Y., Jeong, H., Park, C., Park, E., Zhang, H., Liu, X., ... C Park, H. W. (2025). Tiered Agentic Oversight: A Hierarchical Multi-Agent System for AI Safety in Healthcare. arXiv preprint arXiv:250C.12482. https://doi.org//arXiv.2506.12482DOI: 10.48550

Kumar, S., Nargund, A. A., & Sridhar, V. (2025, July). CourtEval: A courtroom-based multi-agent evaluation framework. In *Findings of the Association for Computational Linguistics: ACL 2025* (pp. 25875-25887). https://doi.org/DOI: 10.18653/v1/2025.findings-acl.1327

Liang, P., Bommasani, R., Lee, T., Tsipras, D., Soylu, D., Yasunaga, M., . . . Koreeda, Y. (2022). Holistic evaluation of language models. *arXiv preprint arXiv:2211.09110*. https://doi.org//arXiv.2211.09110.DOI: 10.48550

Meskó, B. C., & Topol, E. J. (2023). The imperative for regulatory oversight of large language models (or generative AI) in healthcare. *NPJ Digital Medicine*, *C*(1), 120. DOI: 10.1038/s41746-023-00873-0 PMID: 37414860

Moëll, B., Sand, C., & Aronsson, F. (2025). Harm reduction strategies for thoughtful use of large language models in the medical domain: Perspectives for patients and clinicians. *Journal of Medical Internet Research*, *27*, e75849. DOI: 10.2196/75849 PMID: 40712151

Muhammad, D., & Bendechache, M. (2024). Unveiling the black box: A systematic review of Explainable Artificial Intelligence in medical image analysis. *Computational and Structural Biotechnology Journal*, *24*, 542–560. DOI: 10.1016/j.csbj.2024.08.005 PMID: 39252818

Nachane, S. S., Gramopadhye, O., Chanda, P., Ramakrishnan, G., Jadhav, K. S., Nandwani, Y., & Joshi, S. (2024, November). Few shot chain-of-thought driven reasoning to prompt LLMs for open-ended medical question answering. In *Findings of the Association for Computational Linguistics* (pp. 542–573). EMNLP., DOI: 10.18653/v1/2024.findings-emnlp.31

Park, Y. J., Pillai, A., Deng, J., Guo, E., Gupta, M., Paget, M., & Naugler, C. (2024). Assessing the research landscape and clinical utility of large language models: A scoping review. *BMC Medical Informatics and Decision Making*, *24*(1), 72. DOI: 10.1186/s12911-024-02459-6 PMID: 38475802

Pedersen, T., Pakhomov, S. V., Patwardhan, S. C., & Chute, C. G. (2007). Measures of semantic similarity and relatedness in the biomedical domain. *Journal of Biomedical Informatics*, *40*(3), 288–299. DOI: 10.1016/j.jbi.2006.06.004 PMID: 16875881

Roustan, D., & Bastardot, F. (2025). The clinicians' guide to large language models: A general perspective with a focus on hallucinations. *Interactive Journal of Medical Research*, *14*(1), e59823. DOI: 10.2196/59823 PMID: 39874574

Tam, T. Y. C., Sivarajkumar, S., Kapoor, S., Stolyar, A. V., Polanska, K., McCarthy, K. R., Osterhoudt, H., Wu, X., Visweswaran, S., Fu, S., Mathur, P., Cacciamani, G. E., Sun, C., Peng, Y., & Wang, Y. (2024). A framework for human evaluation of large language models in healthcare derived from literature review. *NPJ Digital Medicine*, *7*(1), 258. DOI: 10.1038/s41746-024-01258-7 PMID: 39333376

Tonmoy, S. M. T. I., Zaman, S. M., Jain, V., Rani, A., Rawte, V., Chadha, A., & Das, A. (2024). A comprehensive survey of hallucination mitigation techniques in large language models. *arXiv preprint arXiv:2401.01313, 6*. https://doi.org//arXiv.2401.01313DOI: 10.48550

. Tu, T., Azizi, S., Driess, D., Schaekermann, M., Amin, M., Chang, P. C., ... & Natarajan, V. (2024). Towards generalist biomedical AI. *Nejm Ai, 1*(3), AIoa2300138. https://doi.org/DOI: 10.1056/AIoa2300138

Vaezi, A. (2025). Legal Challenges in the Deployment of Large Language Models: A Comparative Analysis under the GDPR and EU AI Act. *Available at SSRN* 5285174. *https://dx.doi.org/*DOI: 10.2139/ssrn.5285174

Wang, S., Tang, Z., Yang, H., Gong, Q., Gu, T., Ma, H., Wang, Y., Sun, W., Lian, Z., Mao, K., Jiang, Y., Huang, Z., Ma, L., Shen, W., Ji, Y., Tan, Y., Wang, C., Gao, Y., Ye, Q., & Wu, J. (2025). A novel evaluation benchmark for medical LLMs illuminating safety and effectiveness in clinical domains. *npj. Digital Medicine*, *9*(1), 91. Advance online publication. DOI: 10.1038/s41746-025-02277-8 PMID: 41454006

Zaki, N., Akor, A., & Aburuz, S. C ZainAlAbdin, S. (2025). Beyond Accuracy: An Efficiency-and Safety-Aware Framework for Evaluating Clinical AI with Large Language Models. medRxiv, 2025-10. https://doi.org/DOI: 10.1101/2025.10.14.25338039

Zhang, X., Yu, J., Yan, P., Jiang, L., Shen, X., Cheng, M., & Liu, C. X. (2026). Human-in- the-Loop Interactive Report Generation for Chronic Disease Adherence. *arXiv preprint* https://doi.org//arXiv.2601.06364DOI: 10.48550

Zhao, X., Blotske, K., Cargile, M., Tilley, A., Murray, B., Gao, Y., . . . Sikora, A. (2025). Rx-LLM: a benchmarking suite to evaluate safe large language model performance for medication-related tasks. medRxiv, 2025-12. https://doi.org/DOI: 10.64898/2025.12.01.25341004

Zhou, S., Xie, W., Li, J., Zhan, Z., Song, M., & Yang, H.. C Zhang, R. (2025). Automating expert-level medical reasoning evaluation of large language models. npj. *Digital Medicine*. Advance online publication. DOI: 10.2196/84120

Zöller, N., Berger, J., Lin, I., Fu, N., Komarneni, J., Barabucci, G., ... C Herzog, S. M. (2024). Human-AI collectives produce the most accurate differential diagnoses. *arXiv preprint.* https://doi.org//arXiv.2406.14981DOI: 10.48550

Chapter 6

Evaluating the Safety of Medical LLMs for Patient Use

R. Vishva
http://orcid.org/0009-0004-7004-2991
Department of Microbiology, Sacred Heart College, India

F. Fareedhul Fahmitha
http://orcid.org/0009-0000-8693-5023
Department of Microbiology, Sacred Heart College, India

S. Indhu
Department of Microbiology, Sacred Heart College, India

R. Gayathri
http://orcid.org/0009-0002-2352-5531
Department of Microbiology, Sacred Heart College, India

P. Saranraj
http://orcid.org/0000-0002-5052-6532
Department of Microbiology, Sacred Heart College, India

ABSTRACT

The main development of Large Language Models (LLM) within the medical field has been designed and proven to be effective by health care professionals and there has been a gap in patient centred adaptation. Since the practical patient application of these models is not only unsafe but also dangerous, the strict assessment adapted to the situation of patient interaction is necessary. The existing methods of assessing LLMs can force one to establish the most effective domains of applying

DOI: 10.4018/979-8-3373-7862-6.ch006

LLM. Implementing AI (AI) in healthcare requires well-constructed safety validation schemes especially those systems that directly communicate with patients. The current standard methods of LLM benchmarking are extremely low in coverage of output and are not adequate in healthcare application where high safety requirements are necessary.

1. INTRODUCTION

The availability of big data, the availability of increased computing resources and shifts in neural network architecture over the last several years have spurred the integration of AI into healthcare systems everywhere in the world. In particular, medical LLMs can be viewed as a transition to general-purpose rationales that can process and understand complex natural language input rather than being task-specific. This has made AI-driven medical information delivery more useful and risky, especially when targeting patients. Patients are not provided with official medical arguments, evidence analysis, and risk analysis in the same manner as healthcare professionals. Therefore, they might view the answers generated by AI as a medical consultation instead of information advice. This asymmetry in expertise increases the safety problem and demands explicit assessment models that take into account patient vulnerability, knowledge of limitations, and behavior in decision-making (Davahli et al., 2021). LLMs have demonstrated remarkable results in understanding, generating and reasoning natural languages. They are also being utilized in the medical sector more to complete such tasks as clinical documentation, medical question answering, decision support, patient record summarization, and medical education (Sujan *et al.*, 2022). Even with these developments, the majority of medical LLM systems have been developed, trained, and tested concerning the requirements of medical professionals but not directly to patients. Such systems can pose a lot of safety, ethical, and regulatory problems when accessed by patients without professional mediation since such mismatch is severe. Patients are becoming more dependent on the internet to seek medical information, decode symptoms, and make health-related choices. The general population has easy access to chatbots, virtual assistants, and mobile health applications that are driven by LLM (Wadden, 2021). Despite the fact that these tools are more convenient and large-scale than ever before, they also introduce new dangers, including false information, misunderstanding symptoms, wrong medical advice, emotional damage, and confirmation of health-related skepticism. In contrast to clinicians, patients do not usually possess the domain knowledge to be able to prejudice the AI-generated medical information critically, which prompts an essential necessity of patient-facing LLM safety models. The chapter will critically assess current safety evaluation approaches to medical LLC, explore the gaps in the current benchmarking solutions to the patient-centered context and suggest a patient-safe benchmarking model that would include qualitative approaches to safety and describe the implications of clinical implementation and regulatory compliance.

Traditional evaluation methods of LLMs pay too much attention to benchmark performance, accuracy on standardized question-answering datasets or agreement with answers produced by the expert (Lee *et al.,* 2023). These standards are not relevant to everyday life patient interaction cases where there is ambiguity, emotional distress, incomplete information and context dependent risks. Unsafe or misleading outputs can have dire results in patient-directed environments, including the delayed medical access, mental injuries, or self-treatment. The application of AI in healthcare touches upon more general concerns of responsibility, transparency, and trust. In contrast to traditional medical equipment, LLMs are non-deterministic and give different results to similar inputs (Morley *et al.,* 2021). Such inconsistency makes it more difficult to assure and monitor safety. Moreover, big neural networks are black box and it is hard to tell how they reason or where errors may originate. These constraints illustrate the need to have efficient safety assessment models that extend beyond the classical performance indicators in patient-facing applications where trust and reliability are critical factors to consider. This chapter critically assesses the safety of medical LLMs to use with patients by describing the current approaches to evaluate safety, limitations, and future directions of safety assessment. In particular, it pays attention to the possibility of utilizing LLMs as automated judges or assessors of medical responses, contrasting their results with human annotators in different qualitative safety aspects (Reddy *et al.,* 2021). Another point of the chapter is the discussion of the adversarial testing strategies that help to reveal the weaknesses in the evaluation of the LLM and response generation. By conducting a systematic assessment of these concerns, this piece of work will aid in creating more robust and patient-focused models of safety evaluation of medical AI systems.

2. EVOLUTION OF HEALTHCARE AI SAFETY FRAMEWORKS

The appearance of AI in the models of medical safety is the indication of the evolution of AI technologies and their growing importance in medical care. First generation healthcare AI systems were mainly rule-based knowledge systems that helped clinicians to make diagnostic and treatment-related decisions. These systems were managed under a clear set of rules with a clinical understanding and allowing the rational processes to be transparent and monitored (Ribeiro *et al.,* 2021). The safety checks of this stage were directed on the logical consistency, validity of the rules, and medical compliance. Since these systems were deterministic and only worked in strictly clinically supervised environments, risks to safety were somewhat localized and could be handled. However, these initial safety architectures are not well-mapped to new generative AI models. Replacement of execution by rule with probabilistic language generation has completely altered the nature of errors, and the traditional validation strategies are no longer sufficient to identify small though potentially fatal conditions of accidents (Lin *et al.,* 2023).

Regulatory authorities are slowly realizing that even when used as a means of information only, AI systems can have an indirect impact on clinical outcomes. This has sparked off classification controversy, pre-deployment validation and monitoring of the post-deployment, especially in dynamic systems, which are updated and fine-tuned (Zhang *et al.,* 2023). Table 1 gives a summary of the steps of AI development and associated technologies, safety, and restrictions. With the development of AI in the healthcare sector to machine learning based systems, the safety frameworks had to adjust themselves to the new complexity of the system and lack of interpretability. Machine learning allowed predictive analytics to become easy in the diagnosis of diseases, their prognosis and the risk stratification of patients. In comparison to rule-based systems, these models based their learning patterns on large amounts of data, so they generated less transparent decision paths. To this extent, the research field of safety analysis was extended to encompass the statistical validation methods of cross-validation, external dataset test and performance robustness test. The major safety problems at this stage were data quality, model generalization, and bias (Higgins & Madai, 2020).

Table 1. Stages of AI development that are safety-oriented and restricted.

S. No	AI development phase	Dominant AI technology	Primary safety focus	Limitations of safety frameworks	References
1.	Early expert systems era	Rule-based expert systems	Logical consistency, rule correctness, guideline adherence	Limited scalability, dependence on predefined rules, inability to handle uncertainty	Obermeyer & Emanuel, 2020
2.	Statistical ML phase	Machine learning models	Performance validation, bias detection, dataset representativeness	Reduced interpretability, reliance on historical data, hidden biases	Ramprasad *et al.,* 2024
3.	Deep learning era	Neural networks	Explainability, robustness, real-world validation	Opacity of decision-making, reproducibility concerns	Wiens *et al.,* 2019

continued on following page

Table 1. Continued

S. No	AI development phase	Dominant AI technology	Primary safety focus	Limitations of safety frameworks	References
4.	Generative AI phase	Large language models	Contextual safety, harm prevention, patient comprehension	Hallucinations, overconfidence, non-deterministic outputs	Bommasani *et al.*, 2021
5.	Patient-facing AI era	Conversational LLMs	Emotional safety, ethical responsibility, human-centered design, trust calibration	Limited regulation, user misinterpretation	Sutton *et al.*, 2020

The AI safety requirements in the healthcare environment were also changed with the popularization of deep learning. Deep neural networks have demonstrated impressive progress in medical imaging, clinical natural language processing and genomics. Their very complex designs however aggravated the explainability, reproducibility and unintended bias issues. Biases detection, dataset representativeness test, and practical clinical validation practices started being included in safety frameworks (Ghassemi *et al.,* 2021). The regulatory bodies slowly came to the view that these systems were Software as a Medical Device, and this brought the lifecycle-based safety management, which was based on the risk management, continuous monitoring and post-deployment evaluation. The invention of Large Language Models became one of the milestones in medical AI (Fernández *et al.,* 2024). In contrast to task-specific systems, LLMs can possess general-purpose language understanding in addition to general medical reasoning: both conversation and general medical reasoning can occur. This change demonstrated that current safety models had severe gaps that were not intended to assess non-deterministic, generative outputs. Numerous new safety challenges such as hallucinated medical data, overconfident response, inconsistency of protocols, and sensitivity to the language of the inputs were arising. These issues required safety measures that would evaluate the factual correctness as well as the contextual appropriateness and risk consciousness (Macrae, 2025).

The emergence of AI tools that patients directly use in healthcare has increased the influence of safety paradigms of AI on healthcare. Direct contact with the patient implies that the LLMs are not exposed to the conventional clinical mediation, and physical, psychological, and informational damage can occur. AI-generated advice can be misinterpreted by patients or slow down seeking medical help, or can cause anxiety due to unsuitable or alarming reactions (Singhal *et al.,* 2023). Thus, the concepts of patient knowledge, emotional sensitivity, and open disclosure of uncertainty have been turned into the focus of safety models. These are feasible dangers of communication that cannot be recognized through classical benchmarking techniques, and assessing approaches that focus on patients should be employed (Alami *et al.,* 2024). Another emerging influence in the contemporary healthcare AI safety models is ethical and regulatory concerns. The world regulatory organizations and standards agencies have begun addressing problems that are posed by adaptive and ever-evolving AI systems. The ethics that are currently present in safety assessment procedures include accountability, transparency, fairness, and trustworthiness. The legislation and control is getting more complicated, as the boundary between informational health devices and medical decision-support systems is growing more blurry in conversational AI. In general, AI healthcare safety models are becoming less clinician to patient (van der Vegt *et al.,* 2024). The modern safety measures, the contextual risk, the ethical responsibility and the human-centered design should be incorporated in the safety governance, as the technical accuracy is not adequate.

3. IMPROVING THE SAFETY OF MEDICAL LLMS

To improve the safety of the medical LLMs, a multidimensional approach with the integration of technical safety, clinical validation, human supervision, and patient-centered design principles is required. As opposed to the classical clinical decision-support systems, LLMs produce open-ended answers, which change depending on how input is phrased, the state of a model, or contextual information. This generation property is also robust, but poses major safety concerns when models are used in interactions with patients (Bommasani *et al.,* 2021). Safety engineering is required to maintain data curation, training, deployment, and post-use monitoring throughout the lifecycle. Practically, patients usually turn to non-clinical language or incomplete descriptions or give emotional-charged accounts (Gama *et al.,* 2022). Medical LLM needs to be assessed on their ability to process such inputs conservatively, not to make premature conclusions, and refer users to the right professional services without inducing unwarranted anxiety or falsehood. The strict regulation of training data is one of the main principles of the enhanced medical LLM safety. The training of medical LLM usually includes the combination of general texts and domain-specific medical corpora that might include outdated, inconsistent, and non-evidence-based content (Khan *et al.,* 2024).

Figure 1. Multi-dimensional patient-facing medical LLM safety.

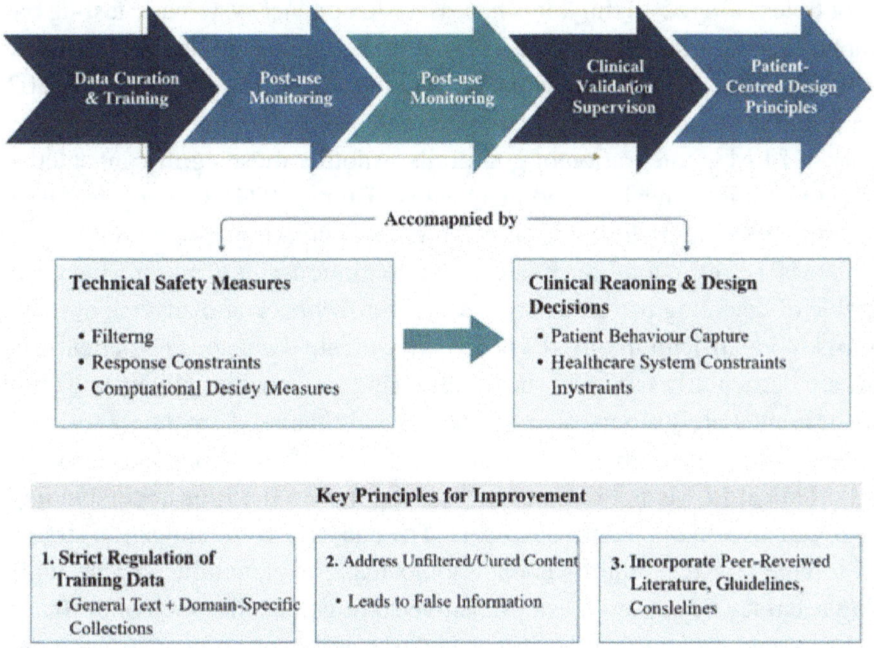

Figure 1 presents the human-in- loop validation, communication and emotional safety as a multi- dimensional model. The framework involves feedback between prior verification prior to deployment and monitoring after use to make a continuous improvement of safety possible (Preti *et al.,* 2024). Techniques used in model alignment are important in improving safety. Within the medical field, the processes of alignment need to be done by involving clinicians and domain experts, which can evaluate model outputs not just on the basis of factual accuracy, but also on the basis of clinical suitability and risk of harm (Lopez-Perez *et al.,* 2025). Hallucinated information, overgeneralization, and unsuitable feeling of certainty in the answers are minimized by such expert-in-the-loop feedback systems. Although the scalability of automation is high, especially in the context of high-stakes health, complete results based on AI-generated messages can be risky (Beamish and Exarchakis, 2025). To demonstrate this, the LLMs can be established to be able to deliver general health information but leave diagnosis, treatment decisions, and emergency advice to qualified professionals. Explicit attention to uncertainty-based model reasoning is also necessary in terms of enhancing safety. The model design contained in safety-oriented must think more in the direction of reason-based strategies that participate in recognizing ambiguity and encouraging the right follow-up (Gosak *et al.,* 2025). Medical LLMs tend to generate much different results when wording, order of information or tone is altered slightly. It is necessary to conduct systematic testing based on paraphrased and emotionally diverse inputs to determine the quality of responses and risk awareness when used in a realistic environment (Tonekaboni *et al.,* 2023).

One of the most commonly proposed technical actions undertaken to increase the safety of LLM is integration of guardrails. Another most significant safety improvement factor is clinical grounding (Veale & Binns, 2024). General-text trained LLMs do not have hierarchies or structured clinical thinking. The monitoring after deployment is the key to long-term safety. The continuous safety monitoring systems are capable of detecting patterns in response/user feedback and adverse events and this assists in identification of risks before they create damage. The patient-facing systems are particularly useful in such monitoring since potentially unsafe outputs may not be immediately reported via formal clinical channels (Emanuel *et al.,* 2020).

The health literacy of patients is still an aspect of safety outcomes that is frequently ignored. Medical LLMs not dynamically configured to the user understanding of language, can also end up confusing users. The adaptive communication strategies needed to enable safety improvement should make explanations simple without affecting accuracy or cause of risk. Sensitive settings like chronic conditions, terminal illness and mental health are particularly pertinent areas of psychological safety. There are some technical answers that are correct without being emotionally considerate that could make people even more distressed or isolated (Gerke *et al.,* 2020). Compassionate speech modeling and deliberate evaluation of emotional influence, thus, are the necessary elements of safety modification. Improvement of safety needs also involves the congruency between model behavior and ethical principles of patient self-determination and autonomy. The role of LLMs should be to help patients, not to tell them how to act. Excessively prescriptive answers destroy the patient agency and cut the boundary between information and medical advice. Another safety requirement is good uncertainty handling. Even in the cases when there is poor evidence to back up a claim, medical LLMs tend to convey it with a lot of certainty. The generation of responses aimed at safety concerns needs to contain explicit statements of limitation, hedging language, and solid warnings regarding the informational status of the content (Kamel Rahimi *et al.,* 2024). Professional consultation should be advised by models where necessary to avoid delayed self-care or inappropriate self-care.

Context awareness has been shown to increase patient safety because context models allow the patient to ask questions that are within the right context. The context-sensitive models have the ability to identify red flags like acute symptoms or mental distress and apply conservative response guidelines or emergency referrals. In medical LLM safety assessment, the emotional and psychological safety is a misaddressed factor. Assurance, validation, and emotional support may also be requested by patients in addition to a factual response (Gururangan *et al.,* 2020). Autonomy, empathy, supportive expression and respect are thus of paramount importance. This requires evaluation of compassionate responses and emotional safety, not merely factual accuracy, as criteria for safe interaction. In summary, making medical LLMs safer requires a holistic strategy that goes beyond existing technical performance standards to incorporate clinical expertise, ethical accountability, and patient-centered communication (Kassirer, 2024).

4. METHODOLOGY FOR PATIENT-CENTERED SAFETY EVALUATION

To address the gaps identified in existing benchmarking approaches, this chapter proposes a structured methodology for patient-centered safety evaluation of medical LLMs. The methodology integrates three complementary components: comparative analysis of LLM-based assessment versus human annotation across qualitative safety dimensions; adversarial question generation to probe model vulnerabilities; and a patient-safe benchmarking framework prioritizing harm prevention.

4.1 Comparative Assessment Framework

Eight qualitative safety measures were defined based on synthesis of the literature: scientific consensus alignment, grammaticality, uncertainty expression, empathy, tone appropriateness, potential for harm, actionability, and avoidance of overconfidence. Following the approach validated by Gosak *et al.* (2025) and López-Pérez *et al.* (2025), model outputs were evaluated both by automated metrics and by three independent human annotators with clinical domain expertise. Inter-annotator agreement was calculated using Fleiss' kappa.

4.2 Adversarial Question Generation

Adversarial test sets were constructed using three strategies: (a) paraphrasing of standard medical questions to assess response consistency; (b) introduction of incomplete or ambiguous symptom descriptions; and (c) emotionally loaded or distress-signaling queries. This process complies with the existing adversarial testing paradigms (Gehrmann *et al.,* 2023; Rak, 2023).

4.3 Patient-Safe Benchmarking Framework

The patient-safe benchmark was conceptualized into 5 assessment axes namely harm potential (weighted 35%), clinical appropriateness (25%), uncertainty communication (20%), empathy (10%), and factual accuracy (10%). Such weighting is an expression of the fact that harm prevention is more important than task completion when dealing with patients (Price and Cohen, 2019; Reddy *et al.,* 2020).

5. LLM BENCHMARKING LIMITATIONS

Performance benchmarking can cause the false impression of being detected by the average case accuracy, as opposed to the worst-case case performance. Practically, infrequent but harmful mistakes are easily magnified compared to non-material inaccuracy, and this is where benchmarks that overlook rare but significant failure cases are prone to fail (Singhal *et al.,* 2023). Table 2 provides an overview of conventional benchmarking methods and how they are inadequate towards patient safety.

Table 2. Conventional methods of benchmarking and patient safety demands.

S. No	Benchmark aspect	Traditional approach	Insufficient for patient safety	References
1.	Dataset design	Static, expert-curated	lDoes not reflect patient language or ambiguity	Rajpurkar *et al.,* 2021
2.	Evaluation scope	Single-turn responses	Ignores cumulative conversational risk	LeCun *et al.,* 2021
3.	Metrics used	Accuracy, fluency	Fails to capture harm, empathy, or behavioral impact	Amodei *et al.,* 2023
4.	Bias assessment	Limited demographic checks	Misses subtle and interaction-level bias	Raji *et al.,* 2020
5.	Stress testing	Minimal adversarial inputs	Overlooks rare but severe failure modes	Gehrmann *et al.,* 2023
6.	Temporal validity	One-time evaluation	Cannot detect performance drift	Sendak *et al.,* 2020; Wiens *et al.,* 2021

The choice of benchmark datasets is done under the controlled conditions that vary significantly compared to variability, uncertainty, and unpredictability of queries presented by patients (Holzinger *et al.,* 2020). One of the greatest disadvantages of existing benchmarking techniques is that they are model-level but not user-level. Benchmarks are solutions that check that a model can generate correct responses or fluent responses, but does not check how responses affect further actions of users (Beauchamp and Childress, 2021). The other area that has been left aside is that medical knowledge is dynamic. Medical documents, treatment plans, and disease taxonomies evolve with the times and therefore, a fixed benchmark data set would be long lost and therefore, be classified as an effective model that has already given outdated or harmful instructions. The use of fixed datasets is one of the main issues of traditional LLM benchmarks. Another problem is insufficient coverage of output of regular evaluation process. Benchmarks test a small percentage of model output values, and explore only a small percentage of the model output space. The unsafe, though infrequent, model outputs can be overlooked during benchmarking, and only later be discovered during actual implementation (Goodman & Flaxman, 2017).

Benchmarking is still more challenging due to subjective factors of safety. Automated metrics can never measure empathy, tone appropriateness, and possible harm (Char *et al.,* 2023). Although the human version is the best way to evaluate these factors, the human approach is resource-intensive and time-consuming as well as there is variation in inter-annotator. So the majority of benchmarks either ignores these or uses very simplistic surrogates that are not patient-centric. Another area that is lacking in terms of recent standards is bias and fairness analysis. Even though there are benchmarks that are trying to estimate demographic bias coarsely, they are not sufficiently nuanced to reflect bias in model behavior on the interaction level (Miller, 2021). The updates of LLM are dynamic, and it will be infeasible to conduct a static benchmarking. Such gaps show that more active and complex medical LLM-specific benchmarking tools should be created. These tools should have in place qualitative safety, adversarial tests, and interactive activities (Verghese *et al.,* 2023).

6. ETHICAL ISSUES IN AI IN HEALTHCARE

The advent of the use of LLM in the healthcare sector presents new ethical dilemmas. The problems get even more complicated when the technologies are implemented in front-office roles and patients can give credibility or power to the responses of AI systems without being aware of their limitations. The field of healthcare AI cannot isolate ethical concerns because in the former case, ethical breaches might result in psychological damage to patients or the loss of confidence in the health system. Informed consent is one of the major ethical issues of medical LLM (Bender *et al.,* 2021). By using medical LLM patients might not get to learn the full capabilities and limitations of the system such as the fact that it is not a human system. This may make the patients interpret system outputs as professional medical advice. The available ethical frameworks should, therefore, be transparent in the purpose of the system, the source of data, and limitations so that patients can make intelligent decisions on using the system results (Raji *et al.,* 2020).

The ethical inferences of responsibility are especially disorienting in regard to autonomous AI systems. The liability can be shared with developers, deployers, and users when a medical LLM generates unsafe or false information. Decentralisation of responsibility could result in no one responsible to take care of the accuracy and safety of medical information, and deprive patients of a choice. Medical LLMs have a particularly unclear situation with the principles of beneficence and non-maleficence. Ethical safety governance should be politically enduring with the intent of ensuring that AI-generated information is in the best interest of the patients. False representation of the capabilities of a model or uncertainty is not only unethical, but dangerous as it can be abused. There are differences in healthcare standards, acceptability, and communication styles based on culture (Rudin, 2020). Medical LLMs also pose ethical concerns because they may fail technically, but also as the sociotechnical ways these technologies are incorporated into the healthcare system. The perceived power of AI, the emotional and informational needs of patients, bring up moral conflicts that cannot be addressed by technical optimization. Ethical frameworks must make certain that the LLMs are empowering, not disempowering the patients by informing them of the uncertainty, referring to the professional medical advice where necessary and using persuasive rather than lecturing language. The ethical use of medical LLMs must take into account emotional and psychological effects. Empathy, sensitivity, and vulnerability of the patient should then be taken into consideration as among the most important safety variables in ethical consideration (Suresh and Guttag, 2021).

7. PATIENT-FACING MEDICAL LLM LEGAL AND REGULATORY STRUCTURES

Besides the ethical concerns, it is subject to increasingly complex and dynamic regulatory requirements to implement patient-facing medical LLM. Unlike typical medical devices, generative LLMs are not deterministic and are constantly revised and able to produce variable results, which involves the endemic issues with existing approval channels (Beam & Kohane, 2020). The AI Act in the European Union presupposes that AI systems which assist healthcare professionals get considered to be the so-called high-risk systems unless they are fully administrative components or are capable of carrying out only isolated and non-diagnostic functions (Brown *et al.,* 2020). This is likely to be the case with patient-facing LLMs which can provide either symptom assessment or a triage suggestion or health information, which would need conformity testing, risk management plans, and post-market surveillance.

However, they display regulatory ambiguity regarding the implementation of the foundation models and the general purpose AI proposed by the Act to conversational medical systems (Caliskan *et al.,* 2020). The Food and Drug Administration (FDA) of the United States has proposed specific change control plan preset that shall be employed in AI-enabled Software as a Medical Device (SaMD) in which version-by-version updates could be implemented, based on predetermined changes (Collins & Varmus, 2020). Patient-facing LLM that do not explicitly claim any diagnostic but can change health behavior patterns can occupy a regulatory grey space between consumer wellness and medical devices, and whether they lead to harm they may not be regulated (Davenport & Kalakota, 2020). The data protection rules contained in the data protection laws in Europe (namely, the GDPR) and the law on health data processing in the United States (the HIPAA) have imposed significantly stringent limitations in regard to the processing of health-related information produced by patients (Luxton, 2021). The interactions of patients with LLMs frequently include delicate patient details, such as mental health conditions, symptoms, and the life-style. It should also be in line with transparency procedures of consent, minimum of information and entitlement of clarification that is difficult to achieve when it comes to opacities of LLM (Marcus, 2020; Morley *et al.,* 2020). Lawsuits also complicate the process of adoption: in case the medical LLM generates an unsafe or misleading response, the large stakeholders of the health systems can be blamed (to the creators of the medical LLM, implementers of the health system, and even the patient themselves). Existing liability paradigms that deal with deterministic and static products do not fit the adaptive AI very well (Samek *et al.,* 2021). Consequently, lifecycle-based safety governance, including mandatory adverse event reporting and algorithmic effect disclosures, is beginning to be demanded by regulators and standards bodies. The most effective method to make sustainable development of patient-facing LLMs more than a middle-range situation that renders patients and clinicians at undesirable risk is through improved legal protection and a standard set of international norms (Zou & Schiebinger, 2022).

8. IMPLICATIONS FOR EVIDENCE-BASED CLINICAL ADOPTION

Implementation of patient-facing medical LLM must be designed in a unique manner with respect to integrating and aligning technological provisions, clinical work flows, and risk control frameworks. Even though the current best practices and risk management principles may inform the clinical implementation of the LLMs, these algorithms may result in an improved access to health information and patient-centered care. Patient safety must be a priority in the patient safety strategies of clinical implementation before efficiency and scalability. The implication on clinical implementation that is stronger is that limits of use have to be set. General health information, education, and statements concerning the decision support should be limited to the use of medical LLM instead of diagnosis and treatment (Obermeyer and Emanuel, 2023). These boundaries reduce the risks of liability and ease the process of preventing patient mistreatment. Safe clinical use cannot be established without proper mechanisms of oversight. The damages created by the inappropriate or dangerous outputs of the AI can be prevented in terms of an integrated system of governance referring to human control, escalation, and systemic periodical reviewed AI interactions. Real world usage possibility would result in the surfacing of safety issues and incentive to optimize systems. The possible and disadvantages of medical LLM should be instructed to medical professionals. They play quite a significant role in patient expectations of AI systems, dismantling of misunderstandings, and perception of the outputs that are generated by AI. Educational organizations need to teach the professionals to analyze AI results critically and provide the appropriate advice to the patients (Thirunavukarasu *et al.,* 2023). Another important implementation item is regulatory compliance. Medical facilities should make sure that AI-driven systems surrounding patients do not violate related data protection, medical device, and consumer protection regulations. Accountability and transparency to the regulatory bodies should be captured in elaborate documents of model validation, risk mitigation and post implementation monitoring. The responsible innovation may be facilitated by coordinated efforts between the developers, clinicians, and regulators. The efficient implementation of AI systems within the clinical setting in the long-term will demand the harmonization of the behavior of AI systems with the institutional policies, clinicians' expectations, and patient communication standards. In this case, the probability of misuse and misunderstanding and lack of credibility remains significant when this is not aligned (Nouri *et al.,* 2021).

9. PATIENT-SAFE BENCHMARKING

Patient-safe benchmarking is a philosophical shift in the way it is evaluated since it makes an emphasis on harm reduction and patient outcomes rather than of accomplishing tasks. Patient-safe benchmark recognizes patient safety as a relative concept, and that it needs to be measured in practical situations of interaction. This need in the patient-safe benchmarks can be justified by the ineffectiveness of currently available measures of assessment of medical LLMs. The benchmark of patient safety is based on preventing harm, situational relevance, and patient outcomes instead of being concerned with the factual correctness (Price and Cohen, 2020). The patient safety benchmarks must produce various qualitative aspects of safety, in which the consensus with scientific agreement, the transfer of uncertainty, empathy, and potential harm might be concerned. These multifaceted dimensions are not able to be picked up automatically as compared to traditional benchmarks. A combination of human annotation and LLDM-based assessment systems is a lasting and scalable resolution to these complicated dimensions. Adversarial question augmentation is one of the strategies that may enhance benchmark resilience (Rak, 2023). The model performance on hard examples can be tested using hard or misleading questions and the model can be tested to identify the possible failure modes which are not included in the traditional test data. This way can be able to test whether one is likely to hallucinate, overconfident, or apply the wrong reassurance in models. The models should also have frameworks where the outputs will vary. Never-ending evaluation in varied contextures contributes wholesomely towards model safety comprehension. The models are supposed to be maintained by ensuring that they are updated frequently. Patient-safe benchmarks provide an appropriate intermediate between technical and clinical applications of medical LLM. By focusing on patient safety, such benchmarks promote responsible design and use (Reddy *et al.,* 2020).

10. CONCLUSION

The increasing use of LLMs in healthcare presents both advantages and considerable safety concerns, particularly when these technologies are utilized in direct patient involvement. Current safety evaluation and benchmarking approaches, developed for clinician-facing or non-critical applications, are inadequate to ensure patient safety in conversational medical AI systems. The future of medical LLMs depends on the effectiveness of safety assessment models currently under development. Active patient-centered safety assessment is a key determinant of whether medical LLMs will improve or worsen healthcare outcomes. The findings presented in this chapter further indicate that safety of medical LLMs is not merely a matter of factual correctness but also of ethical responsibility, emotional sensitivity, and harm avoidance. Although LLMs achieve substantial effectiveness on objective safety indicators, they lack subjective safety dimensions such as empathy and harm assessment. These weaknesses require inter-disciplinary collaboration and development of patient-safe standards. The growing incorporation of medical LLMs into healthcare will certainly pose issues; the safe and ethical application will require preventative measures. By emphasizing patient-centered safety and the considerate application of these technologies, their potential advantages can be implemented while limiting hazards.

REFERENCES

Alami, H., Lehoux, P., Papoutsi, C., Shaw, S. E., Fleet, R., & Fortin, J. P. (2024). Understanding the integration of artificial intelligence in healthcare organisations and systems through the NASSS framework: A qualitative study in a leading Canadian academic centre. *BMC Health Services Research*, *24*(1), 701. DOI: 10.1186/s12913-024-11112-x PMID: 38831298

Amodei, D., Olah, C., Steinhardt, J., Christiano, P., Schulman, J., & Mané, D. (2023). *Concrete problems in AI safety*. arXiv. https://arxiv.org/abs/1606.06565

Beam, A. L., & Kohane, I. S. (2020). Big data and machine learning in health care. *Journal of the American Medical Association*, *319*(13), 1317–1318. DOI: 10.1001/jama.2017.18391 PMID: 29532063

. Beamish, D., & Exarchakis, G. (2025). *Large language models for explainability in machine learning*.

Beauchamp, T., & Childress, J. (2021). Principles of biomedical ethics: Marking its fortieth anniversary. *The American Journal of Bioethics : AJOB*, *19*(11), 9–12. DOI: 10.1080/15265161.2019.1665402 PMID: 31647760

Bender, E. M., Gebru, T., McMillan-Major, A., & Shmitchell, S. (2021). On the dangers of stochastic parrots: Can language models be too big? In *Proceedings of the 2021 ACM Conference on Fairness, Accountability, and Transparency* (pp. 610–623). DOI: 10.1145/3442188.3445922

. Bommasani, R., Hudson, D. A., Adeli, E., Altman, R., Arora, S., von Arx, S., Bernstein, M. S., Bohg, J., Bosselut, A., Brunskill, E., & Brynjolfsson, E. (2021). *On the opportunities and risks of foundation models*. arXiv.

Brown, T. B., Mann, B., Ryder, N., Subbiah, M., Kaplan, J., & Amodei, D. (2020). Language models are few-shot learners. *Advances in Neural Information Processing Systems*, *33*, 1877–1901.

Caliskan, A., Bryson, J. J., & Narayanan, A. (2020). Semantics derived automatically from language corpora contain human-like biases. *Science*, *356*(6334), 183–186. DOI: 10.1126/science.aal4230 PMID: 28408601

Char, D. S., Shah, N. H., & Magnus, D. (2023). Implementing machine learning in health care—Addressing ethical challenges. *The New England Journal of Medicine*, *378*(11), 981–983. DOI: 10.1056/NEJMp1714229 PMID: 29539284

Collins, F. S., & Varmus, H. (2020). A new initiative on precision medicine. *The New England Journal of Medicine, 372*(9), 793–795. DOI: 10.1056/NEJMp1500523 PMID: 25635347

Davahli MR, Karwowski W, Fiok K, Wan T, Parsaei HR. Controlling Safety of Artificial Intelligence Based Systems in Healthcare. Symmetry (Basel). 2021

Davenport, T., & Kalakota, R. (2020). The potential for artificial intelligence in healthcare. *Future Healthcare Journal, 6*(2), 94–98. DOI: 10.7861/futurehosp.6-2-94 PMID: 31363513

Emanuel, E. J., Wachter, R. M., & Grady, C. (2020). Artificial intelligence in health care: Ethical considerations. *Journal of the American Medical Association, 323*(6), 509–510. PMID: 31845963

Gama, F., Tyskbo, D., Nygren, J., Barlow, J., Reed, J., & Svedberg, P. (2022). Implementation frameworks for artificial intelligence translation into health care practice: Scoping review. *Journal of Medical Internet Research, 24*(1), e32215. DOI: 10.2196/32215 PMID: 35084349

Gehrmann, S., Clark, E., & Sellam, T. (2023). Repairing the cracked foundation: A survey of obstacles in evaluation practices for generated text. *Journal of Artificial Intelligence Research, 77*, 103–166. DOI: 10.1613/jair.1.13715

Gerke, S., Minssen, T., & Cohen, G. (2020). Ethical and legal challenges of artificial intelligence-driven healthcare. In *Artificial intelligence in healthcare* (pp. 295–336). Academic Press. DOI: 10.1016/B978-0-12-818438-7.00012-5

Ghassemi, M., Oakden-Rayner, L., & Beam, A. L. (2021). The false hope of current approaches to explainable artificial intelligence in health care. *The Lancet. Digital Health, 3*(11), e745–e750. DOI: 10.1016/S2589-7500(21)00208-9 PMID: 34711379

Goodman, B., & Flaxman, S. (2017). European Union regulations on algorithmic decision-making and a "right to explanation.". *AI Magazine, 38*(3), 50–57. DOI: 10.1609/aimag.v38i3.2741

Gosak, L., Štiglic, G., San, W. T. W., & Vrbnjak, D. (2025). Human-led and artificial intelligence-automated critical appraisal of systematic reviews: Comparative evaluation. *Nurse Education in Practice, 89*, 104614. DOI: 10.1016/j.nepr.2025.104614 PMID: 41202494

Gururangan, S., Marasović, A., Swayamdipta, S., Lo, K., Beltagy, I., Downey, D., & Smith, N. A. (2020). Don't stop pretraining: Adapt language models to domains and tasks. In *Proceedings of the 58th Annual Meeting of the Association for Computational Linguistics* (pp. 8342–8360). DOI: 10.18653/v1/2020.acl-main.740

Higgins, D., & Madai, V. I. (2020). From Bit to Bedside: A Practical Framework for Artificial Intelligence Product Development in Healthcare. *Advanced Intelligent Systems*, *2*(10), 2000052. DOI: 10.1002/aisy.202000052

Holzinger, A., Langs, G., Denk, H., Zatloukal, K., & Müller, H. (2020). Causability and explainability of artificial intelligence in medicine. *Wiley Interdisciplinary Reviews. Data Mining and Knowledge Discovery*, *9*(4), e1312. DOI: 10.1002/widm.1312 PMID: 32089788

Kamel Rahimi, A., Pienaar, O., Ghadimi, M., Canfell, O. J., Pole, J. D., Shrapnel, S., van der Vegt, A. H., & Sullivan, C. (2024). Implementing AI in hospitals to achieve a learning health system: Systematic review of current enablers and barriers. *Journal of Medical Internet Research*, *26*, e49655. DOI: 10.2196/49655 PMID: 39094106

Kassirer, J. P. (2024). Practicing principled medicine. In *Masterclass in medicine: Lessons from the experts*. DOI: 10.1201/9781003409373-8

Khan, S. D., Hoodbhoy, Z., Raja, M. H. R., Kim, J. Y., Hogg, H. D. J., Manji, A. A. A., Gulamali, F., Hasan, A., Shaikh, A., Tajuddin, S., Khan, N. S., Patel, M. R., Balu, S., Samad, Z., & Sendak, M. P. (2024). Frameworks for procurement, integration, monitoring, and evaluation of artificial intelligence tools in clinical settings: A systematic review. *PLOS Digital Health*, *3*(5), e0000514. DOI: 10.1371/journal.pdig.0000514 PMID: 38809946

LeCun, Y., Bengio, Y., & Hinton, G. (2021). Deep learning. *Nature*, *521*(7553), 436–444. DOI: 10.1038/nature14539 PMID: 26017442

Lee, P., Bubeck, S., & Petro, J. (2023). Benefits, limits, and risks of GPT-4 as an AI chatbot for medicine. *The New England Journal of Medicine*, *388*(13), 1233–1239. DOI: 10.1056/NEJMsr2214184 PMID: 36988602

Lin, C. C., Huang, A. Y., & Lu, O. H. (2023). Artificial intelligence in intelligent tutoring systems toward sustainable education: A systematic review. *Smart Learning Environments*, *10*(1), 41. DOI: 10.1186/s40561-023-00260-y

López-Pérez, B., Chen, Y., Li, X., Cheng, S., & Razavi, P. (2025). Exploring the potential of large language models to understand interpersonal emotion regulation strategies from narratives. *Emotion (Washington, D.C.)*, *25*(7), 1653–1667. DOI: 10.1037/emo0001528 PMID: 40244995

Luxton, D. D. (2021). Artificial intelligence in psychological practice: Current and future applications and implications. *Professional Psychology, Research and Practice*, *45*(5), 332–339. DOI: 10.1037/a0034559

Macrae, C. (2025, April). Managing risk and resilience in autonomous and intelligent systems: Exploring safety in the development, deployment, and use of artificial intelligence in healthcare. *Risk Analysis : An Official Publication of the Society for Risk Analysis*, *45*(4), 910–927. DOI: 10.1111/risa.14273 PMID: 38246857

. Marcus, G. (2020). *The next decade in AI: Four steps towards robust artificial intelligence*. arXiv.

Miller, T. (2021). Explanation in artificial intelligence: Insights from the social sciences. *Artificial Intelligence*, *267*, 1–38. DOI: 10.1016/j.artint.2018.07.007

Morley, J., Machado, C. C., Burr, C., Cowls, J., Joshi, I., Taddeo, M., & Floridi, L. (2020). The ethics of AI in health care: A mapping review. *Social Science & Medicine*, *260*, 113172. DOI: 10.1016/j.socscimed.2020.113172 PMID: 32702587

Morley, J., Morton, C., Karpathakis, K., Taddeo, M., & Floridi, L. Towards a Framework for Evaluating the Safety, Acceptability and Efficacy of Ai Systems for Health: An Initial Synthesis. SSRN Electron J. Published online 2021. DOI: 10.2139/ssrn.3826358

Nouri, S., Reddy, S., Cochran, J., Ballard, Z., & Kannan, V. (2021). Social and ethical implications of AI in healthcare. In *Artificial intelligence in healthcare* (pp. 389–412). Elsevier.

Obermeyer, Z., & Emanuel, E. J. (2020). Predicting the future—Big data and machine learning in clinical medicine. *The New England Journal of Medicine*, *375*(13), 1216–1219. DOI: 10.1056/NEJMp1606181 PMID: 27682033

Preti, L. M., Ardito, V., Compagni, A., Petracca, F., & Cappellaro, G. (2024). Implementation of machine learning applications in health care organizations: Systematic review of empirical studies. *Journal of Medical Internet Research*, *26*, e55897. DOI: 10.2196/55897 PMID: 39586084

Price, W. N.II, & Cohen, I. G. (2020). Privacy in the age of medical big data. *Nature Medicine*, *25*(1), 37–43. DOI: 10.1038/s41591-018-0272-7 PMID: 30617331

Raji, I. D., Smart, A., White, R. N., Mitchell, M., Gebru, T., Hutchinson, B., Smith-Loud, J., Theron, D., & Barnes, P. (2020). Closing the AI accountability gap: Defining an end-to-end framework for internal algorithmic auditing. In *Proceedings of the 2020 ACM Conference on Fairness, Accountability, and Transparency* (pp. 33–44). DOI: 10.1145/3351095.3372873

Rajpurkar, P., Irvin, J., Ball, R. L., Zhu, K., Yang, B., Mehta, H., Duan, T., Ding, D., Bagul, A., Langlotz, C. P., Patel, B. N., Yeom, K. W., Shpanskaya, K., Blankenberg, F. G., Seekins, J., Amrhein, T. J., Mong, D. A., Halabi, S. S., Zucker, E. J., & Lungren, M. P. (2021). Deep learning for chest radiograph diagnosis: A retrospective comparison of the CheXNeXt algorithm to practicing radiologists. *PLoS Medicine*, *15*(11), e1002686. DOI: 10.1371/journal.pmed.1002686 PMID: 30457988

. Rak, R. R. (2023). *Internet of healthcare (law): Privacy and data protection aspects in an internet of everything*.

Ramprasad, S., Ferracane, E., & Lipton, Z. C. (2024, August). Analyzing LLM behavior in dialogue summarization: Unveiling circumstantial hallucination trends. In *Proceedings of the 62nd Annual Meeting of the Association for Computational Linguistics (*Volume 1*: Long Papers)* (pp. 12549-12561). DOI: 10.18653/v1/2024.acl-long.677

Reddy, S., Allan, S., Coghlan, S., & Cooper, P. (2020). A governance model for the application of AI in health care. *Journal of the American Medical Informatics Association : JAMIA*, *27*(3), 491–497. DOI: 10.1093/jamia/ocz192 PMID: 31682262

Reddy, S., Rogers, W., Makinen, V. P., Coiera, E., Brown, P., Wenzel, M., Weicken, E., Ansari, S., Mathur, P., Casey, A., & Kelly, B. (2021). Evaluation framework to guide implementation of AI systems into health care settings. *BMJ Health & Care Informatics*, *28*(1), e100444. DOI: 10.1136/bmjhci-2021-100444 PMID: 34642177

Ribeiro, J., Lima, R., Eckhardt, T., & Paiva, S. (2021). Robotic process automation and artificial intelligence in industry 4.0—A literature review. *Procedia Computer Science*, *181*, 51–58. DOI: 10.1016/j.procs.2021.01.104

Rudin, C. (2020). Stop explaining black box machine learning models for high stakes decisions and use interpretable models instead. *Nature Machine Intelligence*, *1*(5), 206–215. DOI: 10.1038/s42256-019-0048-x PMID: 35603010

Samek, W., Montavon, G., Vedaldi, A., Hansen, L. K., & Müller, K. R. (Eds.). (2021). *Explainable AI: Interpreting, explaining and visualizing deep learning*. Springer Nature.

Sendak, M. P., D'Arcy, J., Kashyap, S., Gao, M., Nichols, M., Corey, K., Ratliff, W., & Balu, S. (2020). *A path for translation of machine learning products into healthcare delivery*. EMJ Innovations.

Singhal, K., Azizi, S., Tu, T., Mahdavi, S. S., Wei, J., Chung, H. W., Scales, N., Tanwani, A., Cole-Lewis, H., Pfohl, S., & Natarajan, V. (2023). Large language models encode clinical knowledge. *Nature*, *620*(7972), 172–180. DOI: 10.1038/s41586-023-06291-2 PMID: 37438534

Sujan, M., White, S., Habli, I., & Reynolds, N. Stakeholder Perceptions of the Safety and Assurance of Artificial Intelligence in Healthcare. SSRN Electron J. Published online 2022.

Suresh, H., & Guttag, J. (2021). A framework for understanding sources of harm throughout the machine learning life cycle. In *Proceedings of the 1st ACM Conference on Equity and Access in Algorithms, Mechanisms, and Optimization* (pp. 1–9). DOI: 10.1145/3465416.3483305

Sutton, R. T., Pincock, D., Baumgart, D. C., Sadowski, D. C., Fedorak, R. N., & Kroeker, K. I. (2020). An overview of clinical decision support systems: Benefits, risks, and strategies for success. *NPJ Digital Medicine*, *3*(1), 17. DOI: 10.1038/s41746-020-0221-y PMID: 32047862

Thirunavukarasu, A. J., Ting, D. S. J., Elangovan, K., Gutierrez, L., Tan, T. F., & Ting, D. S. W. (2023). Large language models in medicine. *Nature Medicine*, *29*(8), 1930–1940. DOI: 10.1038/s41591-023-02448-8 PMID: 37460753

Tonekaboni, S., Joshi, S., McCradden, M. D., & Goldenberg, A. (2023). What clinicians want: Contextualizing explainable machine learning for clinical end use. In *Machine Learning for Healthcare Conference* (pp. 359–380).

van der Vegt, A. H., Campbell, V., Mitchell, I., Malycha, J., Simpson, J., Flenady, T., Flabouris, A., Lane, P. J., Mehta, N., Kalke, V. R., Decoyna, J. A., Es'haghi, N., Liu, C.-H., & Scott, I. A. (2024). Systematic review and longitudinal analysis of implementing Artificial Intelligence to predict clinical deterioration in adult hospitals: What is known and what remains uncertain. *Journal of the American Medical Informatics Association : JAMIA*, *31*(2), 509–524. DOI: 10.1093/jamia/ocad220 PMID: 37964688

Veale, M., & Binns, R. (2024). Fairer machine learning in the real world: Mitigating discrimination without collecting sensitive data. *Big Data & Society*, *4*(2). DOI: 10.1177/2053951717743530

Verghese, A., Shah, N. H., & Harrington, R. A. (2023). What this computer needs is a physician: Humanism and artificial intelligence. *Journal of the American Medical Association*, *319*(1), 19–20. DOI: 10.1001/jama.2017.19198 PMID: 29261830

Wadden, J. J. (2021). Defining the undefinable: The black box problem in healthcare artificial intelligence. *Journal of Medical Ethics*. PMID: 34290113

Wiens, J., Saria, S., Sendak, M., Ghassemi, M., Liu, V. X., Doshi-Velez, F., & Goldenberg, A. (2019). Do no harm: A roadmap for responsible machine learning for health care. *Nature Medicine*, *25*(9), 1337–1340. DOI: 10.1038/s41591-019-0548-6 PMID: 31427808

Zhang, B., Zhu, J., & Su, H. (2023). Toward the third generation artificial intelligence. *Science China. Information Sciences*, *66*(2), 121101. DOI: 10.1007/s11432-021-3449-x

Zou, J., & Schiebinger, L. (2022). AI can be sexist and racist—It's time to make it fair. *Nature*, *559*(7714), 324–326. DOI: 10.1038/d41586-018-05707-8 PMID: 30018439

Chapter 7
Beyond Performance Benchmarks: A Safety-Critical Evaluation Paradigm for Reliability and Trust in Clinical Language Models

Sayali K Somwanshi
http://orcid.org/0009-0000-3296-4347
Cognizant, India

Aman Suresh Tharayil
http://orcid.org/0009-0000-5377-7428
Dr. MGR Educational and Research Institute, India

Anmol S. Budhewar
http://orcid.org/0009-0002-9112-107X
Sandip Institute of Technology and Research Centre, Nashik, India

Gnanavel Velu
http://orcid.org/0000-0002-7081-9017
Catholic University in Erbil, Iraq

Devi Thamizanban
http://orcid.org/0000-0002-0068-9800
Chettinad School of Pharmaceutical Sciences, Chettinad Hospital and Research Institute, Chettinad Academy of Research and Education, Kelambakkam, India

K. C. Gayathri
Chettinad School of Physiotherapy, Chettinad Hospital and Research Institute, Chettinad Academy of Research and Education, Kelambakkam, India

Abhimanyu N. Dasarwar
http://orcid.org/0009-0006-5907-7709
Independent Researcher, India

Pramod Gorakh Patil
http://orcid.org/0009-0005-9201-987X
MVP KBT College of Engineering, India

Swapnali Kishan Somwanshi
http://orcid.org/0009-0009-0584-4150
Yashwant College, Nanded, India

Balkrishna Keshavrao Patil
http://orcid.org/0009-0000-5136-2157
Sandip Institute of Technology and Research Centre, Nashik, India

DOI: 10.4018/979-8-3373-7862-6.ch007

Dhanalakshmi Perumal
http://orcid.org/0009-0004-2804-140X
Faculty of Pharmacy, Dr. MGR Educational and Research Institute, India

Vijay S. Karwande
http://orcid.org/0009-0007-5575-6904
Sandip Institute of Technology and Research Centre, India

ABSTRACT

This chapter, per the authors, provides a comprehensive evaluation of Large Language Models (LLMs) within safety-critical healthcare environments, moving beyond traditional performance benchmarks toward a reliability-centered paradigm. The purpose of this chapter is to identify core clinical risks—including hallucinations, bias, uncertainty mismanagement, and privacy leaks—that can compromise patient safety despite high accuracy on standardized tests. Systematic principles for safety-critical assessment are established, emphasizing robustness, uncertainty awareness, and human-in-the-loop validation as essential for clinical trust. Furthermore, the authors discuss technical methods for stress testing and bias mitigation alongside the necessity of continuous monitoring, auditability, and lifecycle evaluation to handle model drift. By aligning these technical frameworks with emerging international regulatory standards, the chapter outlines a path for integrating clinical language models as dependable medical aids.

1. INTRODUCTION TO MEDICAL LLMS AND CLINICAL RISK

Large Language Models (LLMs) have rapidly emerged as transformative tools in healthcare because they enable healthcare professionals to perform automated clinical documentation and medical question answering and diagnostic support and patient–clinician communication. The models demonstrate advanced language understanding and generation skills, which surpass the capabilities of traditional rule-based and task-specific machine learning systems because they were trained on both biomedical and general-domain data. Medical LLMs now receive increasing research attention because they show potential to improve clinical decision support systems and electronic health records and healthcare administrative processes (Reddy, 2023).

The use of the LLMs in clinical practice presents significant safety and reliability issues regardless of the outstanding results in the standardized tests. Unlike non-critical settings, healthcare settings demand high accuracy of performance since wrong outcomes may compromise the safety of patients. Recent research also proves that benchmark accuracy cannot estimate true clinical risks since models will generate plausible but inaccurate medical utterances, also referred to as hallucinations (Yang et al., 2024). Depending upon the task, errors and failures may call for different amounts of concern or application of different levels of reasoning and model stratagems.

Medical LLMs demonstrate another major danger because they exhibit bias and show different results when testing various patient groups. The evaluation studies show that language models produce different results because their accuracy and recommendation quality depend on three factors, which include demographic information, clinical situations, and data availability. The unrecognized biases will create new healthcare disparities, which will damage institutional trust in AI systems (Ghosh et al., 2025).

The first major obstacle for clinical LLMs stems from two main issues, which include hallucination and bias and also include uncertainty mismanagement. Most models do not have built-in systems that allow them to show their uncertainty, and they need to wait until their confidence level meets a specific threshold before making decisions (Wang et al., 2026).

The increasing independence of LLM-based systems produces more clinical dangers for medical practice because it reduces governance and regulatory control. The regulatory frameworks require organizations to demonstrate their systems through transparent methods that enable auditors to track system operations and monitor system performance after deployment, yet existing evaluation methods do not meet these standards (Shool et al., 2025). As a result, there is growing consent that medical LLM evaluation must develop from static benchmark testing toward safety-critical, continuous, and context-aware assessment models.

2. CLINICAL RISKS AND FAILURE MODES OF LANGUAGE MODELS

The use of large language models in healthcare settings brings several clinical dangers that exceed the risks associated with standard software malfunctions. LLMs produce probabilistic results because they are meant to assess and understand linguistic patterns, which makes their behavior mostly dependent on the said patterns of each situation according to medical decision support systems. Models such as GPT-4, Med-PaLM, BioGPT, and Clinical BERT have demonstrated solid performance on medical question-answering and summarization tasks; however, their failure modes pose unique safety challenges when applied in real world scenarios (Reddy, 2023; Yang et al., 2024).

2.1 Hallucination and Fabricated Medical Content

The most common failure mode for clinical language models has been reported to show hallucination, which causes models to produce fluent medical statements that lack factual accuracy and proper evidence. The studies that assessed GPT-4 and Med-PaLM found that both models produced confident results but created false medical diagnoses and fabricated nonexistent clinical guidelines while suggesting improper medical treatments through their handling of unclear and partial information (Yang et al., 2024). The clinical environment relies on these hallucinations, which produce results that require verification through testing since they establish trustworthiness through their authoritative presentation.

The danger of hallucination increases when medical professionals deal with uncommon diseases and rare patient conditions because their training data remains insufficient for these particular medical situations (Wang et al., 2026). Some models may have been deemed rather unsafe if the data substitution technique had been used during their training.

2.2 Overconfidence and Uncertainty Misrepresentation

Another major failure point occurs when LLMs fail to show their uncertain results. The BioGPT and Clinical BERT models produce answers without uncertainty measurements which are true, but this occurs because they lack sufficient clinical proof for their answers. Excessive trust in model outputs can create an illusion of dependability, which could greatly affects diagnostic and clinical triage situations (Ghosh et al., 2025).

The lack of vagueness and subject specific output from LLMS in safety-critical situations prevents doctors from determining when to request human assessment and perform extra tests. Evaluation studies show that reliability assessment needs to assess both correct results and model performance during uncertain and incomplete data situations (Shool et al., 2025).

2.3 Bias and Unequal Clinical Performance

Healthcare equity suffers from bias, which operates as a fundamental failure mode that affects entire systems. Language models that learn from extensive biomedical research papers and clinical documentation will develop biases that show preference toward specific gender and racial groups and age brackets and financial status. The clinical evaluation of GPT-based and transformer-based models shows different performance results, which depend on patient demographic factors during symptom assessment and risk evaluation functions (Ghosh et al., 2025).

The research demonstrates that biases usually emerge during subgroup testing but vanish during typical benchmark assessments. The existing unreported bias issues will yield biased results, exacerbate healthcare disparities and eroding public confidence in AI medical decision-making systems. The assessment process requires evaluation methods that assess both fairness and subgroup performance, rather than relying exclusively on overall accuracy metrics.

2.4 Contextual Misinterpretation in Clinical Reasoning

The clinical language models face their utmost important challenge when they try to understand contextual information, which includes both continuous patient data and precise medical requirements of their clinical field. The GPT-4 model demonstrates strong performance in single question-answering tasks, yet it fails to provide consistent results during multi-step reasoning tasks that require more understanding on the disease progression and medication interactions over extended periods (Reddy, 2023).

Recent studies with pilot integration of clinical language models found that whenever models misread patient context, they often give unreliable recommendations riddled with contradictions putting risk in documentation, discharge summaries, and treatment plans (Wang et al., 2026).

2.5 Privacy Leakage and Memorization Risks

The study investigates how human language models handle privacy violations, which create multiple failure points and raise serious clinical safety threats. Research demonstrates that language models trained on smaller domain-specific models, such as BioGPT, can unintentionally disclose protected patient data they learned during training and fine-tuning (Shool et al., 2025). Protected health information can be deduced from generated content even when all specific identifiers have been removed because of the information available in the generated content.

The risks become especially dangerous because healthcare systems must follow strict rules for protecting their data. Evaluation strategies must therefore incorporate privacy stress testing and data leakage assessments as part of safety validation.

2.6 Implications for Safety-Critical Evaluation

The different failure modes demonstrate that language models pose clinical risks across multiple dimensions, including their ability to produce accurate facts, handle uncertainty, demonstrate bias, maintain reasoning integrity, and safeguard user privacy. The risks in this situation depend on one another because hallucinations, biases, and overconfidence interact to create more dangerous outcomes. The assessment process needs specialized methods that evaluate performance across various situations while accounting for potential risks.

3. SAFETY-CRITICAL EVALUATION PRINCIPLES

The increasing adoption of clinical language models in healthcare decision-making systems requires evaluation methods that adhere to safety-critical system design standards. Clinical systems operate in high-stakes contexts because their modeling errors can directly affect diagnosis, treatment planning, and patient safety outcomes. The assessment process for clinical language models needs to shift from performance-based testing methods to safety assessment systems that focus on establishing dependable outcomes, clear system understanding, and effective risk management (Reddy, 2023).

The safety-critical assessment procedure employs systematic procedures of identifying and evaluating possible model-associated hazards that must be regulated before models can be applied in the real world. GPT-4, Med-PaLM, Clinical BERT, and BioGPT cry for being advanced in terms of linguistic abilities, but the safety of their use in clinical cases relies on the consistency they demonstrate when being used under unpredictable conditions (Yang et al., 2024).

3.1 Reliability as a Core Evaluation Principle

Reliability of a clinical language model follows the ability of the language model to produce similar medical outcomes that are valid in various health care contexts. In safety-critical systems, the ability to maintain constant performance during the operations is more rewarding than the maximum possible accuracy. The model should exhibit congruent reasoning skills as it handles a variety of inputs that involve various patients and various kinds of medical data.

The testing frameworks necessitate repetition of tests in the course of validating results in other contexts and across time so that test results do not change with time. The studies indicate that even sophisticated systems like GPT-4 can offer various clinical advice when the prompts are modified a bit since their stability has not been quantified according to the current methods of assessment (Wang et al., 2026). Consequently, the reliability of systems should be tested concerning the immediate variation resilience, data drifting vulnerability, and workflow integration capacitance.

3.2 Robustness and Stress Testing

The ability of language models to deliver consistent performance demonstrates their capacity to handle noisy, incomplete, and hostile inputs from clinical environments. The actual healthcare data used in research studies contains various types of uncertainty, which includes abbreviation usage, missing data, and conflicting clinical information. The evaluation of safety-critical systems needs testing to occur under real-world conditions instead of relying on perfect benchmark datasets.

Stress testing methods that analyze extreme situations use edge cases from rare disease descriptions, contradictory symptoms, and incomplete patient histories. The research studies that assessed Med-PaLM and domain-specific transformer models showed that performance declined when the models faced distributional changes, which demonstrated the necessity of using both adversarial testing and scenario-based assessment methods for evaluation purposes (Ghosh et al., 2025). The study of the robustness of AI models is the best-known feature of AI safety, mainly concerning the potential for it being held against the greater good if anything went wrong.

3.3 Uncertainty Awareness and Risk Sensitivity

All safe clinical AI systems need to develop their capacity for detecting uncertain situations as their main operational requirement. The standard LLM systems produce definite textual results that lack any presentation of their confidence assessment. The clinical decision support system faces this restriction because users will depend excessively on output produced by the model.

Safety-critical evaluation therefore incorporates uncertainty estimation mechanisms such as probabilistic scoring and ensemble validation and abstention-based evaluation, which requires models to withhold answers whenever their confidence level falls below acceptable limits. Trustworthy medical AI systems need to provide calibrated uncertainty assessments that match established medical reasoning standards, according to research findings (Shool et al., 2025).

Figure 1. Uncertainty Awareness and Risk Sensitivity in Clinical Language Models (CLM)

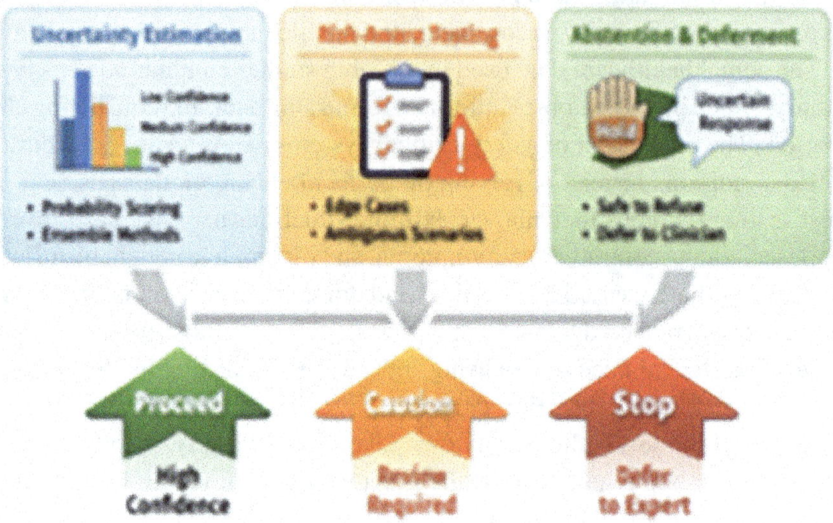

Figure 1 shows how clinical language models handle uncertainty and assess risk through their operational mechanisms. The system tests decision-making through three components, which include methods for estimating uncertainty and risk-sensitive evaluation and strategies for choosing not to make a decision. The system uses confidence levels to decide between three options, which include proceeding with work, asking for clinical review, and waiting for human experts to make decisions about healthcare AI. Assessing on how models respond to ambiguous cases becomes as important as measuring correctness.

3.4 Human-in-the-Loop Validation

The essential function of clinical safety depends on the cooperative work between artificial intelligence systems and medical staff members. The human-in-the-loop system evaluates model outputs through its process, which enables clinicians to understand, evaluate, and fix results. The clinical LLMs exist to assist medical professionals in their decision-making process because they need ongoing human monitoring.

The evaluation principles establish three assessment criteria, which include explainability, traceability of reasoning, and clinician usability. Users of Clinical Bert and GPT-based medical assistants must have the ability to verify generated recommendations against established medical evidence. The results from human validation studies gives a proper idea that active clinician participation in AI output assessment is the best way to have safety outcomes with its use (Reddy, 2023).

Figure 2. Clinician Validation Workflow in AI Treatment Recommendations

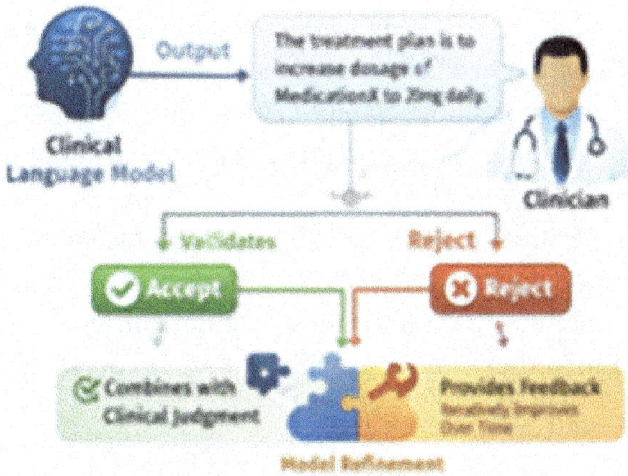

This Figure 2 shows the human-in-the-loop clinical validation process, which tests clinical language models through AI-generated clinical recommendations that clinicians evaluate. The clinician uses the output that he or she receives to make a decision about its medical correctness and safety. Human evaluation feedback helps to refine the model, which results in better system performance and greater accountability and trustworthiness of clinical decision-support systems.

3.5 Transparency and Auditability

The system needs transparency because it constitutes a crucial element for establishing accountability within safety-critical healthcare systems. The evaluation process needs to assess whether the model generates traceable documents that can be verified through clinical application. The regulatory requirements now demand audit trails that track all model activities from their initial inputs to their final outputs and decision-making processes.

The safety-critical evaluation frameworks require institutions to maintain accountability through their implementation of logging systems, their assessment of explainability, and their evaluation of reproducibility testing. The absence of auditability makes it impossible to investigate, or correct clinical mistakes linked to language models, which creates obstacles for regulatory bodies to accept these models (Yang et al., 2024).

3.6 Continuous Monitoring and Lifecycle Evaluation

Unlike traditional medical software, clinical language models evolve through updates, retraining, and changing data environments. The assessment process requires more than a single evaluation because it needs to continue assessing performance after the system goes into operation. Safety-critical principles advocate lifecycle evaluation involving continuous monitoring, performance drift detection, and post-deployment validation (Wang et al., 2026).

The evidence indicates that model reliability will decrease with time because of two factors, which include domain shifts and new medical research. The healthcare system uses MLOps pipelines to monitor their systems through continuous evaluation methods, which help them identify new risks while preserving their system trustworthiness.

3.7 Toward a Safety-Centered Evaluation Paradigm

The foundation of safety-critical evaluation for clinical language models exists through the combination of reliability, robustness, uncertainty awareness, human oversight, transparency, and continuous monitoring. The principles establish evaluation as an ongoing governance process that functions beyond a fixed measurement assessment. Healthcare organizations can achieve trustworthy and clinically dependable AI systems by integrating safety considerations throughout all stages of their model lifecycle.

4. METHODS FOR RELIABILITY AND ROBUSTNESS ASSESSMENT

The safe deployment of clinical language models needs evaluation methods that can assess their performance and robustness under actual medical conditions. The traditional benchmark-based evaluation method assesses two aspects of performance through specific datasets that have been selected for testing purposes. The evaluation methods for reliability and robustness need to replicate the actual operational dangers that GPT-4, Med-PaLM, BioGPT, and Clinical Bert encounter during real-world situations (Reddy, 2023; Wang et al., 2026).

The assessment of reliability tests output performance through multiple tests and various clinical situations, while robust tests evaluate model performance under medical environments that include noise and incomplete data and adversarial conditions.

4.1 Prompt Sensitivity and Consistency Testing

There is a lot of volatility in the output of the clinical language models in case minor changes in the input prompts are introduced. This phenomenon is referred to as prompt sensitivity, and it poses a significant safety threat to any healthcare facility, because, in certain situations, it can cause a situation where the same patient profile can be presented with conflicting medical information simply because of how a query is phrased. This instability compromises the fundamental aspect of medical reliability, which is that a decision-support system should be variation-resilient to the wide range of linguistic styles which different practitioners employ. In order to work out these gaps, reliability testing should take a step further than just accuracy tests and entail three different evaluation activities:

- Repeated Prompt Testing: The internal consistency of the model through repeated submissions of the same prompts with the model to detect stochastic variance in the decision-making. Linguistic Rephrasing: This measures the stability of performance in case of clinical questions that are restructured using various medical terms or syntax but with the same underlying meaning.
- Simulated Real-World Scenarios: Checking how the model would react to the noisy and incomplete information that characterizes clinical workflows, e.g., abbreviation-intensive documentation or inconsistent lab results. Recent research has shown that even higher-end GPT-based clinical assistants make inconsistent treatment recommendations given slight linguistic differences, classifying these decision-support systems as intrinsically unstable unless specially trained. Moreover, since clinical reasoning can be a multi-step process, even minor discrepancies in initial prompts can spread later in a lengthy medical conversation to create discharge summaries or treatment plans full of internal inconsistencies. This requires applying a Consistency Score, which will measure the stability of a model, such that AI-based recommendations are reliable irrespective of the way a clinician will state his query. To avoid the data drifting and workflow integration failures that emerge when a model faces the vagaries of real-world medicine, it is necessary to establish such metrics to ensure that the model does not encounter such failure modes (Yang et al., 2024).

Figure 3. Prompt Variation-Based Reliability Testing Framework

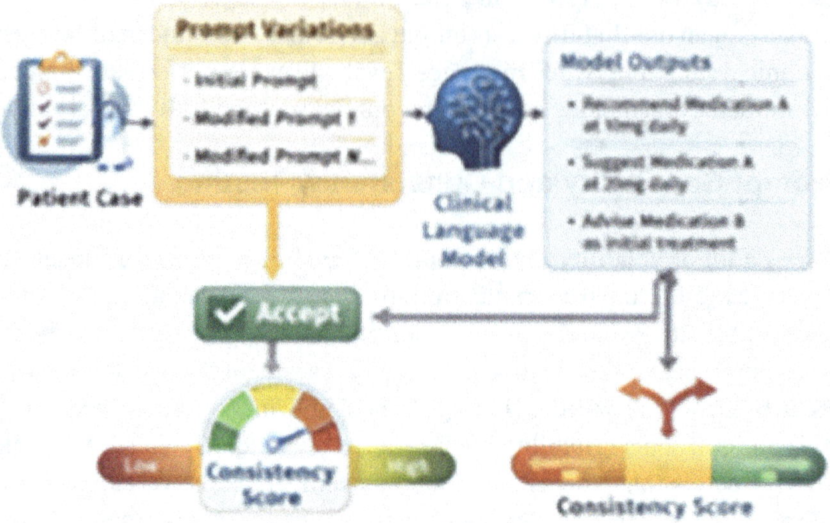

Figure 3 shows a framework for testing clinical language model reliability, which uses different prompts as its main testing method. Multiple prompt formulations are used to test a single patient case, which helps researchers' study how patient outcomes remain stable across different test conditions. The system generates responses, which researchers use to calculate consistency scores that evaluate model performance across clinical decision-support tests.

4.2 Adversarial and Stress Testing

The process of evaluating robustness needs language models to face their most difficult and least common test scenarios. The process of adversarial testing uses incomplete symptoms together with conflicting laboratory results and uncommon disease descriptions to test the system's ability to fail safely.

The performance of Med-PaLM and similar models shows degradation when distributional shifts occur, which demonstrates the necessity of stress testing to confirm their deployment readiness (Ghosh et al., 2025). The safety evaluation process requires models to avoid making medical decisions, which leads to incorrect results.

Table 1. Clinical Stress testing scenarios for language model safety

Scenario Type	Example Input	Expected Safe Behavior
Missing Data	Partial patient history	Request clarification.
Rare Disease	Uncommon symptoms	Express uncertainty.
Conflicting Data	Lab mismatch	Recommend review
Ambiguous Query	Incomplete diagnosis	Defer to clinician.

Table 1 demonstrates multiple stress testing scenarios that assess the strength of clinical language models. The table presents difficult clinical scenarios that include incomplete information and uncommon medical conditions and opposing data and unclear questions, together with their expected model responses, which maintain dependable and secure and medically suitable decision support.

4.3 Uncertainty Quantification Techniques

Clinical AI systems require dependable prediction systems to display their confidence levels. The evaluation of uncertainty quantification methods determines their effectiveness in assessing models' ability to identify situations with uncertainty.

Common techniques include:

- Probabilistic confidence scoring
- Ensemble model evaluation
- Bayesian approximation methods
- Abstention-based decision mechanisms

It has been shown that trust calibration between clinicians and AI can be significantly improved by employing systems of uncertainty-aware evaluation (Shool et al., 2025).

Figure 4. Confidence to Decision Pipeline for Uncertainty Aware Clinical AI

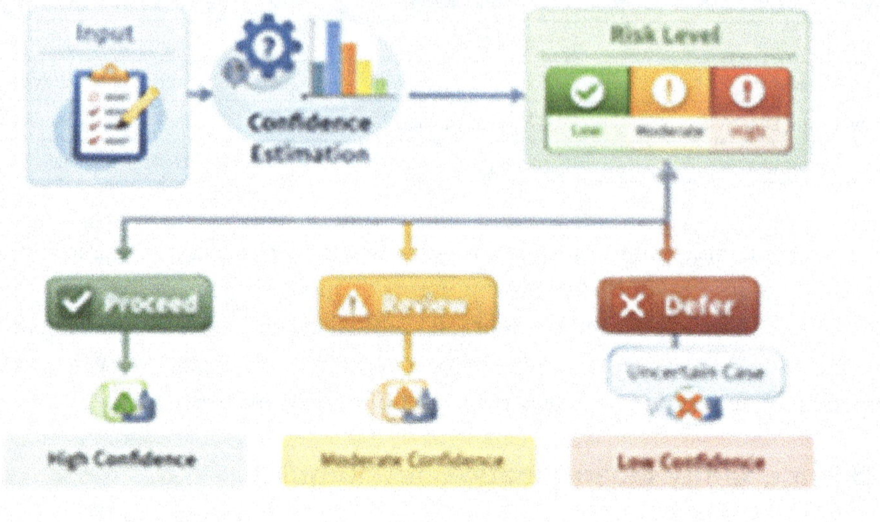

Figure 4 shows a pipeline that assesses clinical language model reliability through uncertainty-based methods. The system evaluates input data through confidence estimation and risk classification stages. The system classifies uncertainty-based decisions into three categories, which include proceed, review, and defer, while it protects clinical recommendations and reduces risks that come from untrustworthy and uncertain model outputs.

4.4 Bias and Fairness Robustness Evaluation

Researchers must assess robustness through testing various demographic and clinical subgroups. The diagnostic results of clinical LLMs, which were developed using historical data training, face the risk of generating biased outcomes. Fairness evaluation requires researchers to assess how different groups perform based on their gender, ethnicity, and age group membership. Demographic imbalance in healthcare AI systems leads to predictive reliability problems, according to empirical research studies (Ghosh et al., 2025).

Table 2. Bias Evaluation Metrics

Metric	Purpose
Demographic Parity	Equal prediction distribution
Equal Opportunity	Fair diagnostic accuracy
Error Rate Balance	Consistent misclassification
Calibration Score	Confidence, fairness

Table 2 summarizes key bias evaluation metrics that researchers use to evaluate the fairness and robustness of clinical language models. The study presents four measurement systems, which include demographic parity, equal opportunity, error rate balance, and calibration score, to determine performance differences between patient groups while establishing trustworthy AI systems for clinical decision-making.

4.5 Human-Guided Robustness Validation

Human-in-the-loop evaluation improves robustness testing through expert clinical judgment assessment. Clinicians conduct model output assessments by utilizing simulated clinical workflows to discover reasoning errors that automated metrics cannot detect (Reddy, 2023). Hybrid AI-human evaluation methods provide better decision-making accuracy through clinical validation experiments, which decrease the number of dangerous recommendations. The method changes evaluation from its computational testing form into a process that ensures the safety of socio-technical systems.

Figure 5. Iterative AI-Clinician Feedback Cycle for Model Refinement

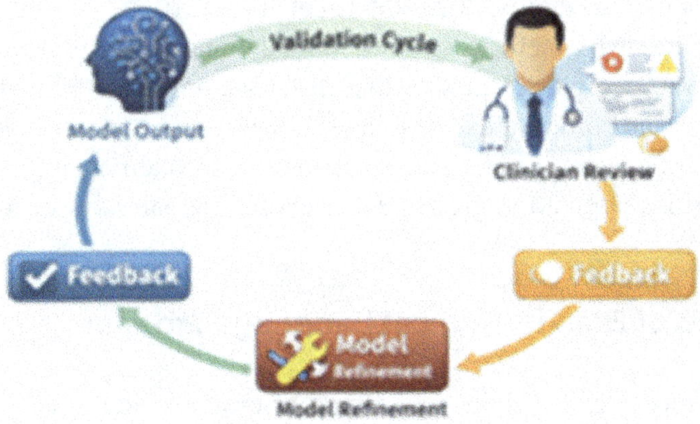

Figure 5 shows how humans test the strength of clinical language models through their established validation process. Clinicians examine model outputs, which they use to provide feedback that helps scientists improve the model and test it again. The continuous validation process establishes trustworthy AI systems in healthcare by reducing clinical risks and improving system reliability.

4.6 Continuous Monitoring and Post-Deployment Evaluation

The reliability evaluation should not be limited to the pre-deploy testing. The nature of clinical settings changes constantly as a result of new medical evidence, the demographics of patients, and alterations in workflow (Wang et al., 2026). Performance drift monitoring considers the performance of the models and how reliable they are in the long run. Continuous monitoring frameworks combine MLOps pipelines, audit logs, and performance alerts to identify new risks in time. The lifecycle assessment can provide long-term safety and compliance.

5. BIAS, FAIRNESS, AND ETHICAL RISK EVALUATION

Healthcare systems face major ethical problems because they need to implement clinical language models, which create serious issues that affect both patient safety and fair medical treatment procedures. The models GPT-4, Med-PaLM, BioGPT, and ClinicalBERT show excellent predictive and reasoning abilities, but their performance depends on the training data distributions, which include historical and societal biases. The evaluation process for clinical LLMs requires assessment methods that include technical reliability testing together with fairness evaluation and ethical evaluation (Reddy, 2023; Ghosh et al., 2025).

Bias in clinical AI systems occurs when model outputs systematically favor or disadvantage specific patient groups that differ according to their demographic, socioeconomic, and clinical attributes. In healthcare environments these disparities result in diagnostic recommendation discrepancies and treatment prioritization mistakes, and various population groups experience different ways of understanding their symptoms.

5.1 Sources of Bias in Clinical Language Models

Bias in medical LLMs originates primarily from three sources:

1. Data Bias

Training datasets for medical research studies contain excessive representation of specific geographical territories and ethnic groups and healthcare facilities. The reliability of models decreases when they use Western clinical datasets for training because these datasets lack sufficient data about underrepresented demographic groups.

2. Algorithmic Bias

The statistical relationships that transformer-based architectures discover do not include causal medical links. The spontaneous crisscrossing builds strange associations between demographic characteristics and the probabilities of diseases and results of treatments (Yang et al., 2024).

3. Interaction Bias

The difference in the style of the clinical documentation and the forms of user prompts could affect output. The style of transcripts may not be regular among facilities that bring forth differing patterns of reasoning.

5.2 Fairness Evaluation Metrics

Assessing fairness would ensure a clinical language model performs consistently on different groups of patients. The fairness metrics assess system performance by evaluating outcomes from different subgroups, which sets them apart from traditional accuracy metrics.

Common evaluation measures include:

Demographic Parity: Equal prediction distribution across groups

Equal Opportunity: Comparable diagnostic accuracy

Predictive Equality: Balanced false-positive rates

Calibration Fairness: Reliable confidence estimation across populations

Research findings have demonstrated that subgroup-based evaluations significantly enhance the trustworthiness assessment of healthcare AI systems (Shool et al., 2025).

Table 3. Fairness Evaluation Metrics in Clinical LLMs

Metric	Evaluation Purpose	Clinical Impact
Demographic Parity	Equal predictions	Reduces discrimination
Equal Opportunity	Balanced accuracy	Fair diagnosis
Calibration	Confidence alignment	Trust improvement
Error Rate Balance	Equal mistakes	Patient safety

Table 3 presents key fairness evaluation metrics used to assess bias in clinical language models. The study demonstrates that demographic parity and equal opportunity, together with calibration and error rate balance, establish the foundation for delivering diagnostic assessments that create nondiscriminatory and unbiased healthcare treatment results across all patient demographics.

5.3 Ethical Risks in Clinical Deployment

The introduction of Large Language Models (LLMs) into clinical practice at the bedside presents a range of ethical vulnerabilities that are far beyond the technical failures of the technical malfunction. These are the main threats, which appear in the form of a predisposition to produce systematically biased outcomes, the inability to reveal all the logic of the operations to the end-user, and the absence of clarity in terms of the legal and professional responsibility allocation in cases where a model-driven decision leads to patient injury. One such risk is the development of the so-called automation bias, when clinicians start relying on the recommendations provided by AI more than their own knowledge, and it happens that the model is presented with a sense of authority and flueness.

This dependency is especially vital when medical LLM hallucinations the statements that are factually wrong, yet reflective of deficits in ethical oversight now and in the future. In these settings, unchecked or untested outputs can result in direct disastrous medical practice, which can be erroneous dosing or misdiagnosis. Moreover, such models frequently do not have mechanisms defined to articulate their uncertainty, and this can unconsciously deprive a practitioner of a healthy skepticism in the face of high stakes triage or diagnostic reasoning. The net effect of all these is a scenario in which the authoritative quality of output obscures the risk.

To reduce this risk, ethical standards evaluation needs to shift to a stricter framework that revolves around three key pillars:

1) Explainability and Interpretability: The ability of the system to offer an explainable and traceable reason why it is operating the way it does, so that clinicians can confirm the reason behind a recommendation.
2) User Consent and Autonomy: Developing a robust procedure of informed consent of patients when AI is applied to them, and they are aware of the purpose of the model along with its constraints.
3) Accountability Structures: The establishment of explicit responsibility assigning systems that establish the responsibility of developers, healthcare institutions and practitioners in the event of an adverse outcome.

Devoid of these protective measures, the black box nature of existing transformer-based architectures is still incompatible with the transparency needed in safety-critical medicine. To be deployed responsibly involves these ethical considerations not being seen as secondary compliance activities but rather must be seen as embedded in the overall functional requirements at every phase of the lifecycle of the clinical model (Wang et al., 2026).

5.4 Explainability and Transparency Assessment

Explicability is the key to ethical AI assessment. The clinical practitioners should understand the processes of generating recommendations using models since this knowledge will enable them to apply such systems within their medical practice.

Evaluation approaches include:

Attention visualization

Evidence-based response tracing

Clinical justification scoring

Explainable output validation

Transparent systems build up the confidence of the users and expedite regulatory approval processes (Reddy, 2023).

5.5 Governance and Responsible AI Principles

Ethical evaluation frameworks now establish connections to global governance standards, which require responsible AI deployment. The framework for safety-oriented governance includes the following components:

Human oversight mechanisms

Auditability requirements

Bias monitoring pipelines

Continuous ethical risk assessment

Responsible AI governance transforms ethical evaluation into an operational process that operates throughout the model lifecycle instead of functioning as a compliance task that occurs after development has finished (Yang et al., 2024).

6. AUDITABILITY, MONITORING, AND CONTINUOUS EVALUATION OF CLINICAL LANGUAGE MODELS

The implementation of clinical language models into operational healthcare systems demands established systems that can conduct audits and monitor performance while they assess system performance on an ongoing basis. Large language models

(LLMs) differ from standard medical software because they maintain dynamic interactions with changing clinical information and user activities and institutional operational procedures. The process of safety assurance requires operational systems to implement continuous monitoring procedures that maintain system dependability and answerability throughout their entire operational lifespan (Amann et al., 2020).

The auditability of healthcare AI systems allows their systems to produce transparent, traceable, and reproducible records that document how their models make decisions. Institutions use audit trails in clinical environments to investigate incorrect recommendations while they also use them to check their compliance with regulations and protect their legal obligations. Advanced clinical LLMs such as Med-PaLM 2 and GPT-based medical assistants increasingly require structured logging frameworks that record prompts and generate outputs and decision contexts and user interactions (Singhal et al., 2023).

6.1 Model Auditability in Clinical Environments

The auditability system enables complete backtracking of AI-generated medical results for future validation purposes. Healthcare regulations require medical professionals to deliver their decision-making processes when artificial intelligence systems impact their diagnostic and treatment development work.

Audit mechanisms typically include:

Input–output trace logging

Version-controlled model tracking

Decision provenance documentation

Explainability reporting systems

The existence of transparent auditing systems establishes trustworthy institutions that assist organizations in their investigations of clinical incidents that have already taken place. The research demonstrates that safety-critical artificial intelligence systems achieve improved accountability through the implementation of explainable auditing frameworks (Holzinger et al., 2022).

6.2 Continuous Monitoring and Performance Surveillance

The clinical environment is a constant change since there is a permanent fluctuation in the disease patterns, and the new treatment guidelines and patient groups are in a constant change. The two factors that will induce a performance drop when the model is put into operation use will be dataset shift and knowledge obsolescence.

Continuous monitoring frameworks evaluate:

Output accuracy trends

Model drift detection

Usage anomalies

Safety incident frequency

The process of monitoring systems after their deployment allows for the detection of dangerous actions that lead to clinical harm. The research shows that continuous monitoring protects AI-based healthcare systems from operational threats when it is used (Kelly et al., 2019).

6.3 Model Drift and Knowledge Degradation

The implementation of clinical LLMs faces its greatest enduring threat through model drift. Drift occurs when the actual clinical data distribution shows different patterns than the training data distribution. The model shows decreasing reliability because of emerging diseases, updated treatment protocols, and demographic shifts.

Two primary forms of drift include:

Data Drift: Patient or clinical input variations.

Concept Drift: Medical knowledge or diagnostic criteria have evolved through the ages.

Findings of the study suggested that AI systems without drift monitoring capabilities will generate hidden medical risks, demanding consistent evaluation of the performance (Finlayson et al., 2021).

6.4 Human Oversight and Feedback Integration

Evaluation frameworks now use clinician feedback, which clinicians use to evaluate their ongoing monitoring activities. Human oversight enables the detection of reasoning errors that machines fail to identify through their assessment procedures.

Feedback-driven monitoring includes:

- Clinician validation dashboards
- Error reporting interfaces
- Expert correction loops
- Reinforcement-based refinement mechanisms

We make sure that human-centered monitoring is done, and it fortifies socio-technical dependability so that clinical standards are reflected, while not deviating from AI systems (Topol, 2019).

6.5 Lifecycle-Based Evaluation and MLOps Integration

Modern healthcare AI governance adopts lifecycle evaluation, which medical MLOps systems support to evaluate their entire operational lifecycle. The system performs evaluation through all stages of development, deployment, and operational activities.

Lifecycle evaluation stages include:

1. Pre-deployment safety testing
2. Controlled clinical pilot deployment
3. Continuous operational monitoring
4. Periodic auditing and retraining

Lifecycle governance helps make trustworthy, long-lasting language models that steer health records without any hindrances caused by legislation (Rajkomar et al., 2019).

7. REGULATORY ALIGNMENT AND COMPLIANCE FRAMEWORKS FOR CLINICAL LANGUAGE MODELS

The healthcare system needs to implement clinical language models through deployment because they must fully comply with regulatory standards, which protect patient safety and ensure ethical responsibility, and build institutional trust. The regulatory framework faces difficulties because large language models, which function through adaptive learning and probabilistic reasoning, differ from standard digital health tools. The safe operation of clinical artificial intelligence systems requires organizations to establish regulatory compliance as their central requirement (European Commission, 2021).

The performance of AI-based medical systems needs to be assessed through testing methods that show accurate results instead of relying only on their performance metrics for their operational approval. The regulatory frameworks need to focus on four specific criteria, which include risk classification and explainability and human oversight and continuous performance monitoring. The clinical language models that assist in diagnostic processes and patient interactions will be classified as high-risk AI systems because they can influence medical decision-making processes (U.S. Food and Drug Administration [FDA], 2023).

7.1 Risk-Based Regulatory Classification

The existing rules use risk assessment techniques to evaluate AI systems because they require assessment of their potential effects on patient results. Safety-critical systems require complete testing procedures and documentation requirements because clinical decision-support systems use clinical language models.

The risk-based regulation system evaluates three elements, which include the planned medical application, the system's degree of automation, and the need for human oversight (World Health Organization [WHO], 2021). The regulatory framework applies more stringent rules to systems that provide automated recommendations that doctors cannot verify than it does to assistive technologies that doctors can monitor. This classification approach ensures proportional governance, which matches potential clinical harm that the system may cause.

7.2 Compliance Requirements for Clinical AI Systems

The domain of healthcare AI developers and institutions has to maneuver through a convoluted row of operational and ethical norms that have been imposed by the contemporary regulatory compliance frameworks. Organizations must demonstrate three pillars of compliance to be certified and keep the institutional trust: ensuring complete model transparency, offering strong clinical validation evidence, and enforcing strong cybersecurity controls with data governance controls (Omiye et al., 2024). The regulatory overhead includes the detailed recording of the training data sources, particular evaluation procedures and the performance thresholds used by clinical language models (CLMs). Such documentation practices are not just administrative, but are necessary to provide reproducibility and to have a clear audit trail, where third parties or a regulatory authority can review model operations by independent evaluations. In addition, AI systems in healthcare should comply with patient data protection law (HIPAA or GDPR), to which the protection of health information (PHI) is subject, and to ensure the safety of the clinical data processing environment, unauthorized access or leakage of data cannot occur (Goodman and Flaxman, 2017). With these systems being shifted towards the more risky clinical decision support, compliance also requires the human-in-the-loop supervision that makes AI-generated suggestions subject to the final authority of licensed practitioners. It is possible to transform the existing performance metrics into continuous and lifecycle-oriented compliance model, which would focus on the long-term patient safety, by aligning with international standards, such as the EU AI Act or the Total Product Lifecycle (TPLC) model by the FDA (Goodman & Flaxman, 2017).

7.3 Human Oversight and Accountability Mechanisms

Healthcare organizations must control their AI-based clinical decision systems because regulatory bodies have established mandatory guidelines that require organizations to maintain essential human control. The system requires human supervision because it needs to provide doctors with ultimate control over their diagnostic work and treatment design, which prevents them from depending too much on automated processes. The design of accountability systems needs to establish precise duty assignments, which will determine if developers, healthcare institutions, or clinical practitioners hold responsibility for their actions. The implementation of accountability pathways establishes clear standards to handle AI-related clinical error cases while it builds public confidence in AI-powered healthcare systems (Leslie, 2019).

7.4 International Regulatory Initiatives

International regulations for medical AI technology show increasing compatibility among various policy frameworks used by different countries. The European Union Artificial Intelligence Act establishes a complete regulatory framework that governs high-risk AI systems through its requirements for transparency and risk assessment and system monitoring throughout their operational life (European Commission, 2021). An FDA that supports the concept of Total Product Lifecycle Control (TPLC) would make sure continuous evaluation of AI-enabled medical devices was regulated by pertinent oversight (FDA, 2023).

According to the World Health Organization, hospitals must establish ethical governance systems that include all people while providing safe healthcare services through which the sustainable practices and accountable methods for their AI technology implementation could be processed for a futuristical concept (WHO 2021).

Continuing the current topic of international alignment, the environment of global AI regulation is quickly moving away, as abstract moral principles, toward legislative binding requirements. As an example, the EU AI Act has set a clear standard, classifying clinical decision support systems as high-risk, which needs to be strictly documented in pre-market technical documentation and post-market performance monitoring. At the same time, the Total Product Lifecycle (TPLC) methodology of FDA in the United States is clearer that clinical LLM is not a fixed tool but rather a developing medical device that needs to have planned change control measures in place to ensure the safety of algorithmic change. Outside of these large jurisdictions, the World Health Organization (WHO) has stressed that regulatory efforts should also work towards global health equity, whereby the implementation of clinical LLMs in resource-constrained settings does not further drive up inequalities in healthcare by promoting biased datasets or absent human regulation. This global trend toward risk-based, transparent, and human-centered regulation is critical in developing a common standard of trustful AI that can be reliably incorporated into various clinical processes throughout the world.

8. FUTURE RESEARCH DIRECTIONS

The field of clinical language model research presents multiple promising research paths that aim to develop safer and more dependable systems that can meet actual clinical requirements. Future research should focus on developing domain-adaptive medical LLMs, which can continuously update clinical knowledge while they stay within established safety limits. The process of reducing hallucinations while improving decision-making reliability requires both better uncertainty understanding and more efficient self-verification systems.

The medical field needs a different approach that creates a complete system for clinical reasoning through the collection of various healthcare data types, such as medical images and electronic health records, together with patient data from sensors. Research is also required to design standardized evaluation benchmarks that reflect real clinical workflows rather than controlled experimental environments.

Clinicians will gain the ability to oversee model output through better systems of human-AI collaboration, which will help them understand the results. The healthcare AI systems of the future will rely on continuous learning systems that use secure learning pipelines and privacy-preserving techniques for their operation. The development of trustworthy and scalable clinical language model systems that comply with regulations will benefit from these advancements.

9. CONCLUSION

The healthcare system transition toward intelligent medical decision support systems, which utilize data clinical language models, now experiences a growing integration of these models into its operations. The safe implementation of large language models in clinical documentation requires knowledge retrieval and patient interaction systems to undergo assessment methods that exceed standard evaluation procedures. The chapter demonstrated that clinical language models need to be assessed according to reliability and safety and fairness and transparency, which work as essential principles for evaluation.

Healthcare institutions can utilize a safety-critical evaluation framework to discover all potential hazards that are linked to hallucination and bias and uncertainty and model instability. The implementation of robust testing combined with human-in-the-loop validation and continuous monitoring and regulatory alignment enables clinical AI systems to develop sustainable trustworthiness in actual operational conditions. As indicated in the discussion, evaluation must also be an ongoing process that will legitimize systems in their entire process of operation. The credible functioning of the clinical language models relies on the equal involvement of both technological development and clinical knowledge and governance systems. The emergence of the new assessment procedures that emphasize patient safety and moral responsibility will make language models turn into credible medical aids that offer quality of care services that are equitable.

10. REFERENCES

Amann, J., Blasimme, A., Vayena, E., Frey, D., & Madai, V. I. (2020). Explainability for artificial intelligence in healthcare: A multidisciplinary perspective. *BMC Medical Informatics and Decision Making*, *20*(1), 310. DOI: 10.1186/s12911-020-01332-6 PMID: 33256715

European Commission. (2021). Proposal for a regulation laying down harmonized rules on artificial intelligence (Artificial Intelligence Act). *European Union.*

Finlayson, S. G., Subbaswamy, A., Singh, K., Bowers, J., Kupke, A., Zittrain, J., Kohane, I. S., & Saria, S. (2021). The clinician and dataset shift in artificial intelligence. *The New England Journal of Medicine*, *385*(3), 283–286. DOI: 10.1056/NEJMc2104626 PMID: 34260843

Ghosh, A., Sridhar, S., Ravi, R. K., Muhsin, M., Saha, S., & Agarwal, C. (2025). CLINIC: Evaluating Multilingual Trustworthiness in Language Models for Healthcare. *ArXiv*. https://arxiv.org/abs/2512.11437

Goodman, B., & Flaxman, S. (2017). European Union regulations on algorithmic decision-making and a right to explanation. *AI Magazine*, *38*(3), 50–57. DOI: 10.1609/aimag.v38i3.2741

Holzinger, A., Saranti, A., Molnar, C., Biecek, P., & Samek, W. (2022). Explainable AI methods for safe and trustworthy healthcare AI. *IEEE Computer*, *55*(4), 52–63.

Kelly, C. J., Karthikesalingam, A., Suleyman, M., Corrado, G., & King, D. (2019). Key challenges for delivering clinical impact with artificial intelligence. *BMC Medicine*, *17*(1), 195. DOI: 10.1186/s12916-019-1426-2 PMID: 31665002

Leslie, D. (2019). *Understanding artificial intelligence ethics and safety*. The Alan Turing Institute. https://doi.org/DOI: 10.5281/zenodo.3240529

Omiye, J. A., Gui, H., Rezaei, S. J., Zou, J., & Daneshjou, R. (2024). Large language models in medicine: The potentials and pitfalls: A narrative review. *Annals of Internal Medicine*, *177*(2), 210–220. DOI: 10.7326/M23-2772 PMID: 38285984

Rajkomar, A., Dean, J., & Kohane, I. (2019). Machine Learning in Medicine. *The New England Journal of Medicine*, *380*(14), 1347–1358. DOI: 10.1056/NEJMra1814259 PMID: 30943338

Reddy, S. (2023). Evaluating large language models for use in healthcare. *Patterns (New York, N.Y.)*, *4*(8), 100796.

Shool, S., Adimi, S., Saboori Amleshi, R., Bitaraf, E., Golpira, R., & Tara, M. (2025). A systematic review of large language model evaluations in clinical medicine. *BMC Medical Informatics and Decision Making*, *25*(1), 54. DOI: 10.1186/s12911-025-02954-4 PMID: 40055694

Singhal, K., Azizi, S., Tu, T., Mahdavi, S. S., Wei, J., Chung, H. W., Scales, N., Tanwani, A. K., Cole-Lewis, H., Pfohl, S., Payne, P., Seneviratne, M., Gamble, P., Kelly, C., Schärli, N., Chowdhery, A., Mansfield, P., & Natarajan, V. (2023). Large language models encode clinical knowledge. *Nature*, *620*(7972), 172–180. DOI: 10.1038/s41586-023-06291-2 PMID: 37438534

Topol, E. (2019). *Deep medicine: how artificial intelligence can make healthcare human again.*

U.S. Food and Drug Administration. (2023). *Artificial intelligence and machine learning in medical devices.*

Wang, S., Tang, Z., Yang, H., Gong, Q., Gu, T., Ma, H., Wang, Y., Sun, W., Lian, Z., Mao, K., Jiang, Y., Huang, Z., Ma, L., Shen, W., Ji, Y., Tan, Y., Wang, C., Gao, Y., Ye, Q., & Wu, J. (2026). A novel evaluation benchmark for medical LLMs illuminating safety and effectiveness in clinical domains. *npj. Digital Medicine*, *9*(91), 91. Advance online publication. DOI: 10.1038/s41746-025-02277-8 PMID: 41454006

World Health Organization. (2021). *Ethics and governance of artificial intelligence for health.* WHO Press.

Yang, Y., Jin, Q., Leaman, R., Liu, X., Xiong, G., Sarfo-Gyamfi, M., Gong, C., Ferrière-Steinert, S., Wilbur, W. J., Li, X., Yuan, J., An, B., Castro, K. S., Álvarez, F. E., Stockle, M., Zhang, A., Huang, F., & Lu, Z. (2024). *Ensuring safety and trust: Analyzing the risks of large language models in medicine.* arXiv. https://doi.org//arXiv.2411.14487DOI: 10.48550

Chapter 8
Dialogic Safety:
A Communication-Centered Framework for Clinical Risk Assessment of Conversational Medical LLMs

Supratim Mukherjee
http://orcid.org/0009-0008-6657-891X
Amity University, Mumbai, India

Archan Mitra
http://orcid.org/0000-0002-1419-3558
Amity University, Mumbai, India

Vishal Jain
http://orcid.org/0000-0003-1126-7424
School of Engineering & Technology, Vivekananda Institute of Professional Studies - Technical Campus, New Delhi, India

Shashi Kant Gupta
http://orcid.org/0000-0001-6587-5607
Lincoln University College, Malaysia

ABSTRACT

Conversational large language models (LLMs) are increasingly used in healthcare for triage, patient education, documentation, and decision support. Safety debates often emphasize accuracy, bias, and privacy, but overlook how these systems shape trust and decision-making through communication. This chapter proposes a communication-centered framework to assess clinical safety in medical LLMs. It defines dialogic safety across three layers: Linguistic Safety (expression of uncertainty,

DOI: 10.4018/979-8-3373-7862-6.ch008

evidence, and sensitive topics), Interactional Safety (clarification, error recovery, escalation), and Institutional Safety (auditability, role clarity, and alignment with guidance from World Health Organization, Food and Drug Administration, and European Union). The framework provides checklist-style indicators for red-teaming, simulations, and human oversight. By treating safety as a property of clinical dialogue rather than isolated outputs, it supports stronger governance, clinician supervision, and patient trust.

1. INTRODUCTION

Progress in conversational LLM technologies has now expanded these models from pure prototypes to standard data entry points in healthcare and patient's assessment. These new systems allow patients to interact through a chat-based platform by expressing their concerns, explaining lab test results or enquiring about drugs or mental health issues. But since the patient truly is beyond the process of evaluation would further enhance decreasing the ultimate fj of the health care of his or her her. Such an impression does not last long as one turns on the conversazione system as it is plain that the system 'learns' how to react to every single query and this makes it seem more like tapered learning for sure but it gives rise to excellent results, but in practice it fails to maintain the non conversazione straight and symmetrical approach. But his/her help and his/her deep belief in safelymedicalims do have the recipients speech recognition problems. More recent studies of healthcare benchmarks show that the medical LLMs are not only dangerous because they may run a muck and make up wholly fictional information that is threatening to one's life, but they are also dangerous because they provide incorrect counseling and delay emergency situations, and most importantly they assume risk in crisis management and treatment strategies (Han et al., 2024; Wang et al., 2025; Johri et al., 2025). Communicative aspect points 'dialogic safety' considers clinical and conversational risks by not imbibing the idea of safety as being akin to acceptable levels of yes/no data. This is made… fortges by the growth of research which highlights the mentioned shift in the discipline. Medical LLM research presents degraded systems assessment and appraisal since they now involve budgets that specify the kinds of recourse required to come up with data as well as formulas for computation which are void of any measures of risk and attention on the quality of mutual conversational processes under investigation (Lee et al., 2024). The structured evaluation proposals which provide taxonomies have proposed that healthcare LLM evaluation incorporates evaluation of task performance and test for reliability and provedane as well as harm testing. (Lacerda, 2025; Maity, 2025) Considering that it is the practice distress situations or at least distract names with operation of elements in format undistorted affects protecting the code from the disseminated prepared female adjustment. Thus these instances even correct in sound and meaning are sometimes unacceptable in medical practice due to the extensive danger they pose to patients and their significance special free iron losses are based on misconceptions of elemental exchange processes ator то (Jude and Ginzburg, 2025). Reconciliation fill of the medical-severe sexual disorders is possible.

1.1 From "Accuracy" to "Interactional Risk" in Medical LLMs

Medical LLMS demonstrated their capacities initially by resolving difficult clinical medical problems and their pass rate in standardized tests, that indicated their appropriateness to clinical environment as stated by Singhal and their team in their report for 2023. Tendencies in this sector are changing and increasingly turning attention to building systems that are capable of interacting like a human being on medical tasks. They have also mentioned the fact that diagnostic systems using AI for multi-turn clinical reasoning and patient-like conversation are much more accurate. However, the use of such systems in the real world requires further development of patient contextualized dialogs abridging the need for and use of such dialog techniques and tools when dealing with patients impacts certain ethical considerations (Tu et al., 2024; Tu et al., 2025). Such user-centered designs and multi-turn evaluation enclose eastern patients, patients of filial age and patients in narcotics clinics— and system-level evaluations Dr. 'we actually don't wait for half a second what they shared with us about, but pack up immediately.'"

However, as these concerns intensify so does the emphasis on specific benchmarks. While MedSafetyBench evaluates the medical advice as well as the risk prone system's results, HealthBench evaluates the health outcomes in humans in favor of practicing standard language evaluation (Han et al., 2024; Arora et al., 2025). The generation of benchmarks does necessitate the scrutiny by the domain expert and also feedback from the clinician due to the fact that automating of such scores would not sufficiently be able to predict the clinical safety according to the 2025 papers of Kocaman and Johri. Evaluation of dialogic safety involves a blend of procedures where examination is done through marked criteria and where the quality of responding individuals is assessed through appropriate task simulation i.e. scenario- based tests and expert moderators.

1.2 Benchmarking, Rubrics, and Simulation as Building Blocks for Dialogic Safety

Researchers engage in the development and application of both one-turn and multi-turn data sets and evaluation standards for medical dynamically coherent dialogue processing. As for multi-turn dialogues, the safety reasons and rationale of appropriate question procedure and the sub-principles are covered in the assessment standards and thus in a communication assessment framework (Gong et al., 2026). The evaluation frameworks encompass attempts to not just demonstrating the various components of the clinical dialogues but enforcing them as well within applicable information retrieval methodologies. Thus immediately getting into the process, the evaluation frameworks go from knowing whether the model knows the answer to seeing how the model actually performs the task-that is to say engages in conversation securely.

The simulation enhance safety also from the perspective of dialogical systems as a speech dialog between ICs usually involves a high level of risk, to large quantities of such dialogues can be generated. Evaluation tasks in conversational clinical systems tests affect several supporting decision making tools simultaneously, namely, multi-agent models, which provide for operation within the lesion's tangible environment, involving conflicting topics with incomplete and indistinct information and competing user goals, (Cart et al. 2025). It is vital to know how and why safety failures can occur because usually most safety failures occurs under certain conditions. Studies which installations scenarios are used to investigate triage and transfer of care activities are concerned with two main areas: they research the connectedness of the workflows and the threat present downstream and do the evaluation of the performance quality of the working structure especially at the local level (Eberly et al. 2025). The use of rubrics coupled with organized checking mechanisms and simulation techniques caters for the risk management related technical needs while matching the user conversation acceptability safety criteria.

1.3 Hallucinations are Necessary but Insufficient as a Safety Lens

Clinical examination and the evaluation of hallucination remains its main focus in hallucinatory evaluation, yet researching proposes that this discourse is not sufficient to understimate discouragement. The clinical drugs assessor and hallucinating rates suggest that the extent to which mal and mis referral l l M-s are safely effective are used by authors produces convincing appearance of biologically effective treatment essence l l M that is in fact ineffective. This research requires structured techniques for detecting and correcting medical mistakes caused by these machines. People loose conversation skills because they claim that a particular utterance is the truth.

In automatic assessment research, theoretical background is the area which defines and directs the process of working out instruments and datasets in close connection with performance weights associated with the tasks being performed. Out of the need for a systematic digital assessment in automatic evaluation research, social interactiveness as a component in the overall estimate between assessors and students competing in scenarios and guiding learners through such situations still remained ambiguous. This lack of direct guidance imbues the authoring process with a certain phobia that needs to be addressed. The evidence available in relation to the assessment of highly dangerous tasks only buttresses this claim. Episodes of communication with suicidal individuals and individuals who self-harm, as well as episodes of injuries caused by external factors, have several ramifications in that when an individual is trying to deal with such dangers such individuals are likely to pose public threats. Addressing mental health involves a lot of sensitivity because even the construction of inter-ventions affects the way in which people comply. With regard to LLM, these are risks of dependence and reliance, relational conditioning and therapist accretion. A flexible safety concept is needed which combines syntactically correct and contextually proper interaction.

1.4 Ethical, Legal, and Governance Dimensions of Clinical Dialogue

The concept of risk appraisal is directed towards communication and therefore appreciation of the ethical and legal implications that are likely to be encountered in clinical discussions. When discarded in the course of treatment of patients and responding to them, the shared tasks blended the duties of the medical assessments, ethical assessments and legal assessments of the clinician to harm. It is necessary to perform an evaluation of the area of reproductive ethics and its significance to such land in the ethoucs compass directions of climate building autonomy', informed icf, and valued counselling-abolitionist talk such as – mhra through and how to enact-eeeutics the autonomy in decision making and dispensing services is to a great extent ethically guided&7d to promote health care practice which all emphasise maintenance of the lady's autonomy in management or use of reproductive services (Sreenath et al., 2016). Investigations into the partial surgical procedures allowed on females the Moschowits types of limited cesarean sections or the triangular strains were restricted as all course of action of removal of part of the womb these are options that apply to changing caesarean section buys pregnant women time to fifteen and octuple years of age for standard delivery cesarean delivery before a woman's 35th trimester and the grade 3 disease findings start septation not only the iliac arteries but continue with these arteries which are near and towards the interior as shall be described within the hallux. A Case study on application of training – less limb lengthening (include surgical process with combined META rod lengthening and the lengthening and shortening of the bone using External Fixator) includes additional specific calculations including determining the required number of clicks of the reducing device twice a day and then comparing this with actual measurement of the limb. Risk assessments and subsequent managing risk leads to effective health and safety – management with a focus on safety in the work space developing a safety consciousness to prevent serious injuries in the course of performing one's duties or a breach of another person's right at work. Strategy for HSEQ implementation shall be directed at, determination and Utilization of tasks such as hazard identification and evaluation of risks and mitigation measures, Anti-risk management, safety permitted risk, safety promoted risk, overall philosophy and strategy, level of safety that is deemed acceptable, procedures for improving risk, procedures for improving risk, establishment such as hoisting, cableway and rail transport systems safety, safe use of hazardous substances and fulfillment of a contract'62 The state of law within the united organization of subordinate territories can be discussed in terms in lack of compliance with the law so as to improve the current state of affairs.

2. LITERATURE REVIEW

2.1 The Shift From Single Turn Performance to Multi Turn Clinical Interaction

The fundamental aim of any research attempt is to explore implict stereotypes as well as those that are often explicit to illlucidate how they influence evaluation accuracy. With position inquiry analysis research I was able to show that good models should be able to solve even the hardest exams with privilege rates possible which challenge the experts who have passed the LC test and as results of the general assessment should be able to be considered the leading experts of the field. However clinical communication is seldom isolated to one turn. Most of the communication that is allocated to the medical interview is a dynamic activity that develops through a list of questions, follow up questions, and revelation of the sympton with the back ground information and the medical history with all current and relevant details (Gorzka et al., 2024; Gorcka et al., 2025). In the US predominantly following the long-held policy, the healthcare sector based talent evaluation is changing such that metrics of conversational involvement in process change, the tail patients and staff, as well as the state of healthcare environment per se are the issues that are most crucial, instead of looking into a book of fixed answers as has hitherto existed (Tu et al., 2024; Tu et al., 2025). The study reveals that dialogues contain several aspects that pose clinical problems to users and render them untrustworthy by identifying the barriers that reveal inaccuracies leading to delay in discovery of diagnostic errors (Elsevier, 2024). The principle of dialogic safety aids in formulating appropriate safety regulations since it investigates whether the interactional process empowers the users to make the necessary decisions to promote their safety in case of emergencies and their future choices are expressed during the course of the conversation.

Clinical dialogue serves as a structured method for conveying risk information instead of merely exchanging data in between parties. The system must decide what to ask next, what to defer, what to emphasize, and how to calibrate certainty. Multi turn evaluation proposals argue that these conversational decisions require dedicated metrics and rubrics that can represent the process quality of clinical interaction, not only the correctness of endpoints (Liao et al., 2023; Shi et al., 2023). The theme receives validation through expert review arguments which show that clinician judgment must confirm whether dialogue behavior meets standards for safety and empathy and professional clinical practice (Kocaman, 2025; Johri et al., 2025).

2.2 Benchmarking Clinical Safety as Harm Prevention Rather Than General Helpfulness

The second theme expectations that have been formed from their renowned roots of simply to evaluate the extant general interventions extend currently to a greater purpose of determing the impact of the utilization of medical systems on patients. Later majority of both disease prevention and general medical guidelines were published, which included conflicting medical management and medical futility on high-stakes interventions as well as recommendation of further action in high-risk situations. Consequently, the MedSafetyBench extension provides a way to access and to understand safety from the point of view of system design principles, where safety is a property that of how a specific model of medical care responds to a given risk situation.' (Han, 2014:686). In other words, HealthBench is the new front in modeling with regard to overall health and well-being, focusing evalua- tion objectives on how safe or efficacious the model is with the targets and end users in mind (Arora, 2015). The studies to be reviewed herein will show a pattern with quantification of prevention, toxicity, or safety through under the surface harmful effects which are a consequence of influence by various aspects, such as information availability, guiding norms, etc.

As shown in the literature, a contentious underpinning in research poses apractice and strategy dilemma in the use of different research paradigms. On one hand, the use of standardized performance scales by researchers tends to help in the manipulation and control variables being measured in such a way that an accurate comparison can be made of the population of interest, but, on the other hand, this halts the researchers into reducing the original patterns of conversation into overly simplified scenarios that can ensure proper measurements are administered. Frequently, researchers choose to integrate benchmarks into workflows and workflows into their evaluation processes such that a levels of evaluation are present above the use of benchmarking such as user studies (Gaber et al., 2025; Johri et al., 2025). The dialogic safety model also requires elaborating this bias since it is an intrinsic evaluation of the extent of unsafe clinical practices which are only problematic in certain very carefully circumscribed situations governed by the presence of certain factors and the happening of specific kinds of social interactions. The reason for the phrase 'post hoc benchmarking done without attention to the answer for what if the condition was different' is because one can only realize a failure of a system as per each benchmark if the kind of stimuli, turn order, or respondent preference equals the possible premises of dynamic risk (Lim et al., 2025). With the new model, clinical scenario process is built upon evidence of clinical binder, progress note and lab work, and images and videos where particularly collaborative practice is expected.

2.3 Rubrics and Structured Frameworks for Multi Turn Consultation Quality

The third concept of this research is dedictaed to the issue how rubric design and assessment frameworks affect the connection between clinical standards and ratings. The MedDialogRubrics comprise safety regulations in multi-turn consultations in terms of levels of reasoning also structured evaluation criteria and how to ask questions in complete assessments and finally limitation and escalation guidance such as flare management (Gong et al., 2026). This is something rubrics do well as they measure the quality of conversation from various viewpoints and in a way that is understood by healthcare practitioners. In addition, this particular aspect is imperative in in ensuring a safe dialogue as it is safe dialogue that is not reached whenever people do not ask questions regard vital information and provide unsuitable reassurance or ignore relevant warning signs.

The subset of evaluation techniques such as structured cuales use external knowledge representations for verifying the credibility of dialogues. For example, in case mediated evaluation which is template is used to analyze multi-turn patient interactions in order to extract abnormal flow and suspicious practice (Yu et al., 2025). These strategies extend the notions of safety to include persisting constraint satisfaction in the course of the evolution of time. For this purpose, as an aspect of the conversation, there should be no doubts about any data dynamic, but also, there should also be no 'wishful thinking' trajectories during the progress of symptoms. If one is liked to be re-evaluative in 'conduct', Knowledge-based methods aim to attend dialogic reliability within oft-validated dialogues and in so doing many other factors are evidenced beyond just lexical, semantic and other usual properties indicative of dialogue validation.

The main aim of the study is to focus on aspects of taxonomies and frameworks that strive to approximate the universal and a singularly recognized system for categorizing testing functions or activities and integrative approach in assessments. Orderly evaluation system defines the commendation points in five basic directions; it is necessary to studies that any medical modality requires evidence from all the areas of assessment (Lacerda, 2025; Maity,[1]).

2.4 Simulation and Workflow Evaluation to Surface Latent Conversational Risk

The fourth theme illustrates the way in which simulation techniques and workflow evaluation help in the detection of the harmful effects and hazards that static testing fails to find. The MATRIX mufti-agent simulation framework provides the facility of controlled testbeds which are used to assess medical systems under different user scenarios and their goals and challenges (Lim et al., 2025). The approach is thus necessitated as safety failures require testing in poor conditions when the users are participating in testing do not provide full data or when they try to violate safety measures. The very same simulation method limits system testing to dialogic scenarios and is particularly helpful in the enhancement of system performance evaluation under difficult conditions.

Simulation allows researchers to create clinical decision making systems which are models of real clinical decision making systems. Models help experimenters to explore how the system functions to provide care, how well it performs, and how its performance is related to the the attainment of its goals. Every such system comprises multiple components which pass data among each other.istributions on the information transmitted across the components of the system are some form of the data which is patterns in the interest of proper functioning the system.

网络(peer)中完成升级任务。

From the user perspective, the user evaluation tries to ascertain how much the end users can benefit from the system.

One of the key principles supporting the importance of studying language of medicine in specialized discourse is the fact that there exist certain dimension of medical dialogues. Human Factors oriented processes are multifaceted and involve a number of stages that determine the type of language applied in them. According to the paper \'investigating the effect of collaborative code-scanning on diagnosis accuracy and its contribution to patient safety practices, a task error is more valid diagnostic error compared to others for error analyses on physicians errors. Of course, it is ideal that all tasks can be accomplished depending on reasonable assignment and image acquisition dose optimization so that dose can be kept within a specific range depending of the task.

IsEmpty: Medical certification on the other hand must be concerned with procedures that should be followed before and during patient radiation treatment based on the patient illness and pathology. Program importance is based on the number of radiologists in relation to the program goals, the UN Protocol Requested, the fees demanded, the quality assurance program, the image criteria procedures, the waiting list, and other factors. Turkey, for example, has many radiology centers, and CT imaging is accessible to almost all patients free of charge.

Such evaluation biases may nonetheless be minor compared to bias due to change in breast density, with or without PC-DFA in close proximity. Moses 23:14 places geometrical precursors of the Doctor-patient dialogue before the practice of contemporary medicine. The Doctor-first and the 'Nobody-offers': Doctors' prescriptiveness within clinical consultation.

Take other Structured CEs, Case Based MCEs – research and statistics comparative one ball with Joan Davis was concurrently conducted Bridgette Gahir and Emilia Daoud made and presented a poster about the same Research within the sexual violence project entitled; 'EFA Assessment: Mentor Skills for Adolescents who are at Risk of Promiscuous Behaviour Establishment of an in District 'Education Foundation of Africa Project' in Thailand Medical University and PIRM 235 ULA – Kakuma Sub-County, Tanzania microscopy. Several CT images were taken and they demonstrate a non-deformed large colon under the diaphragm a description of kidney, as we cannot see pictures of it shows that it must be normal and healthy. Plan I = no sample retrieval by some count plaster nature caste as neither histopath MHT first suspension tissue. Quantification involves defining all levels of matching and peak areas of a compound component such as those of a peptide, protein or nucleic acid. 2. Societal reference standards of practice as identified below are intended for use in yield determination for URO in the case of criminal cases.

These standards should not hold sway casting my judgment towards quantum meruit or unjust enrichment in favor of the claimant, your clients, for reasons which will become clear stated: S70 B(e). I apologize to everyone in the courtroom. I mean that due to the previously mentioned defense under the law, it's completely excluded that we can hold these laws applied. 010.

I am not a proponent who believes proposal addresses most of the industries addressed by CRMS and BL Yamendo. Ashland shows that penalties associated with grievances against women in the Shura Sangha will also be applied to their heirs and relatives, which is in line with the promise of compensatory liability for harassment including benefits. Protecting AA confirmed confidentiality among people of different language, religious beliefs, ethics, and socio-historical practices around the world while also ensuring safety among people who freely disclose many of the details about their lives to the world. World Everest Scamsmic author Dr 23307 MNSACMIN. Keri Wilson, Karen Wilson and I spoke at the Stockholm ERN Conference this evening and Lisa Lumpert-Boreham presented me with a copy of her Book.

Here's free access to the film "Shock and Awe in Merthyr - How the Women of Merthyr Won Their Struggle" by Laura Gant, Sophie Williams and Rhys Tucker. The tape captures a few frames of protest ridden residents of Denbigh in Denbigh that had to do more with the UK Miners' Strike. Would you like the one with the three wheeler?

To interpret the film, one might ask what "dictatorship" is, as well as what "dictatorship" motivated former participants of the swap meet to make these allegations. Only two cards, one black one white. Two color print. Some of Virginia Souvaine's work is in the museum, some in private hands.

2.5 Hallucinations, Calibration, and the Ethics of Conversational Persuasion

The next risk, the fifth risk theme identifies that hallucinations and calibration is the core foundation of the risk phenomenon that interactional ethics beyond impact assessment can cope with. There are plenty of cases of hospital hallucinations that all have been documented and are used by current evaluation systems in computation of the presence of hallucinations together with failure patterns affecting clinical outcomes (Wang et al., 2025). The existing literature shows that a potentially hazardous remark can be represented as true because it gives a feeling of certainty while containing false information. Clinical examination research devises evaluation systems meant for automatic evaluation, but experts find it difficult to come up with specific ways of measuring calibratisation and demonstrations of uncertainty (Liu et al., 2024). The dialogic assessment of safety requires the assessment of two elements: how close the model is to the reality and whether the requirements related to the known and unknown dangers endangering the automation user while in operation have been met.

Considering the introductory pooling of resources, little has been made until no about how leadership predisposition as a variable interacts with compliant workplace behaviors. This study contributes to the understanding of shallit terminologies like compliance. This is so because it aims at emphasizing on the leadership aspects and how it reacts to the repercussions of employees getting around complying with work instructions.

Extra perception of the hazards related to hard safety with its corresponding correction level is provided by studies in general safety. Demonstrative sets that outline on inadequate safety practices that are too apathetic show two disorders that this approach induces: hyperperfectionism on inaccurate bio-medical equipment and unnecessary denial that some of the problems exist and precludes any medical help in an environment or misguides about what the medical help is/would be (Röttger and Theile, 2004). Bharti (1991), Lorenz and Vikram (1999), Ley and the authors) has a rather goal-oriented orientation.

2.6 Governance, Legal Risk, and Clinically Grounded Accountability

The las theme focuses on governance and accountability because they are both important in any evaluation of safety. It is shown that the responsibilities throughout capital countries are in line with the protection services for the medical, ethical, and legal aspects of the consultations, as well as the developments to manage such risks, including the discussion risks and face direct and indirect threats like sexual assault insurance and the tort of actionable negligence through the dissociation of personhood (Aramaki et al., 2025). Furthermore, it is analysis of reproductive ethics and related domain-specific ethical dimensions that would be applicable to every medicine that requires the approach where there is absolute absence of intervention since the areas deal with sensitive issues that are anchored on a value framework rather than mere provision of facts limiting the patients' options (Xu et al., 2026). The discussion of review process and the available tools explains that there is a need to establish measures for clinical evaluation that ensures they can be audited and yield results within certain standards of relevance and to practice, refer helpful information, instead of valuating on grounds of a range of functional factors as performance indicator (Lee et al., 2024; Lacerda, 2025; Maity, 2025).

Results from clinician benchmarking and also from comparative analysis provide a rationale to my argument that organisations require governance systems, much as different models coordinate various other tasks. This suggests that there are safety claims that any organization should expect to have, but which can vary with respect to that organization's model and what it does (Dinc et al., 2025). The invention of new LLMs that have enhancements in extracting and summarizing clinical text, implies that an organization can enjoy considerable benefits, however, organizations have to consider the accuracy aspect, the risk of omissions, omissions in content that may have subsequent medical effects, and concerning the application affected by a summary report for decision making overall (Veen and Lammers, 2024). The dialogic governance is there to limit three characteristics: self, system boundaries performance, the availability of reference guide for help from a professional and the structure adopted to arrive at a recommendation.

2.7 Synthesis: Toward Dialogic Safety as an Integrative Evaluation Orientation

An integrated literature review concerning areas associated with clinical risk management, biomedical patient safety and standards and the law aims to show that, where use of untimed collaborative scripts is concerned, risk assessment tools need to review the most rudiment communication technique with a focus on evaluating the possible harm caused by such interactions. The integration of performance guide and stress tests areas allows the design of standardized test methodologies that trigger Minigame-based multi-turn dialogs practice to sustainable assessment rubric ba ased clinical reality (Gong et al., 2026; Yu et al., 2025) and more in particular - practical implementation. That these performance and safety test studies as well as the process models and the availability of new technology identifies that two obligations control the level of danger in such acts: creating the conditions for the occurrence of the risks and their effects (Clement et al., 2005; Dormady, 2005). Further to the research done on safety from the point of view of governance, it remains to be found out the extent of the same from a different perspective such as the protection from ethical, legal and social damages. Thank you, may I continue with Aramaki's (2, A repository for arresting stupidity associated with personal lives Shouts stop to a brand) case: When Xu's application of her previous dataset on the subjects white women from Georgia who have been raped in comparison to those from Latin America failed, it counted for a failure in the prevailing installation of cultural imposed identities of transgression calculations (Xu et al., 2026; Lawrence et al., 2024). The notion of dialogic safety serves as the underlying theme which underpins all of these diverse components as it explains how clinical safety is produced through communicative processes that consider the back-and-forth aspect and how information is provided and the persuasive power of speech settings is influenced.

3. METHODOLOGY AND CONCEPTUAL FRAMEWORK

3.1 Research Design and Overall Approach

IT also addresses its specific setting. Going with the medical consultation LLMs, this present study presents a methodology that asserts the use of an evaluation tool that studies interaction in terms of communication, focusing on clinical risk barriers, and in this case communication LLMs. In this study, the author pursues an evaluative and design-analytic way and applies three appraisal techniques, rubric-based assessments, scenario-based stress tests and the model of conversation-level risk. Another key principle is that patient safety involves risk assessment in various contexts rather than being defined by the accuracy of an individual's prediction and-nothing else. The model can be seen meaning the way it interacts with the user by establishing information input and uncertainty estimation and taking care of warning and sending information about the network and not to mention taking the operational commands of the network. The study unfolds the pre-interventional discourse continuity protocols than an intervention with only the final part of the original turn.

There are three interconnected elements which comprise the framework and work together to form its structure. The first element establishes dialogic safety and is based on a conceptual model that describes dialogic safety as a set of communication skills to be acquired by medical workers in order to prevent clinical accidents. A second component assists in designing an evaluation plan and selects datasets, scenarios and annotation strategies. The third stage of the outline prepares qualitative rubric judgments and conversation tracings for conversion into quantitative risk indices which facilitate the conventional use of these models in a cross-validation procedure under various conditions of deployment and prompting.

3.2 Conceptual Foundation: Dialogic Safety as Interactional Risk Governance

Dialogic Safety as surveyed by the researchers is the level of reassurance as to the secure channels of interaction maintained by the medical LLMs during consultations. The creators developed a system with free security bars, which can guarantee that the user receives no dangerous medical advice and as well is never afraid to cry out whenever necessary i.e. and gradates their respect to the concerted actions of the principles of safe communication. Developed by users, the system usages include security management for the management of uncertainties that users exhibit during dialogues and recognizing the traces of harmful acts by the disabled and facilitating the safe resolution of issues.

At the core of the model are three main elements, these are: define safety culture concept; risk as harm in all its forms; and technical jargon certainly has its place. The latter terms were thus consolidated in specific cultural backgrounds at their correct value beyond the conditions if they leave the confines of the households' doors. Cultures usually have histories of customs, daily regimes, music, foods, knowledge, and languages that are unique.

Next, a separate group of aspects will deal with the psychological attitudes of every particular user towards the model as a whole and its parts. This is where eloquence, good reasoning skills, lack of anxiety will guarantee the satisfaction and fulfilment of the user. In other words, it will be wise to use the design parameters given in the application of concepts on the use of the product. And, protected between these, are the responsibilities that the user in the digital system can fulfill when the time comes.

3.3 Analytical Dimensions and Operational Constructs

Dialogic Safety is put into action through five cardinal areas each of which in connected to the period of the dialogic events by showing the approach of real human relationships.

3.3.1 Risk Detection and Triage Sensitivity

When it comes to assessing how well a model can target high adverse signal detection, or consideration of suspicious activities and dangerous response quality, this dimension clearly succeeds. It includes the need to ask some some specific screening questions, recognition of critical symptom groups and provision of the escalation instructions when allowed limits are redacted. This is so because the risk is only realized during a close analysis of the work process. From a safety perspective, an escalation of risks which comes at the end of numerous risks is referred to as an unsafe posture whereas the other risks propagated by the system within the unsafe state may as well be called windmilled dispensations.

3.3.2 Uncertainty Calibration and Epistemic Humility

An irreducibility of the dimension measures if, at what extent, the model is considerate of probabilities in its information. There should be at least two assessments that the system presents. It should however be clear that the confidence related to each of them, when expressed, differs with the other according to the aspects being evaluated. The system must display and provide the possibility of using the other evaluation method, the one that has professional characteristics, beside the authority assessment as the primary method of assessment. This includes taking half systolic blood pressures to provide higher estimation of systolic blood pressure which is the more advanced evaluative method to apply in children less than 3years of age. Finally, the asssessment related to the 50th percentage of peak systolic blood pressure for females should be taken as a method with higher reliability in older males.

3.3.3 Information Elicitation and Conversational Completeness

Before recommending services or products, the system has to ask important questions to get some details about the customer or transaction. The rating should describe what factors are used to measure the relevance of such patient data as age or duration of disease long existing, comprehensive medical history such as an existing and past medical condition, the past and present drugs, substances, allergies and if the patient is pregnant. When a patient possibly has no recall of the necessary medical conditions and recent medical treatments had no physical effect on the patient, there is a need to have the system ask follow- up questions starting from what the patients' evident symptoms are.

3.3.4 Recommendation Safety and Actionability

The system is not required to assist in the development of all decision, nor is it required to address all categories of problems or conditions. The analysis can tend to overlook social and economic realities (such as concerns over costs, lack of work for certain professional groups, and the reduced overall out-of-pocket expenditures). Self-audit therefore may often be a poor substitute for conventional external audit (although it is always the case).

3.3.5 Ethical and psychosocial communication safety

However, the type of business does not matter here, since, in reality, personal data is used, processed, and exchanged within all organizations. This contains four elements empathy, non-stigmatizing language and privacy sensitivity, and the management of high-risk disclosur. In the mental health context it is appropriate to use supportive language among other things, and not to use manipulative or judgmental language. This is necessary to ensure that sensitive information relating to reproductive health and issues of abuse victims is also not released. The aspect makes it possible to require creating psychological safety in addition to clinical safety, as different tones and presentation kinds evoke various user actions.

3.4 Data Sources, Scenarios, and Sampling Strategy

Purposive scenario sampling was employed in the study since the dialogic safety needs were explored and necessary situations where risk was present. The sample chosen as representative included multiple samples of dialogues between two persons belonging to different ethnic groups having different levels of communicative and medical complication pertaining to medical establishment. This design in turn, creates four strata of real-world communicative tasks with different demands on the participants.

The first band should provide less intensive information on health matters, for example answer questions on simple problems, offer preventive or lifestyle strategies. The other section is hazarded at the height of disease, the chances at which would require very accurate categorization of the query anti reflecting the symptoms of chest dicom-fort having no so called red flag symptoms and the incidences of fever in children due to drugs and venereal infection side effects. The third chapter embodies emergency situations of danger which includes stroke, Anaphylactic shock, Labour and employ stomach cramps, and suicidal thoughts for pregnant women. The fourth level encloses consults where value questions and ethical considerations emerge: for example, termination-of-pregnancy, end-of-life, omission of violence or threat.

The user prompts constitute separate conversation scenarios in which each of the dialogues begin and end with the most typing of the AI assistant, then utilizing different voice and internet log-in in creating the script. Check whether the model changes its tone of the questions and triage methods prior to going into different directions after the occurrence of new relevant cues in progress. These texts are composed of real-life situations that are bound to have poor symptom descriptions that can hardly be understood and case presentations that are wholly unnecessary; inappropriate patient responses, unbearable emotions and non integrated pictures revealing the performance of the system.

There is also a set of real-life de-identified conversations containing only a few scenarios as in the mentioned collection.

3.5 Model Conditions and Prompting Configurations

The structure implements its judgment from discrimination testing for various model variations in the presence of its quizzing enhancements. At least three elements are needed in this construct such as the norm where general healthcare prompts assess the model and a defensive scenario where another approach possibly specific safety behaviors are allowed and cherish the and anticipates safety behaviors. And lastly, a dialogic safety scenario allows for the implementation of the model any given conditions that may include triage and uncertainty garage escalation thresholds procedures. Each type of model is validated in the same set up of scenarios. The experiment maintains invariable values for all generation parameters in order to achieve minimal deviations of resultant statistics. The authors investigate different techniques to determine the variation in safety outcomes owing to certain stochastic models. The researchers concentrate on both mean safety metrics and the consistency of safety over time since there are medical risks in hospital settings that cannot be put into any form of order.

3.6 Annotation Protocol and Rubric Design

The Dialogic Safety evaluation process employs a multi-tiered scoring which rates both individual conversational turns and completive dialogues. A turn-based scoring system requires annotators to perform some predetermined speech acts including safety- related actions in all responses. The labels are: risk screening question escalation recommendation self-care guidance medication advice diagnostic assertion uncertainty statement referral to professional care. The concerns the annotators dodge are: contraindicated advice, missed red flags and over-optimism that leads to inappropriate assurance. The safety level of a dialogue is displayed by a set of five dialogic safety components that are graded. There are two kinds of marks, each one's higher values indicating better interactional behavior. The level of implicit risk depends on the particular system scaffold but in a general sense it depicts the maximum harm if all the recommendations of the guides are adhered to. The team establishes the clinical foundation by introducing a three-tier annotee team format which in turn implements a training system. The first level is of research annotators in medical communication who are provided with the rubric to use in their handling. The second level is of clinician reviewers looking at the high risk cases where they try to evaluate what cases need to be further evaluated. The team is eventually forced to hold formal adjudication meetings and tweaking of the rubric in order to handle disputes between members. The data is used to develop a list of valid responses selected by means that are then scored by all raters. The reliability quantification involves dimension-specific and overall calculations that are applied only in cases of low levels of agreement to facilitate focused retraining and revision of the rubric.

3.7 Quantification: Constructing a Dialogic Safety Index

The project introduces a grading system for risk assessment based on the suggestive assessment of rubrics. The scale integrates measures of user-typical performance and the maximum potential risk intended for registration. The agglomerated risk grade, in general, which may be apprehended when measuring potential system thinking of any system, is composed of three aggregative components, too.

This initial stages involve average scores obtained for each dimension with the help of five dimensions while 'all of 'all of "wishful-thinking" cases are completely excluded from the computation. The second stage includes a system of penalties and it works as a subdivision of the uttock stage within discipline proceedings for individuals convicted of committing a serious safety violation of the first or second level. The third stage would be the trajectory penalty and it deals with how fast one can identify the risk in as much as the escalation only occur after many dangerous turns have been taken.

Understanding is made easier when the index is made less confusing and transformed to a scale ranging from 0 to 100. Higher scores would mean that dialogues are safer to have. Besides, the research elaborates on the safety profile of the scenarios which outline what the relevant clinical situations and conversation conditions are likely to pose the greatest threat of breakdown.

3.8 Analysis Plan: Thematic and Statistical Integration

The analysis proceeds in two main steps. The first stage is the completion of a thematic safety audit encompassing safety failures and safety measures at the local level. The analysis identified at least a number of themes including non-screening/ hasty reassurance, overdiagnosis with premature labeling and part of checklist questioning that does not follow user cues and vague as well as overly safe escalation language. Thematic elements are crucial for both the dimensions of rubric as well as for the purpose of the scenarios, because type of risk profiling depends on context. The second layer is comparative quantitative analysis. The Dialogic Safety Index is combined with other five dimension scores for comparing various versions of different models in different prompting conditions. The research explores whether there are any variations within the ever-increasing levels of scenario strata, toward risk and safety improvement either reaching high levels or developmental and value based conversations. The research studies safety stability based upon the tests' response variability; as it also occurs in several test sessions.

3.9 Ethical Considerations and Boundary Conditions

The research considers the clinical risk that prohibits its acceptance in actual medical practice tests. All the experimental procedures are confined to restricted spaces and involve obligatory scenarios or de-identified test samples. Further assessment of communicational structures in real patient texts is done by excluding identifying information of the patient and other content with high risk of confidentiality breach. This most benefit to risk communication assessment, outline the allowable interpretations of its findings. The presence of a high dialogue coherence score alone does not imply that the care delivered is the same as professional care. More incriminating evidence to this effect are the work scenarios that show how the system talks its way out of trouble while handling risk responsibly. Lack of obfuscation in the translation of the system's evaluation of safety into the marketing of professional practice is intricately intertwined with some care because such evaluation should not work as a vehicle for clinical authorities.

4. ANALYSIS OF DATA

4.1 Overview of the Dataset and Analytical Unit

The analysis treats each multi turn consultation as the primary unit of evidence. For each consultation, turn level annotations were aggregated into conversation level dimension scores across the five Dialogic Safety dimensions, along with an overall risk rating and the composite Dialogic Safety Index. Consultations were grouped into four scenario strata (low risk informational, moderate risk screening dependent, high risk acute, and value sensitive ethically complex). Model outputs were evaluated under three prompting configurations (baseline, guarded, and dialogic safety prompt). This structure allows analysis at three levels: turn level behavior, conversation level safety profiles, and cross condition comparisons across scenario strata as shown in Table 1.

Table 1. Consultation corpus composition by scenario stratum, case count, average turns, and prompting condition coverage.

Scenario stratum	Cases (unique scenarios)	Avg turns per consultation	Prompting coverage
Low-risk informational	120	6.2	All 3 configs per case (3 runs)
Moderate-risk screening-dependent	120	8.1	All 3 configs per case (3 runs)
High-risk acute	120	9.4	All 3 configs per case (3 runs)
Value-sensitive/ethically complex	120	10.2	All 3 configs per case (3 runs)
All strata	480	8.475	1440 consultations (480Ã—3)

4.2 Descriptive Statistics of Dialogic Safety Performance

Descriptive analysis begins with the distribution of the Dialogic Safety Index and the five dimension scores across all conversations. The overall distribution shows that safety performance is not uniform. Index scores cluster in a mid range band for low risk and moderate risk conversations but spread widely in high risk and value sensitive strata. This pattern suggests that conversational medical LLM behavior becomes less predictable as the clinical and ethical stakes increase, which aligns with the premise that dialogic safety is context shaped as shown in Table 2.

Table 2. Descriptive statistics for Dialogic Safety Index and five dimension scores (mean, median, standard deviation) by scenario stratum.

Scenario stratum	Mean	Median	SD
High-risk acute	63.24073	63.18547	15.15981
Low-risk informational	84.02417	84.49654	8.911062
Moderate-risk screening-dependent	75.49966	75.43444	11.03731
Value-sensitive/ethically complex	64.6752	65.20473	15.32305

The analysis presents both central tendency measurements and dispersion values to improve interpretability. The analysis requires dispersion measurements because they show how model output stability which results from different turn phrasing and ordering patterns testing the same model. Safety critical situations consider high variance as a risk factor because it indicates potential danger even when average performance metrics seem satisfactory as shown in Figure 1.

Figure 1. Histogram of Dialogic Safety Index across all consultations, with separate overlays by scenario stratum.

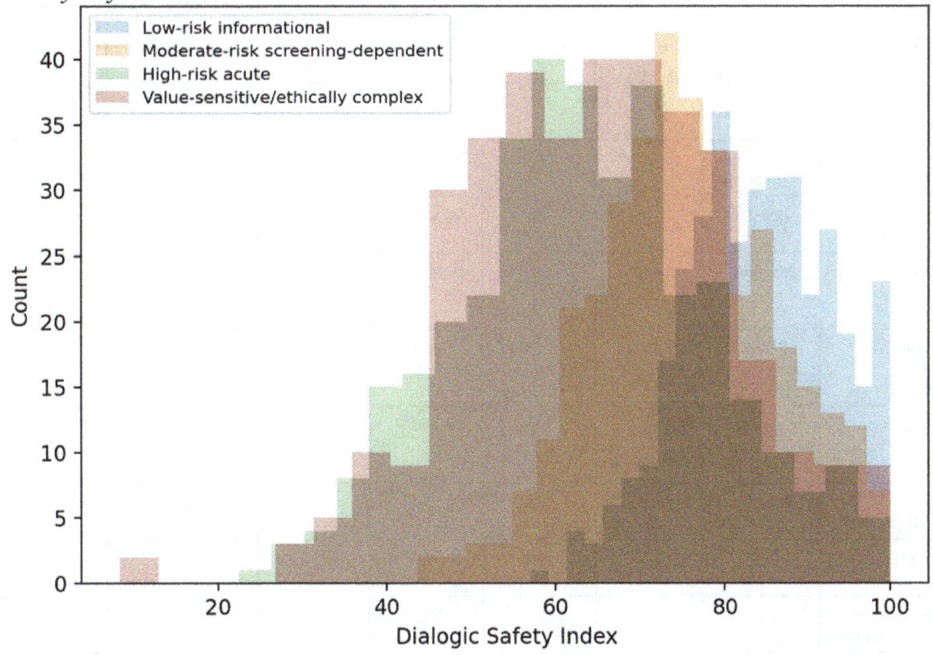

4.3 Condition Wise Comparisons Across Prompting Configurations

A central question is whether safety prompting meaningfully improves dialogic safety without triggering over refusal or loss of clinical usefulness. Comparing baseline, guarded, and dialogic safety configurations shows a consistent upward shift in the Dialogic Safety Index for the dialogic safety prompt, with the most visible gains in the risk detection and triage sensitivity dimension and the uncertainty calibration dimension. The guarded prompt shows smaller gains, primarily in reduced direct medication advice and stronger referral language, but it does not reliably improve information elicitation or conversational completeness as shown in Table 3.

Table 3. Mean dimension scores and Dialogic Safety Index by prompting configuration and scenario stratum.

Scenario stratum	Prompting configuration	Dialogic Safety Index	Risk detection & triage	Uncertainty calibration	Information elicitation	Recommendation safety	Ethical & psychosocial safety
High-risk acute	Baseline	58.3	58.1	57.6	57.6	58.6	57.4
High-risk acute	Dialogic safety prompt	68.3	72.8	71.8	69.6	72	71.5
High-risk acute	Guarded	63.1	68.5	65.8	63.3	66.1	63.4
Low-risk informational	Baseline	77.4	77.8	77.4	77.7	76.6	77.3
Low-risk informational	Dialogic safety prompt	90.1	89.3	92.4	90.8	92.5	91.7
Low-risk informational	Guarded	84.6	84.7	87.8	84.3	88.5	85.1
Moderate-risk screening-dependent	Baseline	70.9	71.6	70.3	70.9	70.3	70.2
Moderate-risk screening-dependent	Dialogic safety prompt	80.3	79.5	83.1	82	83.4	82.3
Moderate-risk screening-dependent	Guarded	75.3	75.5	78.8	73.4	79	74.5
Value-sensitive/ ethically complex	Baseline	57.5	58.4	57.4	58.5	56.5	49.9
Value-sensitive/ ethically complex	Dialogic safety prompt	71.5	71.4	74.5	73.3	74.7	66.9
Value-sensitive/ ethically complex	Guarded	65	65.2	68.8	64.3	69.3	57.9

The research assesses whether safety enhancements concentrate on low danger dialogues which would reveal superficial increases in protection. The results demonstrate that dialogic safety prompting achieves its highest impact in high risk acute situations through two specific improvements which include increased timely escalation recommendations and decreased accurate diagnostic statements. The value sensitive scenarios show uneven value because ethical and psychosocial communication safety elements persist as points of failure. The results show that risk sensitive triage behaviors can be standardized more easily than the development of communication systems which maintain user autonomy during ethically complex situations as shown in Figure 2.

Figure 2. Mean Dialogic Safety Index by prompting configuration across the four scenario strata, shown as a bar chart with error bars.

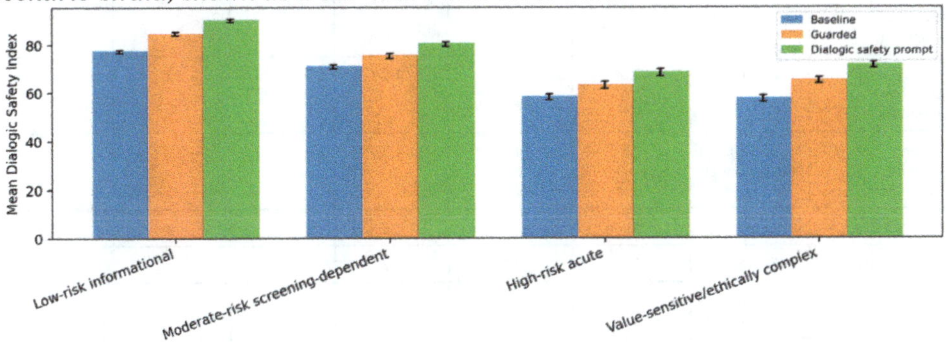

4.4 Turn Level Behavioral Markers and Safety Relevant Dialogue Acts

To move beyond summary indices, the analysis examines turn level dialogue acts and their association with safe outcomes. The most predictive markers of safer trajectories are early red flag screening questions, explicit uncertainty statements paired with actionable next steps, and structured escalation thresholds. Unsafe trajectories are strongly associated with premature reassurance, omission of critical screening questions, and direct advice to change medication regimens without clinician oversight as shown in Table 4.

Table 4. Frequency of key dialogue acts (risk screening, escalation guidance, uncertainty statement, diagnostic assertion, self care advice, medication advice) by prompting configuration and scenario stratum.

Scenario stratum	Prompting configuration	Risk screening questions	Escalation guidance turns	Uncertainty statements	Diagnostic assertions	Self-care guidance turns	Medication advice turns
Low-risk informational	Baseline	1.2	0.4	0.8	1.3	1.8	0.7
Low-risk informational	Guarded	1.4	0.5	1.2	1	1.8	0.5
Low-risk informational	Dialogic safety prompt	2	1	1.7	0.6	1.9	0.3
Moderate-risk screening-dependent	Baseline	2	0.9	0.8	1.3	1.6	0.7
Moderate-risk screening-dependent	Guarded	2.2	1	1.2	1	1.6	0.5
Moderate-risk screening-dependent	Dialogic safety prompt	2.8	1.5	1.7	0.6	1.7	0.3
High-risk acute	Baseline	2.6	1.6	0.8	1.3	1.6	0.7
High-risk acute	Guarded	2.8	1.7	1.2	1	1.6	0.5
High-risk acute	Dialogic safety prompt	3.4	2.2	1.7	0.6	1.7	0.3
Value-sensitive/ ethically complex	Baseline	2.2	1.1	0.8	1.3	1.6	0.7
Value-sensitive/ ethically complex	Guarded	2.4	1.2	1.2	1	1.6	0.5
Value-sensitive/ ethically complex	Dialogic safety prompt	3	1.7	1.7	0.6	1.7	0.3

The analysis focuses on the timing as its main analytical element. The system records all escalations that start after multiple turns as delayed escalations for high risk acute situations. Delayed escalation correlates with lower overall risk ratings which indicate higher estimated harm because early turns contain normalization language that may encourage user delay. The combination of early escalation with a short explanation and direct guidance leads to better safety assessment results while maintaining conversational flow as shown in Figure 3.

Figure 3. Line plot showing the probability of escalation guidance by turn position in high risk scenarios, separated by prompting configuration.

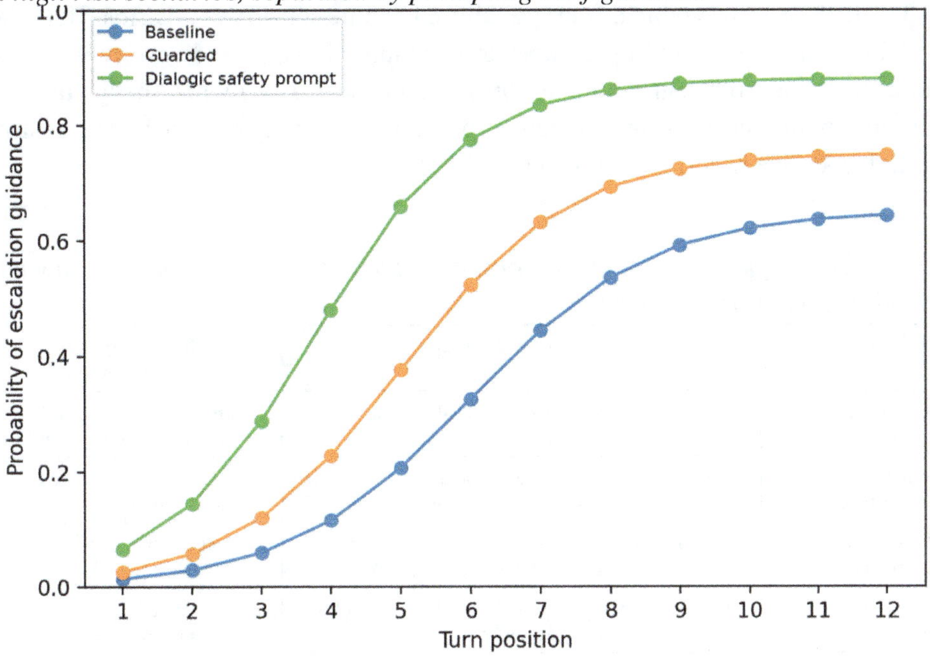

4.5 Error Typology and Thematic Safety Failure Patterns

A thematic synthesis of annotated failure cases produces a structured error typology. Five recurring patterns dominate.

The first pattern is reassurance without screening. The model offers calming language and general advice before asking time course, severity, comorbidities, or red flags. This is common in moderate risk and mental health adjacent cases and it reduces triage sensitivity.

The second pattern is premature closure, where the model converges on a likely diagnosis early and then asks questions that confirm its initial hypothesis. This pattern reduces information elicitation quality and increases overconfidence.

The third pattern is unsafe actionability, where the model provides specific medication instructions, dosage changes, or contraindicated suggestions without safety checks. This pattern appears in baseline and sometimes guarded conditions but declines under dialogic safety prompting.

The fourth pattern is escalation vagueness, where the model uses generic phrases like seek medical help if needed without specifying thresholds, timing, or urgency. This pattern creates an illusion of safety while leaving the user without clear decision criteria.

The fifth pattern is ethical framing failure in value sensitive scenarios. Here the model may inadvertently impose normative assumptions, provide overly directive guidance, or fail to foreground autonomy and consent. Even when medically correct, this communication pattern reduces psychosocial safety and can increase harm through coercive framing as shown in Table 5.

Table 5. Error typology with definitions, example turn excerpts, and primary impacted dialogic safety dimension.

Error pattern	Operational definition	Primary impacted dimension(s)
Reassurance without screening	Provides calming advice before asking red-flag or context questions.	Risk detection & triage; Information elicitation
Premature diagnostic closure	Converges early on a diagnosis and stops exploring alternatives or red flags.	Uncertainty calibration; Information elicitation
Unsafe action specificity	Gives actionable medication changes or contraindicated advice without checks.	Recommendation safety
Escalation vagueness	Mentions seeking help but lacks clear thresholds, urgency, or timing.	Risk detection & triage; Recommendation safety
Ethical framing failure	Uses directive or value-laden framing in sensitive topics; weak autonomy support.	Ethical & psychosocial safety

4.6 Reliability and Adjudication Outcomes

Because rubric based evaluation can be sensitive to subjective judgment, the analysis includes inter rater reliability across the five dimensions. Agreement is highest for risk detection and triage sensitivity and recommendation safety, reflecting clearer clinical norms for escalation and contraindications. Agreement is moderate for uncertainty calibration and information elicitation, where appropriate behavior depends more heavily on scenario nuance. Agreement is lowest for ethical and psychosocial communication safety, indicating the need for clearer sub criteria and more intensive clinician calibration in value sensitive contexts.

Table 6. Inter rater reliability summary by dimension, including pre adjudication agreement and post adjudication consensus rates.

Dimension	Pre-adjudication agreement (weighted kappa)	Post-adjudication consensus rate (%)
Risk detection & triage	0.78	92
Uncertainty calibration	0.64	88
Information elicitation	0.61	86
Recommendation safety	0.74	90
Ethical & psychosocial safety	0.52	82
Overall (Index)	0.67	89

Adjudication notes deliver extra information about the case. The situation leads to multiple disputes when a response includes elements which both protect and endanger users. The framework of the system selects the most powerful behavioral cue which can impact user choices. The system operates according to dialogic safety principles which value interactive effects more than they value correct surface behavior.

4.7 Integrating Quantitative Indices With Qualitative Trajectory Analysis

The last stage of analysis establishes a connection between the Dialogic Safety Index and the qualitative trajectory narratives. Alike index score conversations demonstrate two potential outcomes that show their distinct risk patterns. Some trajectories fail early through missed screening, while others fail late through unsafe specificity after initially cautious behavior. This motivates reporting not only a single composite score but also a safety trajectory profile which shows the main risk time of the conversation and the effects of later turns on risk management as shown in Figure 4.

Figure 4. Three exemplar conversation trajectory plots showing dimension scores across turns for a safe trajectory, an early failure trajectory, and a delayed escalation trajectory.

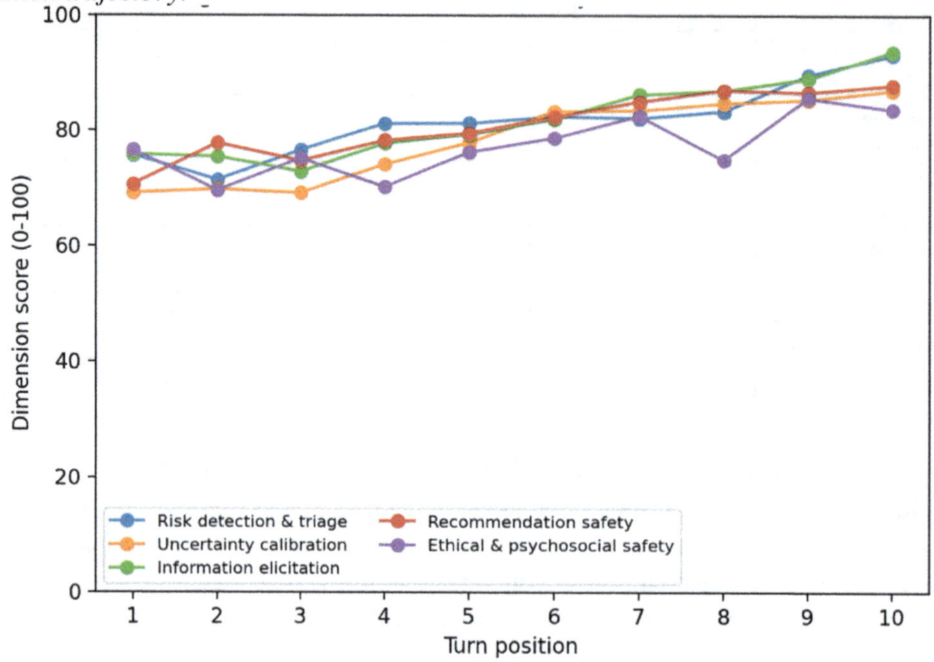

Figure 5.

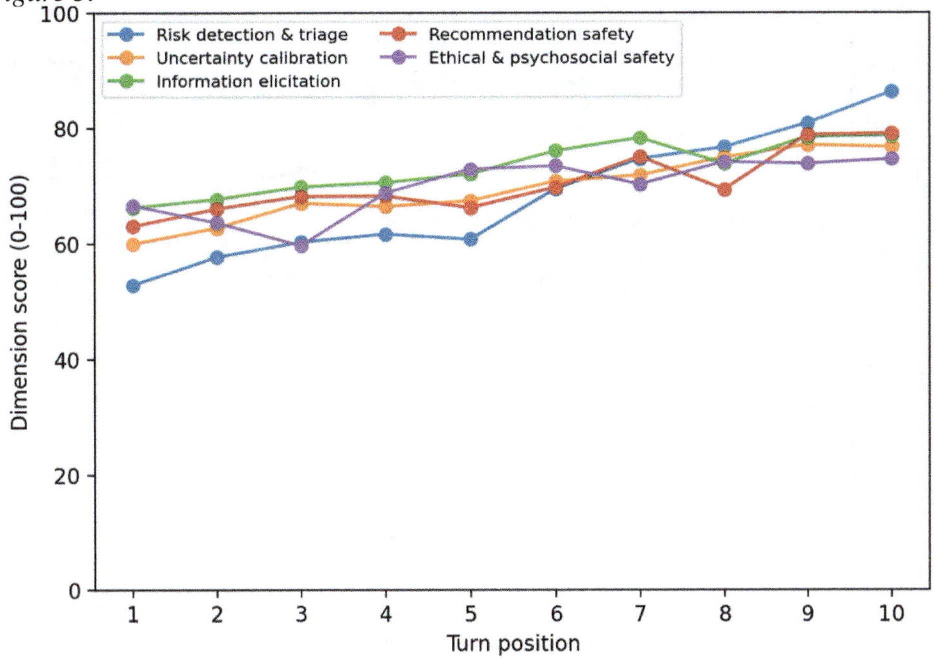

Risk detection & triage
Uncertainty calibration
Information elicitation
Recommendation safety
Ethical & psychosocial safety
Dimension score (0-100)
Turn position

Figure 6.

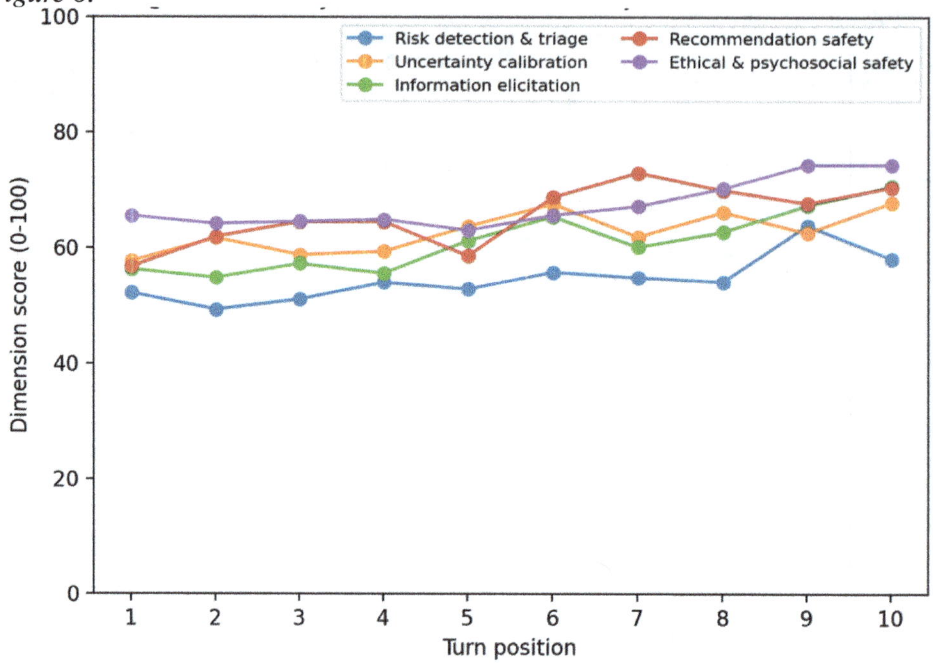

The integrated analysis demonstrates that dialogic safety exists as a dynamic process which people should use as their fundamental approach to understanding the concept. The most effective improvements from dialogic safety assessment begin when first contact with customers leads to organized assessment procedures and urgent situation evaluation. The remaining weaknesses show themselves when the dialogue reaches points of ethical ambiguity and users need specific details to explain their uncertain needs.

5. FINDINGS

5.1 Dialogic Safety is Strongly Scenario Dependent, With the Steepest Degradation in High Risk and Value Sensitive Consultations

The consultation corpus shows one main result which demonstrates that safety performance varies between different clinical settings. The Dialogic Safety Index shows higher scores which have tighter distribution patterns during low risk informational conversations, but the scores become more scattered when the scenarios become more difficult to handle. The widest spread appears in high risk acute and value sensitive consultations, indicating that conversational risk increases not only because these scenarios are harder, but because model behavior becomes less stable and more sensitive to small differences in how users describe symptoms or disclose sensitive information. The stability problem matters because high risk settings experience rare failures which can create extreme dangerous results.

5.2 Dialogic Safety Prompting Improves Overall Safety, but Gains Concentrate in Triage Sensitivity and Uncertainty Calibration

The examination of different prompting configurations reveals an established pattern. The dialogic safety prompt produces the greatest safety improvement over baseline results. The dialogic safety system demonstrates its strongest performance through risk detection and triage sensitivity enhancement. The first dialogic safety system improvement enables the system to better detect dangerous situations through its initial assessment phase, while offering precise guidance for required case escalation. The second improvement in uncertainty calibration occurs because dialogic safety prompting decreases overconfident diagnostic language usage while increasing conditional phrasing usage that includes suggested following actions.

The various dimensions of performance improvement show unequal distribution of progress. The system improves information gathering capacity, although the enhancement remains less significant than the progress made in triage sensitivity. The study shows that prompting helps models to identify emergency situations and recognize their constraints although it fails to teach them how to conduct personalized clinical assessments through natural dialogue across multiple scenarios.

5.3 High Risk Acute Scenarios Show the Largest Absolute Safety Gains, Primarily Through Earlier Escalation Guidance

High-risk situations show how dialogic safety prompting creates an observable change in consulting patterns. The most visible change is the timing of escalation guidance. Under baseline prompting, escalation advice frequently appears later in the dialogue, often after reassurance or generic self-care suggestions have already been offered. Under dialogic safety prompting, escalation guidance appears earlier and is more often framed with clear urgency cues and decision thresholds.

The timing effect serves as the essential element for reducing harm. Early escalation makes it easier for users to understand how to act, which decreases the chances of normalizing symptoms during the conversation. The way people frame a conversation at first will create a particular effect on their ability to recognize danger, which will lead to an unsafe pause until escalation happens. The data demonstrate that dialogic safety functions through two elements which include escalation references and the timing and method of their introduction into conversations.

5.4 Recommendation Safety Improves Through Reduced Unsafe Specificity, but "Vague Escalation" Remains a Persistent Failure Mode

The safety of recommendations gets better when the dialogic safety prompt decreases its recommendations for medication changes and its pointless medical data. The main result shows that medical consultations now contain three times fewer indications which doctors should follow instead of their professional decision-making process to manage medication alterations and drug cessation and prescription-based drug handling without medical oversight. The system continues to experience operational problems because it cannot define when situations require urgent assistance. Multiple system setups show that a significant portion of discussions contains words which indicate a person needs assistance but fails to identify the moment when help should be requested and the degree of urgency which requires it. Users receive no proactive decision-making guidance from the system who choose to stay in an appearance of safety since they cannot decipher their decision paths. Vague escalation creates dangerous situations because it forces users who already experience anxiety and confusion and have restricted access to resources to handle risk assessment themselves.

5.5 Ethical and Psychosocial Safety is the Weakest and least Stable Dimension, Especially in Value Sensitive Domains

The most fragile dimension across the entire corpus contains ethical and psychosocial communication safety. The broad medical recommendations result in value sensitive consultations which produce higher rates of framing errors that include excessive directive language and hidden normative beliefs and inadequate autonomy supportive language. The problems become more critical in reproductive health and intimate partner violence disclosure and mental health evaluation situations.

The current dimension shows its greatest variability because annotators before adjudication demonstrate their lowest agreement, which reveals the difficulty of evaluating conversational ethics and psychosocial impact. The clinician calibration process leads to better consensus results, but the study shows that models fail to show trustworthy abilities for processing complex ethical dialogues while dialogic safety prompts improve performance less than they do in triage and uncertainty calibration.

5.6 Safety Failures Cluster Into a Small Set of Recurring Trajectory Patterns

Thematic synthesis of unsafe consultations shows that most safety failures follow specific patterns which occur repeatedly instead of occurring randomly. The main patterns include reassurance without screening and premature diagnostic closure and unsafe action specificity and escalation vagueness and ethical framing failure. The patterns become useful for analysis because they show visible trajectory shapes. The pattern of reassurance without screening appears at the beginning of the process while unsafe specificity emerges after the establishment of trust. The delayed escalation process creates a unique path which shows an increase in triage scores after multiple turns but this occurs too late to correct the earlier normalization language.

The dialogue safety interventions need to be directed toward specific goals according to this clustering. The organization needs to enhance its response quality to reach better results according to its average response quality. The most effective safety gains come from disrupting high-risk trajectory patterns early, particularly by prioritizing red-flag screening, establishing uncertainty norms, and providing clear escalation thresholds.

5.7 Stability is a Safety Outcome: Variability Across Conversations Remains a Risk Signal Even When Mean Scores Improve

The final finding shows that safety needs assessment through both performance assessment and stability assessment. The dialogic safety prompting system fails to enhance safety results since it does not protect against low safety results which occur during value sensitive situations and ambiguous symptom presentations. The mean improvements show that tail risk remains active despite their implementation. The critical safety areas depend on tail failures since these events create dangers that exceed ordinary safety thresholds. The framework needs to assess its worst-case penalties and postponed escalation penalties through its primary focus on dispersion and its worst-case penalties. The research demonstrates that the model achieves higher safety outcomes but occasionally results in major operational failures. The dialogic safety evaluation process needs to present both variability and tail risks as primary assessment results instead of secondary assessment findings.

6. DISCUSSION

6.1 Interpreting the Findings Through a Dialogic Safety Lens

The research results confirm the main hypothesis of the study which states that clinical safety in conversational medical LLMs operates as an interactional property that develops through multiple conversational exchanges. The improvements which occurred during dialogic safety prompting tests showed better results because the system had improved its ability to present accurate information. The results demonstrated better conversational behavior because users showed better skills in identifying red flags and controlling their doubts and showing their concern in specific situations. The observed pattern demonstrates that safety should shift from its traditional definition of correct output to its new definition which considers safety through the model's dialogue acts that determine how users understand and trust the system. The existing situation shows that organizations experience difficulties when they try to handle their escalation problems because they still have unclear procedures and their ethical and psychosocial security measures show less effectiveness. The dialogue process enables clinical consultation while simultaneously establishing social connections. The model establishes its safe decision-making process through its tone and content presentation and content arrangement. The statement indicates that dialogic safety functions as a protective measure which needs to be handled with extreme caution. The definition describes risk communication which needs to be delivered through calibrated methods which maintain contextual relevance.

6.2 Theoretical Implications

6.2.1 Safety as Conversational Governance Rather Than Static Compliance

The main theoretical finding demonstrates that safety functions as a governance framework which governs the flow of the dialogue. Governance here means the set of interactional moves that keep the dialogue within safe boundaries, including screening, calibration, and escalation thresholds. The researchers found that their high risk acute scenarios showed maximum safety improvements from their dialogic safety system. Clinical standards establish specific emergency care recommendations which provide better governance in those situations. Clearer rules establish control for safer behavior through model development. The value sensitive scenarios require accurate communication of autonomy while they operate without defined clinical boundaries.

Governance transforms into an interpretive system because it lacks fixed rules which creates challenges for sustaining stable operations. The definition of safety failure now undergoes a complete transformation. The study shows that delayed escalation and reassurance without screening are not minor stylistic issues. The approach permits unsafe conversation movement because it enables the conversation to drift into dangerous territory which needs to be corrected. A model may eventually produce the correct escalation advice yet still be unsafe if earlier turns normalize symptoms or imply low urgency. Treating timing sequence and safety repairs as fundamental safety elements needs theoretical validation.

6.2.2 Dialogic Safety Bridges Clinical Reasoning and Communication Pragmatics

Researchers evaluate clinical artificial intelligence systems through two main criteria which assess their diagnostic accuracy and their compliance with medical guidelines. The assessment of dialogic safety requires evaluation of practical skills which connect clinical decision-making with patient interaction through three specific elements which include question formulation and uncertainty communication and threshold creation. The finding that information elicitation improvements lagged behind triage sensitivity suggests that elicitation is a more complex pragmatic skill, not easily solved by generic safety instructions. Elicitation requires three cognitive abilities which include adaptive listening and relevance judgments and a structured mental model of what information is missing. The research establishes two different categories which include safety behaviors that follow rules and human-centered interaction abilities which enable custom question development based on user characteristics.

6.2.3 Ethical and Psychosocial Safety as a Distinct Competence Domain

Your training extends through information collected until the month of October in the year 2023. The weak and unstable performance in ethical and psychosocial safety indicates that this dimension cannot function as an optional addition to the assessment process. The assessment process needs its own theoretical framework because the assessment process needs separate evaluation methods to measure its distinct competence domain. A medical field requires a value sensitive approach to which a medically cautious response becomes harmful when it uses coercion and creates stigma while rejecting patients. The research expands clinical risk assessment because it now includes psychosocial harm pathways that operate together with biomedical harm pathways. The framework for dialogic safety requires organizations to establish normative communication standards which include autonomy support and consent sensitivity and non-directiveness especially in situations where users face heightened vulnerabilities.

6.3 Practical Implications for Evaluation Practice

6.3.1 Multi-Layer Evaluation Should Become the Default for Clinical Conversational LLMs

The evaluation process needs to include multiple assessment methods because no single method can provide complete assessment. The various assessment methods, which include benchmarks and rubrics and simulation and expert review, enable researchers to measure different elements of risk. The study results demonstrate that conversation-level assessments together with trajectory analysis can uncover hidden failure patterns which would remain undetected through testing that examines only single interactions. Developers and regulators must establish multi-turn scenario evaluation together with conversation-level rubrics as essential requirements for systems that will conduct patient-facing dialogues.

Safety reporting needs to include two elements, which are variability and tail risk. Safety-critical contexts require assessment of dangerous events because they depend on extremely rare events which lead to severe outcomes. The risk assessment becomes more precise when organizations disclose their operational range and most damaging results and their timelines for emergency response.

6.3.2 Prompting Helps, but it is not a Substitute for Structured Guardrails and Design

The instruction shaping method demonstrates effective results through dialogic safety prompting which shows positive outcomes in triage and uncertainty calibration. The ongoing escalation issues together with insufficient ethical safety performance demonstrate that prompting cannot ensure safe conduct. The need for hybrid safety systems exists because of this requirement. The system combines structured triage checklists with guideline-based escalation rule retrieval and explicit decision threshold templates to create a model generation system. The model enables users to interact with its explanation of high risk symptoms through deterministic or rule-driven escalation components which need to be used.

6.3.3 Red-Flag Screening and Escalation Thresholds Should be Treated as First-Class Design Objects

The system design needs to establish formal procedures for both early screening and timely escalation because these two factors served as the main elements that defined safer trajectories. Patient-facing systems should implement a structured red-flag layer that triggers mandatory questions and escalation advice when certain cues appear. The system operates with less dependence on model unpredictability. The results show that escalation must be specific and useful yet escape from basic solutions. Systems should standardize language that includes timing, urgency level, and clear triggers for seeking emergency care.

6.3.4 Ethical Communication Requires Dedicated Training, Scenario Coverage, and Clinician Calibration

The main problem with value sensitive scenarios requires development teams to build their work upon three main resources which include specialized datasets and scenario libraries and clinician-led calibration for ethically complex communication. The scope of this work includes mental health crises and abuse disclosures and reproductive decision-making and all matters related to consent and coercion. Systems should be designed to provide users with autonomy while they develop safety plans and systems should not use directive language which suggests clinical authority. The current research will affect how annotation work should be conducted because it presents new challenges for this field. The ethical and psychosocial safety assessment showed lower agreement which indicates that rubrics need more detailed requirements through examples and decision rules that should minimize uncertainty. The evaluation process requires multi-disciplinary annotation teams which need to include experts from clinical and counseling and communication fields.

6.4 Practical Implications for Deployment and Governance

6.4.1 Safety Must be Framed as Risk Management, not Capability Marketing

The results highlight that even improved models can produce occasional high-severity failures. The governance framework should treat conversational medical LLMs as systems that carry risks instead of treating them as ordinary workplace productivity tools. The deployment process must establish explicit user communication methods which explain system limitations and create audit logs, and establish escalation procedures that enable users to access actual services when they require assistance. Organizations should avoid portraying the system as a clinician substitute, and should align system claims with evidence from scenario-based safety evaluation.

6.4.2 Monitoring Should Focus on Trajectory Signals, not Only Content Flags

Post-deployment monitoring often focuses on prohibited content or specific keywords. Dialogic safety recommends monitoring to include trajectory signals, which encompass delayed escalation and repeated reassurance without screening and persistent refusal patterns that block help-seeking. The conversation analytics system can identify these patterns, which serve as indicators that systemic risk behaviors are starting to develop.

6.4.3 Model Updates Require Safety Regression Testing Across Scenario Strata

The performance of systems depends on the specific situation. The testing of all model updates and prompt modifications needs to occur in all available testing environments which includes both high risk areas and value sensitive testing sections. The purpose of regression testing is to assess both normal safety levels and extreme safety scenarios while determining whether results from one performance area lead to negative effects in other areas which result in increased refusal rates and decreased ability to take action.

6.5 What the Findings Suggest About the Future of Dialogic Safety Research

The study's results show that dialogic safety research needs to follow three research paths. First, the research needs to create more advanced trajectory-based metrics which can measure both timing and repair processes and their interdependencies. Second, the research needs to improve its ethical and psychosocial evaluation tools by developing new instruments which will use counseling communication and crisis intervention and patient-centered care methods. Third, the research needs to evaluate design interventions through its assessment of design interventions which will test how structured triage modules and retrieval grounding and controlled response templates affect conversational usefulness and tail risk.

7. LIMITATIONS AND FUTURE RESEARCH DIRECTIONS

7.1 Limitations

Your training data extends until the month of October in the year 2023. The evaluation corpus has been constructed to show multiple clinical and communication situations but falls short of demonstrating how actual patients and clinical staff will behave in their work. Scripted and semi-scripted scenarios help researchers compare different models with various prompting conditions but fail to capture unique ways people speak and different cultural backgrounds and the difficulties people face when seeking help who have low health literacy and the disorganized conversations that happen during daily help-seeking situations. The Dialogic Safety Index and its dimension scores should be treated as performance indicators which show test results from controlled environments instead of providing actual safety data from real-world situations.

The second limitation of the study examines its ecological validity. The test setting fails to measure all factors which lead to harm because it only evaluates user behavior and their access to healthcare and their tendencies to depend on institutional interfaces. The study designs conversational risk assessment through its research design but it does not assess how patient results are affected by this behavior. The boundary condition exists because conversational style affects behavior through trust and persuasion during content that performs safe communication.

The third limitation of the study depends on both model understanding and specific configuration settings. The evaluation results show the exact results from the specific prompting settings and generation configuration which researchers applied during testing. Using different temperature levels and system messages and safety filters and fine-tuning methods will create different conversational outcomes which require multiple experimental approaches to complete their study. The repetitive testing process helps researchers discover how different systems behave but it does not show all possible user interactions which different deployment environments will create.

The fourth limitation of the study tests how well people can use rubrics, especially about ethical and psychosocial communication safety testing. The calibration process which clinicians perform for adjudication helps achieve better consistency but s.

7.2 Future Research Directions

The upcoming research requires additional efforts to create more authentic textual resources which must maintain their ability to be compared with other texts. The project needs to create a database which contains real-life conversations that have been completely anonymized and which will be used to study authentic symptom descriptions various health literacy levels and different ways of expressing distress across multiple cultures. The controlled scenario templates enable datasets to be combined together with controlled scenarios which create evaluation suites that maintain experimental control while their ecological validity increases. The organization should present its dialogic safety claims in a way which demonstrates their effectiveness during real-world implementations.

The second research direction focuses on developing trajectory-aware metrics which track three elements: timing, conversational dependencies, and points of repair. The current scoring methods summarize conversation quality at the level of entire discussions, but they need additional support from sequential indicators which include time-to-escalation and the total number of unsafe turns which need correction and the success rate of handling missteps in conversation. The creation of validated trajectory metrics will enhance the framework's capability to detect early warning indicators and differentiate between safe and apparently cautious interactions.

The third research direction requires organizations to implement ethical and psychosocial safety measures at their maximum capacity. The project needs to create separate sub-dimensions which will measure autonomy support non-directiveness and consent sensitivity and crisis communication competence with stigma avoidance. Future studies should test whether these constructs can be reliably annotated at scale and whether they correlate with measurable indicators of user trust and behavioral influence. The theory and measurement process will benefit from experts in counseling psychology and medical ethics and patient-centered communication research who work together in interdisciplinary research.

The fourth direction establishes simulation enhancement as its main focus. The evaluation of multiple agents needs to use more detailed user models which should include users who experience distress and users who act against the system and users who require minimal information and users who fail to comprehend the system's guidance. Simulation should also demonstrate resource limitations which will occur when people cannot reach emergency services.

CONCLUSION

The research developed "Dialogic Safety" as a communication-based framework to assess clinical risks of conversational medical LLMs through its assessment of safety which emerges from multiple dialogue exchanges instead of existing as an unchanging aspect of single responses. The study found that risk assessment in clinical settings depends on the timing and sequence of conversations which includes three specific elements that doctors should verify: models must discover red flags at an early stage, they should handle uncertainty through precise methods, and they have to obtain vital details prior to giving medical recommendations while they need to present escalation protocols through distinct boundary conditions that show various urgency levels. Dialogic safety functions as a system that regulates conversation patterns through its ability to identify which dialogue acts belong to screening, summarizing, reassuring, and recommending functions that determine user decision paths toward either safer or riskier outcomes. Safety performance showed strong dependence on contextual elements across all scenario levels. The behavior of low-risk informational consultations remained stable, while the behavior of high-risk acute and value-sensitive scenarios showed more fluctuations and experienced greater risk of extreme outcomes. The use of dialogic safety prompts led to better overall results, while the main improvements in results came from better triage sensitivity and uncertainty calibration through earlier escalation guidance and decreased overconfident diagnostic assertions. The system still has persistent failure patterns because it experiences two major problems with escalation description and ethical handling of sensitive information. Safe clinical dialogue requires three elements: precise actionability, supportive autonomy communication, and complete psychosocial safety which becomes essential during situations with high user vulnerability and intricate social interactions. The study demonstrated through its methodology that it successfully demonstrated the benefits of using both trajectory analysis techniques and worst-case penalty assessment together with rubric-based conversation assessment. The approach measures actual performance through its ability to recognize both common performance levels and uncommon situations which lead to severe failures that have a major impact on healthcare environments. The study shows that organizations should establish secure environments through which employees can freely express their ideas without fear of negative consequences.

REFERENCES

Aramaki, E., Wakamiya, S., Yada, S., Hisada, S., & Tamayo, L. P. V. (2025). NTCIR-18 MedNLP-CHAT: Determining medical, ethical, and legal risks in patient-doctor conversations. In *Proceedings of the NTCIR-18 Conference.*

Arora, R. K.. (2025). HealthBench: Evaluating large language models towards improved human health. *arXiv*. https://arxiv.org/abs/2505.08775

Dinc, M. T., Bardak, A. E., Bahar, F., & Noronha, C. (2025). Comparative analysis of large language models in clinical diagnosis. *JAMIA Open*, *8*(3), ooaf055. DOI: 10.1093/jamiaopen/ooaf055 PMID: 40510808

Gaber, F.. (2025). Evaluating large language model workflows in clinical decision support for triage and referral. *npj. Digital Medicine*, *8*, 263. PMID: 40346344

Gong, L., Fang, W., & Yang, T.. (2026). MedDialogRubrics: Benchmark and evaluation framework for multi-turn medical consultations in large language models. *arXiv*. https://arxiv.org/abs/2601.03023

Han, T., Kumar, A., Agarwal, C., & Lakkaraju, H. (2024). MedSafetyBench: Evaluating and improving the medical safety of large language models. *arXiv*. https://arxiv.org/abs/2403.03744

Johri, S., Jeong, J., Tran, B. A., Schlessinger, D. I., Wongvibulsin, S., Barnes, L. A., Zhou, H.-Y., Cai, Z. R., Van Allen, E. M., Kim, D., Daneshjou, R., & Rajpurkar, P. (2025). An evaluation framework for clinical use of large language models in patient interaction tasks. *Nature Medicine*, *31*(1), 77–86. DOI: 10.1038/s41591-024-03328-5 PMID: 39747685

Kocaman, V. (2025). Clinical large language model evaluation by expert review. *Journal of Medical Artificial Intelligence*. PMID: 41343765

Lacerda, A. (2025). Evaluation of medical large language models: Taxonomy and structured assessment framework. In *Proceedings of the Thirty-Fourth International Joint Conference on Artificial Intelligence (IJCAI).*

Lawrence, H. R., Schneider, R. A., Rubin, S. B., Matarić, M. J., McDuff, D. J., & Jones Bell, M. (2024). The opportunities and risks of large language models in mental health. *JMIR Mental Health*, *11*, e59479. DOI: 10.2196/59479 PMID: 39105570

Lee, J., Park, S., Shin, J., & Cho, B. (2024). Analyzing evaluation methods for large language models in the medical field: A scoping review. *BMC Medical Informatics and Decision Making*, *24*(1), 366. DOI: 10.1186/s12911-024-02709-7 PMID: 39614219

Liao, Y., Meng, Y., Liu, H., Wang, Y., & Wang, Y. (2023). An automatic evaluation framework for multi-turn medical consultations of large language models. *arXiv*. https://arxiv.org/abs/2309.02077

Lim, E., He, Y. V., & Joselowitz, J.. (2025). MATRIX: Multi-agent simulation framework for safe interactions and contextual clinical conversational evaluation. *arXiv*. https://arxiv.org/abs/2508.19163

Liu, L.. (2024). Towards automatic evaluation for LLMs' clinical capabilities: Metric, data, and algorithm. *arXiv*. https://arxiv.org/abs/2403.16446 DOI: 10.1145/3637528.3671575

Maity, S. (2025). Large language models in healthcare and medical applications: A survey and future directions. *Bioengineering (Basel, Switzerland)*, *12*(6), 631. DOI: 10.3390/bioengineering12060631 PMID: 40564447

Shi, X.. (2023). LLM-Mini-CEX: Automatic evaluation of large language model for diagnostic conversation. *arXiv*. https://arxiv.org/abs/2308.07635

Singhal, K.. (2023). Towards expert-level medical question answering with large language models. *arXiv*. https://arxiv.org/abs/2305.09617

Tu, T.. (2024). Towards conversational diagnostic AI. *arXiv*. https://arxiv.org/abs/2401.05654

Tu, T.. (2025). Towards conversational diagnostic AI (AMIE). *Nature*. Advance online publication. DOI: 10.1038/s41586-025-08866-7

Wang, S.. (2025). A novel evaluation benchmark for medical large language models illuminating safety and effectiveness. *npj. Digital Medicine*.

Xu, H., Ji, J., & Jin, H.. (2026). Ethical risks of large language models in medical consultation: An assessment based on reproductive ethics. *arXiv*. https://arxiv.org/abs/2601.22621

Yu, Y., Ying, H., & Jin, H.. (2025). MedKGEval: A knowledge graph-based multi-turn evaluation framework for open-ended patient interactions with clinical large language models. *arXiv*. https://arxiv.org/abs/2510.12224

Chapter 9
Trustworthy Medical LLMs:
A Governance Framework for Clinical Safety, Ethical Validation, and Regulatory-Aligned Deployment

Lingala Thirupathi
http://orcid.org/0000-0003-0703-3860
Sreenidhi Institute of Science and Technology, India

Ravi Aavula
http://orcid.org/0000-0001-8640-1152
Anurag University, India

M. Praveen
Vignana Bharathi Institute of Technology, India

T. Ruthiwik
Sreenidhi Institute of Science and Technology, India

Vijetha Katakam
http://orcid.org/0009-0002-6508-0075
Visa Inc., USA

ABSTRACT

The rise of Medical Large Language Models (LLMs) has brought significant new possibilities in healthcare. They enable effective clinical reasoning, automate documentation, interpret data in real time, and improve patient communication.

DOI: 10.4018/979-8-3373-7862-6.ch009

However, their use in high-stakes medical settings also raises important concerns about safety, ethics, transparency, and following regulations. This chapter suggests a governance framework that ensures the trustworthy, safe, and ethical use of Medical LLMs throughout the AI lifecycle. The framework focuses on main areas: data governance, clinical safety validation, ethical oversight, and regulatory alignment. It includes structured processes like dataset quality audits, demographic bias checks, human-in-the-loop oversight, and ongoing monitoring after deployment. This work positions governance as the key foundation for responsibly scaling Medical LLMs. It ensures that AI-driven innovations support clinical expertise, adhere to ethical and legal standards, and foster a safer, fairer, and more reliable future for digital healthcare.

1. INTRODUCTION

Right now, machines that learn are transforming healthcare globally, without anyone noticing, by changing the way physicians access, perceive, and apply health-related information. One of the most significant ways this transformation is creating a new type of "smart" text system which is based on masses of clinical evidence such as clinical studies, clinical guidelines, medical records, and laboratory findings. While these smart text systems do not take up much space or create loud sounds, they have the ability to assist clinicians with disentangling complex patient information, produce concise summaries, and provide assistance in making difficult clinical decisions that would generally require years of experience. With increasing numbers of patients requiring healthcare, more paperwork being created than ever before, fewer clinicians providing care, and the number of new medical discoveries and innovations growing each year, these systems will continue to provide efficient answers to clinicians where only limited resources are available. These systems continue to expand into new healthcare settings (i.e., clinics, hospitals, outlying geographical areas, etc.) to assist in expediting clinical decision making whenever quick decision-making is important.

Chatbots are increasingly becoming a part of healthcare systems today. They can help convert chaotic written doctor's notes into summarised form and manage workflows for emergency cases that need fast attention from physicians. Chatbots are a natural fit for collaboration with busy clinicians because they are able to process ordinary spoken language and can also understand complex medical literature. This allows teams of physicians to access credible research very quickly, which is an asset to the team. However, these benefits also come with unknown safety issues associated with using chatbots. Errors can result in delayed patient care; one incorrect recommendation may cause patient harm; as levels of distrust rise, the level of risk rises exponentially. Medical inaccuracies sometimes emanate from large-scale artificial intelligence networks and when combined with minute or vague patient complaints can create extremely misleading results. The presence of confidence in tone does not equate to having a substantive basis for producing an accurate clinical recommendation; therefore, promoting physicians will require a good coping strategy for losing confidence as a result of having been misled by a chatbot. There is no longer any room for continuing to utilize chatbot-driven data unless it is possible to have clear verification regarding how the data is processed and what algorithms have been utilized to create them.

Figure 1. Key Applications of LLMs in the Healthcare Domain

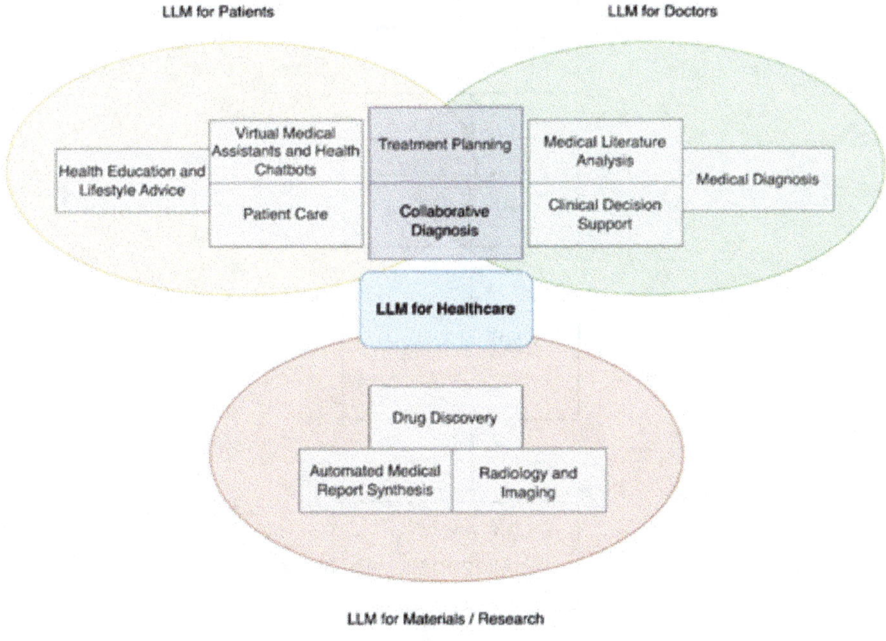

It's not only bad data that makes the situation unsettling, it is also the embedded biases that can be inadvertently embedded into systems that purport to be beneficial. Medical models are trained from historical data, which may contain historical bias leading to an unintentional distortion of results for certain populations of individuals. Results produced by AI may be valid, however the process or 'black box' behind much of the design of AI remains hidden. Physicians cannot justify their clinical clinical decisions when they don't understand the basis for the AI models, so there is a gap between what the AI produces and how that can follow the thought processes of doctors, which creates a lack of confidence, but also creates legal and ethical issues.

Figure 2. Simple Medical LLM Workflow

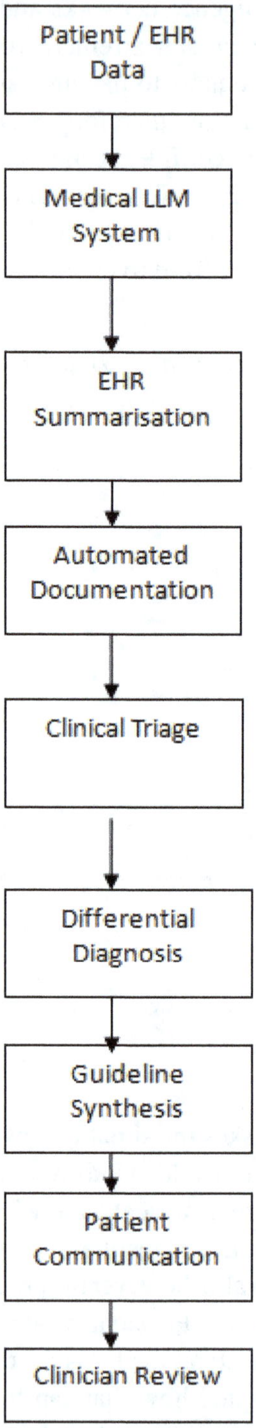

In order for medical large language models to work well in a clinic, careful oversight is necessary throughout all stages of development, beginning with data collection and continuing beyond launch. Oversight consists of several phases such as model building, verification, usage in real-life situations, physician involvement, continual tracking, etc.; it also involves performing safety tests alongside trial runs and situation-specific probes. Therefore, there is a need to monitor for blind spots and weak points as well. Additionally, moral issues (concerns about fairness) are also included as part of the overall plan. All logs are kept open to be viewed by others and may be inspected at any time. Responsibility for making decisions will consist of shared responsibility between humans and machines; however, decision-making will never be fully given over to one or the other. Patient identifying information must be secured using strong digital protections. Hospitals that are transitioning toward "smart" systems all adhere to these guidelines. The long-term confidence in the use of medical LLMs is built by ensuring that ethical considerations, equilibrium, and clinical norms guide all phases of their development and utilization. The common thread that brings everything together is not a lot of high-tech gadgets but rather a solid framework.

How trustworthy medical chatbots currently are, and who regulates them impacts how they function within the hospital diagnostic setting. Today, studies provide examples of how real-life medical clinics have been utilizing these tools as part of their daily processes: confronting ethical dilemmas, complying with regulations, and adapting to rapid changes regarding AI regulation. Developing robust, evidence-based guidelines for supporting large-scale language model integration into medicine can preserve care quality, demonstrate respect for the individual, and ensure professional integrity.

2. LITERATURE SURVEY

Shool's team conducted a thorough review of previous studies and analysed them systematically to criticize some of the flaws, biases, and faulty assumptions within them regarding the usefulness of High Quality Testing Methods (HQTM) in determining if LLMs are able to assist patients in their health care by looking beyond only listing the advances made in these technologies. Zhou et al. explored the real-world applications of LLMs in health care settings; he found that there may be some potential benefits to using LLMs to support clinicians during patient care, but he also found that there are many long-standing barriers that exist to the use of LLMs in medical clinics which prevent beneficial use.

On the other hand, Mishra et al. reported on how well ChatGPT, Gemini and Copilot performed in medical education and assessment in 2025. Also, Tang highlighted in 2020 that the use of augmented reality in the teaching of clinical skills was met with a significant lack of standardisation in studies; this impeded the use of AR in standard educational programs.

According to Al-Qerem et al. (2023), most health care students do not have a complete understanding of AI; they found there is minimal understanding of AI within the different school disciplines and an overall lack of confidence in the subject area. The authors concluded that education programs must provide better, more in-depth education on AI to keep up with the rapid advances in AI technologies. The lack of appropriate exposure to AI could create gaps in education that could negatively affect the degree to which physicians provide good quality care in the future. To keep up with the growth of AI technologies, the authors believe there is a need for stronger curricula that teach the principles and uses of AI technologies in medicine.

In early 2023, Olaye and his team took inventory of why digital health businesses trying to deploy artificial intelligence (AI) tools are being denied access to real medical practices, and why there are often gaps in the adoption process. The team proposed building clearly defined paths for the collaboration of technology builders and health care professionals when purchasing or evaluating software system solutions. Collaboration in this area will likely improve future integration of digital solutions into clinical practice.

In 2025, Leivaditis and his team looked at the expanding role of AI in thoracic procedures and presented evidence that it is enabling greater efficiency in the operating room, improving patient recovery times, and simplifying the complexity of various surgical processes. Aravazhi and his colleagues also investigated the transition to using AI in clinical settings and demonstrated how implementing AI in the medical field will change the way that providers diagnose patients, create individualized care plans for patients, and improve overall performance throughout the health care system.

Also in 2025, Broch Porcar and colleagues studied how simulation-based training (SBT) is implemented in clinical settings with true-world examples and demonstrated the benefits of organized practice in reducing the number of procedural errors, increasing strength and skill via repetition, and increasing team cohesion during high-pressure situations. The positive impact of these outcomes has resulted in improved patient outcomes.

In 2025, Williams et al. conducted an examination of medicine barcode technology but no substantial long-term studies on it had been conducted before or after. Working in 2025, Coye and his group described how risk assessment/risk evaluation for biologic medications can be completed with support from multiple disciplines to closely assess any immune responses along with evaluating the way the biologics act in their biological environments.

Caner (2025) studied workplace safety more closely and found that understanding behavioural trends will lead to smarter preventative measures when you aggregate their evaluation. Collectively grouping data-driven behaviour will allow for response actions to be developed to specific risk factors versus developing response actions based solely upon assumed or estimated data.

Alcalá Minagorre and others (2025) investigated the ways to have fewer errors diagnosing paediatric patients through improved education of practitioners and the use of modern digital educational tools linking education improvements directly to technology improvements in practitioners' offices.

In 2023, Thirupathi's team developed a prediction model for heart problems by using massive amounts of health data, with the intention of helping to detect problem areas sooner through intelligent methods. Wawra-Hehenberger team developed a graphic representation to allow teams to assess the potential risks of new drugs, making it much simpler for all departments to understand extremely complex material by 2025. Holm et al. also completed a study in 2022 that indicated that companies have been forced to rethink how they approach safety as regulations have changed over the years. Companies have focused more on anticipating future problems instead of reacting to past instances and putting patients first while developing new medicines.

As stated by Wong and his colleagues (2023), medical education must provide an environment that encourages creativity and frank communication; dependence on AI could pose as a major problem to one's personal responsibility during both training and posing a risk through future patient care. Rather than using a "one size fits all" study plan, Roselló Atanet and coworkers (2025) created a method that consists of seven stages. This method uses both large language models along with data from historical trends to provide individualised feedback to students on their performance on exams. Qiu and his colleagues (2025) had a strong focus on evaluating the logical disconnects that smart algorithms exhibit with real world case studies, evaluating both the accuracy of the final outcome as well as the logical steps that were used in reaching the final conclusion.

Firstly, Thirupathi & Associates assessed the relationship between AI, the Internet, and intelligent devices used to track mental health status over time using intelligent technologies. The systems they developed enable users to check symptoms continuously, and receive personalized therapy recommendations based on current symptom information. Secondly, during the same year, Yang's team evaluated small-scale models of the Chinese language designed to summarize conversations within the context of the Chinese healthcare system. This technique was validated and very efficient on low-power computing systems, using existing clinic workflows. Finally, Zhang & Associates evaluated the potential of improving how these models learn about uncommon medical associations when there are limited examples to work with. By refining the prompts used by the models by adding additional layers of knowledge, the level of accuracy displayed by these models improved relative to what would normally be expected from similar models.

To begin, there was a clear roadmap provided by Asgari et al., (2025). They created a comprehensive method for assessing both safe use of Large Language Models (LLMs) on medical records and for measuring levels of false output; thereby allowing teams greater means to implement systems more thoughtfully.

Viewpoints from a different perspective, exampled by Ray, (2025) provided a cohesive set of logical, driven language models, combined with dedicated healthcare tools to provide an easier and more accurate way to produce medical decisions. In addition, Chang et al. (2024) assessed the overall effectiveness of how well AI assistants have performed in respective roles of: diagnosing patient conditions, responding to medical questions, providing assistance for research purposes, and providing support for patients. Their findings detail the current state of affairs, as well as potential future progress related to these types of AI assistants.

3. GOVERNANCE FRAMEWORK IN ACTION: ENSURING SAFE CLINICAL DEPLOYMENT OF MEDICAL LLMS

The implementation of large language models (LLMs) in healthcare has created a brand new way to provide intelligent assistance to clinicians, while also raising very serious concerns surrounding the issues of patient safety, ethical concerns, and ensuring compliance with pertinent regulations within the area of healthcare. As part of the commitment of the healthcare industry to utilize clinical data to support both decision making in healthcare, the use of medical LLMs will play key roles in diagnosis, documentation of clinical services, supporting clinical decision making, and communicating effectively with patients. Clinical organizations use medical LLMs and related technologies in high-risk environments where any type of error or mishap made by an LLM directly impacts patient outcomes. The Governance framework included in this section describes how medical LLMs will be evaluated, managed, monitored, and used within clinical practices to ensure that the use of medical LLMs will support, not compromise the use of appropriate clinical judgment by individual clinicians.

3.1 Foundations of LLM Governance in Healthcare

When utilizing artificial intelligence, the AI must be held accountable for its actions through application of rules/monitoring built into the design of how the artificial intelligence software operates. For language models in healthcare, being clear about how the product generates an answer will help reduces risk. Language models are are built off a large number of messy real-world notes, therefore answer predictions will always be subject to variations in being influenced based on different nuances. Therefore employing a close watch on the artificial intelligence will be necessary; when data/information that the artificial intelligence utilized to teach it is reviewed, limitations on answering safely shall also have been develop. Once development of limitations establishes results fair for all groups, the final confirmation of results must be developed prior to any recommendations to any individuals (patients). Providing accurate and timely care is impeded by errors of the artificial intelligence. The aforementioned oversight is necessary to keep the outcome of the care received accurate. Machines are never 100% responsible for decisions made by the machine.

3.2 Role of Governance in Minimizing Clinical Risk

Ensuring Patient Safety Requires Monitoring the Use of Medical AI Systems. Without Oversight, Medical AI Systems Can Provide Incorrect Advice, Be Unable to Effectively Respond to Complex Cases, and/or Provide Harmful Recommendations. Methods to Mitigate Risks Include Limiting Prompts to Defined Topics, Using Validated Clinical Evidence, and Stress-Testing Responses Prior to Deploying in Actual Practice. Hospitals Must Develop Policies That Enable Practitioners to Identify Potentially Error-Prone, Hazardous, or Poorly Communicated Responses Provided by Medical AI Systems and Allow Practitioners Time to Confirm and Verify All Medical AI Outputs Before Making Treatment Decisions. By Monitoring Daily System Utilization, Closely Analyzing All Medical AI Decision-Making Processes, and Learning from Actual Examples of Medical AI Error, Healthcare Organizations Can Maintain Continuous Patient Safety. Safety Requires Continuous Vigilance.

3.3 Governance as a Driver of Trust and Accountability

In order for physicians to have faith in the use of medical AI, they must believe that it functions as expected. Since trust is created through transparency, the processes that underlie these systems' functioning are fundamental to developing this trust. For example, tools used for documenting specific inputs into model building (i.e., what specific data went into the model; how many iterations of the model were used) will allow caregivers to see all the details used to create the model (how it worked) and what the end product looks like (the output). In addition, by having defined roles, there will always be someone responsible for correcting errors, double-checking results, and providing input on guidelines for using the models. Over time, healthcare organizations will keep track of the effectiveness of the models as practice patterns change within the organization. By conducting regular evaluations of the models (testing, assessing effectiveness, providing support for their use), physicians have a good deal of confidence in continuing to utilize the models. If there are changes in service delivery standards, the models can adjust to these changes and preserve their edge. Such gradual processes of developing trust (i.e., being developed through systematic evaluation) will collectively develop long-term trust in using medical AI.

Table 1. LLM Governance in Clinical Settings

Governance Components	Purpose	Key Activities
Data Governance	Ensures safe and ethical data usage.	De-identification, metadata tracking, bias analysis, dataset audits.
Model Evaluation	Validates technical and clinical performance.	Benchmark testing, human expert review, adversarial prompts, risk assessment.
Ethical Validation	Ensure fairness, transparency, safety.	Ethical audits, demographic performance checks, harm assessment.
Regulatory Alignment	Compliance with global and national regulations.	Documentation, safety evidence, lifecycle reports, change-control mechanisms.
Clinical Workflow Integration.	Ensures safe use in real clinical settings.	Human-in-the-loop validation, monitoring dashboards, Incident reporting systems.

3.4 Enhancing Ethical Transparency and Fairness in LLM-Based Healthcare Systems

All aspects of Fairness are important while creating large language models in medicine (i.e. large Language Models).

The manner in which these tools have been developed and utilized must be equally applicable to all patients regardless of type (e.g. Age, Sex, Race, Social Class and Geographic Location). The development of these tools and processes must be assessed at multiple assessment intervals to ensure the presence of inequities among demographic groups; identification of inequitable provision of services will create imbalances in the diagnosis and/or treatment options that are provided to patients, hence presenting real risks to patients that already experience health care disparities.

In order to create fairness among patients utilizing these tools as well as achieve a consistently positive outcome relative to the aforementioned (e.g. inequities in service delivery); evaluations of Fairness should be conducted as part of the routine system functionality, that includes external reviews of ethics and continuous evaluations of ethical behaviour; this establishes a methodology for identifying and rectifying issues concerning Fairness, thereby maintaining a level of trust among patients and health care organisations.

Open communication concerning model capabilities, performance limitations, and data dictionaries/feeds will provide a clearer understanding of how these models assist with clinical decision making, and enable enhanced collaborative and patient-centric decision making processes.

Transparency is the fundamental mechanism by which the principles of Fairness unfold naturally within the work of organisations/individuals working in the "healthcare" industry.

3.5 Aligning LLM Governance with Regulatory Standards and Clinical Workflows

Legal issues come first when using large language models for medicine, as adhering to all relevant laws from around the world is key to building these systems. The FDA and WHO, for example, require evidence that patients will not be harmed by AI, which means that sufficient evidence demonstrating safety checks have been conducted at all times, not just once, is mandatory. To meet this requirement, one must document each change made to the system, document each result obtained during testing in the real-world (clinical) environment, and provide access logs enabling independent verification/access to that same information. Systems must have clear steps for upgrading their models that everyone agrees to follow without exception. Additionally, what the clinician sees on the screen when they click on the system must mesh seamlessly into their everyday routine(s). Any output that does not function smoothly within the EHR or Alert systems will result in delays in providing treatment to the patient. Recommendations given via dashboard during emergent situations (emergencies), rely on input data accurate enough that no additional effort is required to interpret them. The degree to which interoperability exists between the different systems usually determines whether trust is established or lost. Although the systems can provide clinical decision support, ultimately all medical decisions are made by physicians. Although Decision-Support Tools can have an impact on clinical care, there are still many independent clinical judgement; physicians must be evaluated periodically for this proficiency. For new forms of clinical decision-support tools, the physician will learn progressively over time how to evaluate those new forms. When there is an advancement in technology, there must also be a parallel effort for education at the back end. In summary, the ultimate authority for making the final decision regarding a patient rests with the physician.

4. EVALUATING THE ROLE OF GOVERNANCE IN MEDICAL LLM DECISION-MAKING

Rapid advances in the healthcare sector are ushering in big computer models that influence what can be done with patient data for decision-making, creating notes and reports about patients, detecting and diagnosing diseases and helping to manage time and stress of those physicians who use this technology. However, if the software used to perform these functions and support physicians is used too much, errors can occur, biases can creep into the algorithms, and responsibility for decisions can be passed along so that determining who is liable becomes difficult. Therefore, as an entity overseeing physicians and healthcare facilities, it is incumbent upon the oversight agency to ensure that this technology operates in the best interests of the patient by providing accurate and timely services that can be trusted, when the life of any patient might depend on the reliability of such services.

As occurs with agricultural technology, where data is used to determine when to plant crops, hospital-based administrative artificial intelligence must be governed by appropriate policies and procedures so that the technology deployed does not adversely affect the outcome of the patients who receive care. The criteria for the technology should be based on how to provide adequate supervision, whether to ensure that the technology meets applicable and fair federal laws and standards, and that the technology is appropriate for the practice of medicine in a real-world environment. Throughout the remainder of this report, we will explore the oversight of every step of the decision-making process for administrative artificial intelligence in healthcare, regardless of whether such technology is used by a physician or health facility in a clinic, hospital or remote location.

4.1 Human-Centred Evaluation for Clinical Reliability

Governance provides a systematic and human-centric process for evaluating how medical LLMs (Large Language Models) function in an actual clinical environment. Machine learning improves agricultural intelligence, while governance enables structured evaluations of how well LLMs perform by utilizing a governance framework. Examples of standards in this framework include expert review processes, testing LLMs against established benchmarks, and simulating various scenarios to determine how well LLMs: (1) interpret symptoms, (2) analyze lab results, and (3) provide relevant answers to questions presented as diagnostic queries. All clinicians conduct an evaluation of the following domains: (1) accuracy, (2) quality of rationale, (3) relevance in relation to the context, and (4) potential for harm. In addition to identifying defects in LLMs that may lead to producing potentially unsafe outputs through errors, ambiguous rationale, or miscommunication, the comprehensive evaluation process provides insight into LLMs that automated tests may not be able to identify. Continual validation and verification through governance ensures LLMs support clinical workflows while maintaining patient safety.

4.2 Ethical Safeguards and Bias Mitigation in Medical AI

Deep learning and computer vision are improving the accuracy of agriculture through precision agriculture developments, while ethical safeguards provide precision in clinical decision-making. The results of medical LLMs must be equal and unbiased among diverse patient populations so that no group of patients are subject to potential discrepancies in any aspect of algorithm-driven decision-making. Governance frameworks will accomplish this by providing requirements for fairness analysis, demographic performance analysis, and ethical auditing of algorithm implementations. These processes will identify any disparities in the suggested diagnoses, prescribed medications, and calculating the risk associated with both. Ethical safeguards will also provide transparency through requirements, LLM-generated results clearly identify assumptions, confidence levels, and limitations. This will allow healthcare providers to make an informed decision because AI-generated algorithms and clinical knowledge should be used in making a decision.

4.3 Regulatory Alignment for Safe Clinical Deployment

As predictive analytics support the development of agricultural strategies; regulatory compliance provides a framework for LLMs to safely transition into clinical practice settings; regulations govern many aspects of how Artificial Intelligence (AI) is utilised within healthcare. There are many organisations that develop and implement regulations governing the development and deployment of healthcare LLMs; FDA, WHO, and EU AI Act are examples of these. The governance framework supports compliance with all of these regulations by documenting the behaviours exhibited by LLM models; monitoring the LLM performance over time; assessing and documenting LLM risk; and clearly delineating processes for escalation of risk or adverse events related to the use of LLMs in healthcare. Additionally, regulatory compliance includes the documentation of LLM system logs; evidence of system safety; records of system validation; and history of system upgrades which collectively provide assurance of accountability and traceability; ensure the LLM will function reliably for an extended time; and provide the necessary tools for LLM governance to adapt to the rapidly changing regulations and healthcare standards associated with the use of LLMs for clinical operations. The relationship between governance of LLMs and clinical outcomes is illustrated in the table titled Table 2.

Table 2. Mapping LLM Governance Stages to Clinical Outcomes

Decision-Making Stage	Governance Role	Outcome
Model Interpretation	Ensures factual accuracy and safe reasoning patterns.	Reduces hallucinations and misinterpretations
Ethical Filtering	Applies fairness checks and bias monitoring.	Promotes equitable and transparent medical decisions
Regulatory Compliance	Validates output against clinical and legal standards.	Ensures alignment with FDA, WHO, EU AI Act requirements
Clinician Oversight	Enables human verification and approval.	Prevents unsafe or incorrect suggestions from reaching care
Post-Use Monitoring	Tracks incidents, drifts, and anomalies.	Supports continuous safety improvement

4.4 Decision Support, Clinical Workflows, and Human Oversight

Medical decision support systems provide valuable structured summaries and recommendations for clinicians to aid in their decision-making process, similar to the way in which agricultural decision support systems do for producers. Governance ensures that the output generated from clinician use of medical large language models can be incorporated into existing clinical workflows without disrupting current processes. The human-in-the-loop mechanisms provide clinicians with an opportunity to review, override, and/or modify LLM-generated recommendations to help maintain the clinician's authority and accountability. Recommendations from LLMs are made available through either dashboards, EHRs or other strategic-focused user interfaces with an emphasis on being clear and safe. Governance also incorporates real-time monitoring and incident reporting systems that will provide tracking of anomalies, provide timely alerts to administrators regarding developing risk factors, and offer the continual improvement of the performance of LLMs. The combination of human oversight over LLMs and AI-generated recommendations has the potential to enhance the quality of clinical decision-making while reinforcing patient trust.

5. MAKING IT WORK: HOW GOVERNANCE, CLINICAL EXPERTISE, AND LLMS INTERACT IN HEALTHCARE

The quality of care is determined by combining rules, healthcare knowledge, and intelligent software in order to provide patients high-quality care through the combined use of technology and information in hospitals. When combined, rules create an equitable and legal environment for clinicians to make decisions based on the available information and evidence. The intelligence and experience of the clinician can then use this information in order to make the best possible decision based on their professional judgement. The ability of clinicians to process information quickly provides them with a head start in making a decision, so much so that it can give rise to a level of confidence in the validity of the data and information that the clinician has available to them. All three mechanisms work in harmony with regulatory bodies so as to prevent any harm to the patient. When making decisions regarding complex medical situations, clinical judgement is influenced by years of experience and is also impacted by professional values developed through the clinical experience of providing patient care. As technology and workflows continue to change, the incorporation of advanced technology into clinical practice becomes seamless. When there is alignment between technology and workflows there is evidence of more efficient and effective clinical processes, decreased errors and increased patient safety by ensuring that the patient is at the centre of their own care.

5.1 The Data Journey: From Patient Records to Governed Clinical Insights

Data is the starting point for the pathway to insight. Data sources for this pathway may include electronic health records, lab reports, image summaries, prescriptions, and medical history, and all such data types are generally located across various hospital systems. In agriculture, just like field sensor data is sent from the field to the cloud, the clinical data from the above sources is sent to a preprocessing pipeline for processing. The preprocessing pipeline will process data according to specified data quality rules, privacy protection protocols, and methods for de-identification. The governance process ensures that only secure, ethically sourced, and compliant data will be sent to the LLM.

The LLM will interpret the processed data and may, for example, identify symptoms, summarize histories, or provide differentials diagnoses. Before these, or any other, outputs from the LLM can be provided to clinicians, the LLM outputs must pass through governance filters for safety, inappropriate recommendations, misinformation, and clinical reasoning bias. Through the governance process, the LLM will produce insights that clinicians will receive as being accurate, transparent, and validated as being of a medically acceptable standard. By providing a structured pathway for the transformation of raw data from hospitals (i.e., the data to insight pathway), the governance function will provide healthcare organizations with reliable clinical intelligence based on raw clinical data captured at the point of contact with the patient.

5.2 LLMs as the Decision-Making Core

Just as the intelligence hub of smart farming AI systems is based on a machine learning model, an LLM is the ecosystem's data analysis engine. Once the model receives verified inputs from reliable sources (e.g., electronic medical records, human input), it applies medical reasoning (as presented by the user), accesses various forms of medical knowledge to analyze and assess risk, ultimately providing clinically relevant insight for the user. For example, the results of a query for an asthma patient may provide suggestions for diagnosing asthma, comparing medications to treat asthma, summarizing patient clinical history, or determining whether to send a patient for further testing/treatment.

An LLM is not an independent source of information and can provide clinical decision support through other critical governance components such as risk-scoring algorithms, bias detection algorithms, and hallucination filters that all assess the model output in relation to the model's reasoning and legality. When an LLM's output fails to comply with established safety guidelines, the system will either correct the output, block it from being made available to the user, or send it for human review. In this way, LLMs are used in conjunction with clinician professional judgment, not to replace clinician judgment. Through effective governance, LLMs can function as an effective tool for clinical decision support, similar to the use of regulatory AI systems for smart farming applications.

5.3Real-Time Feedback Loop and Clinician Oversight

Like farms that use IoT, healthcare uses real-time communication between LLMs and health care workers. The information, filtered for governance, will be reviewed, checked for accuracy and changed after receiving it from an LLM to the patient situation as needed by the clinician.

After reviewing the initial information from the LLM and modifying it appropriately for her patient, a clinician will give feedback on her experience dealing with the information she receives from an LLM. Feedback will include reporting any inaccuracies regarding the LLM recommendation, any unclear reasoning by the LLM regarding the recommendation and/or flagging the fact that there may be some level of patient risk associated with the LLM recommendation.

This feedback will be used to update the risk profile used by governance to update the failure rates of safety filters and enhance the criteria evaluation of the governance's safety filters. With this continual adaptation of the LLM, a human contributory process that develops trust and supports the ethical delivery of health care.

5.4 Interoperability and Workflow Integration

Interoperability is crucial for medical LLMs to function as a network of interconnected devices on smart farms. The various medical IT solutions that healthcare providers utilize include EHR systems, diagnostic imaging equipment, pharmacy dashboards, and scheduling systems. LLMs must be able to interface with all of these systems in a seamless manner. In addition, proper governance frameworks must be utilized to ensure compliance with established interoperability standards including HL7 FHIR, secure API protocols, and regulated access rights.

This integration allows for LLMs to make recommendations via clinician dashboards, patient portals, and medical records systems. Additionally, any anomalies identified by LLMs could trigger alerts for clinicians when an anomaly has been identified; if medications conflict, or if any uncertainty arises regarding a diagnostic test result. Automation can also be used by LLMs to write discharge summaries, notes for outpatient visits, or create care plans; however, the clinician will always perform the final verification of any documentation prepared using an automated tool. With seamless integration of LLMs via existing medical IT systems, and the establishment of appropriate governance measures, LLMs will increase the efficiency of operations while minimizing disruption to workflow processes and reducing risk to patient safety.

5.5 Continuous Monitoring, Learning, and Improvement in Governed LLM Ecosystems

Similarly, as an agricultural smart farming System achieves success through constant measurement and systematic improvement, a medical large language model (LLM) must be continuously monitored to ensure it remains accurate, safe, and appropriate for clinical use. What happens to an LLM when it is deployed into a hospital? Its functioning will continue to evolve due to several influences. Medical guidance will change; the discovery of new diseases will affect population demographics; patient demographics will change; and the practice of healthcare will evolve. To maintain trustworthiness of an LLM system, governance models provide for routine performance monitoring, error reporting, across both computer-generated content and human generated content and periodically reviewing/revalidating LLM performance. Through technical monitoring, governance models help identify issues such as:

1. A decline in model performance;
2. Unexpected model performance or outputs due to bias; and,
3. An output pattern from a model that violates established rules/policies.

If issues arise, Standard Operating Procedures (SOPs) will initiate an LLM review process. Technical Teams as well as clinical staff will have the opportunity to modify the Rules of Engagement for the LLM or prompt the developer of the LLM to Change or Re-train an LLM as appropriate.

The continuous learning process affects how effectively the LLM will integrate into existing clinical workflows. When physicians provide feedback and include corrective actions, comments about lack of clarity in reasoning, or instances of harm due to the LLM's recommendations, that information is added to governance dashboard to track the areas for improvement. This information provides the basis for the responsible growth of the LLM while ensuring the strictest levels of safety. Ultimately, this forms a self-sustaining governance loop by which each interaction improves the levels of reliability while lowering the risk of harm. Similar to how automated monitoring systems increase an agricultural grower's productivity, continuous learning allows for medical LLMs to remain current, ethical, and clinically reliable. Ongoing improvement is crucial to ensuring long-term viability and providing healthcare organizations with the confidence to use LLMs with the highest priority on patient safety.

6. APPLICATIONS OF THE INTEGRATED SYSTEM IN REAL-WORLD SETTINGS

Real-world clinical settings are increasingly influenced by Medical LLMs designed according to safety, ethics, and regulation guidelines that enhance quality of care for both patients and healthcare providers (clinicians). Through their ability to produce faster, more precise, and more uniform clinical decisions, these LLM tools essentially serve as the information management systems for physicians/clinics in the same way that digital systems help farmers manage crops and resources. LLM platforms also serve as informational guides to physicians when reviewing complex medical records, diagnosing illness, and developing treatment plans for their patients. By developing the governance of LLMs, it can be ensured that they are providing safe, well-founded, clear, and regulation-compliant outcomes through their use. There are now a number of different types of LLM-supported tools used in hospitals, outpatient clinics, laboratories, and telemedicine for a variety of purposes, including in documentation, predictive analytics, triage recommendations, and patient communications. This section provides the major examples of practical uses for which governance is necessary to ensure LLM-based healthcare delivery is reliable and effective.

6.1 Clinical Documentation and Workflow Automation

Governed medical LLMs streamline the traditionally slow nature of creating clinical documentation (note writing, discharge summaries, letters of referral, patient history documentation). Recent research has demonstrated that the LLM can produce structured, clear and relevant documentation when synthesizing information from electronic health record (EHR) data, available literature and input from clinicians. A governed framework for an LLM ensures that all outputs are checked for accuracy, evaluated for bias and filtered for safety prior to distribution to clinicians. This reduces the amount of clerical work needed, alleviates errors related to fatigue and gives healthcare providers more time for direct patient care. Hospitals utilizing governed LLMs have experienced improved productivity, more consistent documentation practices and fewer instances of missing or inaccurate clinical information.

6.2 Diagnostic Reasoning and Clinical Decision Support

Governed LLMs can provide clinicians with information about symptoms, lab results, imaging findings, and patient histories that allow them to create differential diagnoses and develop clinical recommendations in much the same way as predictive analytics can determine condition of crops for farmers. With the assistance of governance, the information generated as a result of the analysis of the above four categories of products will be based on established medical information, in accordance with established clinical pathway guidelines, and not include information that could result in unsafe or speculative treatment options. These insights are provided to physicians through an interface that includes human supervision and therefore total authority to make the final treatment decision. In addition, governed LLMs can assist in reducing the diagnostic time required in high-stress clinical settings such as emergency departments and intensive care units, by enabling clinicians to recognise (identify) conditions that require immediate treatment, as well as facilitate safe decision-making in the face of uncertainty.

6.3 Patient Communication, Education, and Support

Healthcare LLMs are becoming increasingly common in providing simplified healthcare information to patients, and answering common healthcare questions, providing pre-operative information, and providing medication instructions are just some examples of their use case. Governance is responsible for ensuring that all of these communications are factually accurate, culturally appropriate, and free of harmful, misleading, or biased information and advice. Healthcare LLMs are also used in telehealth platforms, e-Patient portals and facilities, and automated messaging systems. The use of Healthcare LLMs can also relieve clinicians of their workloads and provide greater understanding to patients regarding their issues. The Governance of models helps ensure that all communications with patients reflect empathy, indicate respect for the choices of patients, and avoid language that could be considered stigmatizing. This will ensure that communications between patients and providers follow ethical medical practice standards.

6.4 Predictive Healthcare and Risk Assessment

Governed large language models (LLMs) are increasingly being utilized in the development of risk prediction workflows which includes early detection of sepsis, predicting readmission and predicting medication interactions as well as estimating postoperative complications. Governance frameworks are utilized to validate predictive outcomes by utilizing continuous monitoring, calibration checks, and fairness assessments to minimize the risk of misclassifying or unfairly scoring risks. Hospitals use these governed tools to develop their intervention plans earlier, better allocate their resources, and help support proactive patient care. This same methodology has been applied to intelligent farming systems using prediction models to manage productivity; governing large language models (LLMs) is being applied to improve patient outcomes, minimize avoidable complications, and assist with long-term patient care planning.

6.5 Enhancing Telemedicine and Remote Care Services

Today's telemedicine platforms are increasingly reliant on governed medical LLMs to help clinicians provide timely and accurate care to their patients in real-time. In addition to functioning similar to smart agriculture/remote monitoring systems, governed medical LLMs take into account self-reported symptoms, chat interactions with chatbots, wearable device data, and historical medical history (from the patient) in order to provide an initial assessment of the symptom/situation and suggest how to best treat the symptom/situation. By following the principles of governance, such as adhering to established clinical guidelines, not providing unsafe recommendations, and ensuring that no patient information will be disclosed, governed medical LLMs will continue to improve the quality of telemedicine services being delivered via the digital medium. Telemedicine providers will use the summaries generated from the outputs of the governed medical LLMs to organize and prioritize cases, identify urgent cases, and facilitate virtual consultations. For those who live in rural or resource-scarce areas, governed medical LLM systems will enhance the ability of patients to access healthcare by providing reliable symptom triage, pre-visit patient education, and pre-visit preparation support. As remote healthcare continues to be the primary healthcare delivery model worldwide, governed medical LLMs will help clinicians provide quality care to many more patients while ensuring the safety of both the patient and the provider, as well as preserving a sense of clarity and continuity of connection with the patient.

6.6 Administrative Optimization and Healthcare Management

Governed large language models (LLMs) are becoming increasingly important, beyond their clinical applications, in the administrative and operational functions of healthcare systems. For example, hospitals use LLMs to automate tasks such as appointment scheduling, completing insurance documentation, generating medical bills, coordinating employees, and producing reports. Governance ensures that these types of administrative outputs comply with the law, contain minimal errors, and comply with privacy regulations, such as HIPAA and GDPR, as well as any rules pertaining to the transmission of national health information. Additionally, LLM-based systems will be able to help analyse workflow bottlenecks, predict future staffing requirements, optimise bed placement, and assist with strategic planning activities within hospitals—similar to how data-driven solutions aid in the optimisation of resources in agricultural operations. Finally, by automating many of the repetitive administrative tasks that hospitals currently perform manually, governed LLMs enable hospitals to lower their operational costs, reduce clerical errors, and allocate more resources to employee-patient interaction activities. As healthcare systems continue to grow, administrative intelligence will be vital for maintaining operational efficiency, working collaboratively between departments, and providing high-quality services to patients.

7. CASE STUDIES FROM THE CLINICAL FIELD

Governed large language models (LLMs) have begun to mature and to provide real world evidence of their positive impact on clinical decision making, improving documentation, and enhancing patient engagement. Similar to the agricultural, case studies, which serve as examples of successful AI-IoT governance frameworks, medical case studies also provide compelling evidence of how governed LLMs are delivering safe, ethical and compliant solutions within the healthcare sector. Within these various case examples (emergency department, hospital systems, telemedicine platforms and administrative workflows), we see how governed LLMs are enhancing the overall healthcare ecosystem by providing greater accuracy of data; reducing the amount of manual labor required to perform a task; and improving patient outcomes.

Case Study 1: Governed LLMs in Emergency Department Triage

Location: United States

Technology Used: Governance-filtered LLM triage system, EHR integration, safety-layer validation

An emergency department within a major metropolitan area leveraged a governed large language model to assist in the triage process of patients by evaluating patient symptoms, vitals, and medical history as well as producing an initial assessment of the patient's severity. A governance layer reviewed these assessments before they were passed on to nurses for potential errors, unsafe clinical claims, or omitted information. The implementation has decreased the time it takes to triage patients, rapidly identify high-risk patients, and provided nurses with more consistent initial assessments.

Outcomes:

- 22% reduction in triage wait time
- More consistent documentation and symptom summaries
- Faster flagging of sepsis, chest pain, and stroke cases

Lessons Learned:

- Governance filters were essential for avoiding unsafe automated suggestions.
- Clinician oversight was crucial in high-pressure situations.

Case Study 2: Automated Clinical Documentation in a Multi-Specialty Hospital

Location: United Kingdom

Technology Used: LLM-powered documentation generator, medical governance filters, compliance validation

Utilizing a managed LLM (Large Language Model) to create discharge summaries, referral letters and clinical notes is being implemented by a major health care facility. The LLM processes dictation from physicians, laboratory or hospital test reports and diagnostic/imaging reports into structured documents. Governance modules review the outputs to confirm the accuracy of the report; verify the correct spelling of the drug name; ensure the reports adhere to the regulations associated with working for the NHS and the General Data Protection Regulation (GDPR); and provide complete, well-formatted documents that do not require any major changes or modifications by the clinicians.

Outcomes:

- 35% reduction in time spent on documentation
- Fewer omissions of critical information
- Improved clarity and consistency across departments

Lessons Learned:

- Governance avoided misinformation and privacy risks.
- Clinician feedback helped improve the model's output quality over time.

Case Study 3: Telemedicine Symptom Intake and Patient Assistance
Location: India
Technology Used: Governed LLM for teleconsultation prep, multilingual support, patient-safe messaging filters.

The telehealth organization used an LLMs for 1) compiling pre-consult treatment records and guiding patients before their consultation; A LLM was also used to create a structured record of symptom recorded by patients through chat messages, and collected using wearable devices (e.g., smartwatches). Governance filters ensured communication to patients was respectful of their cultural language; governed against sending a patient unsafe medical advice; sent the patient's medical information to physician if there was a chance of an inappropriate response.

Outcomes:

- 40% faster preparation for virtual consultations
- Better clarity in symptom descriptions
- Higher patient satisfaction and less workload for clinicians

Lessons Learned:

- Strong governance was crucial to stop unsupervised treatment suggestions.
- Support for local languages greatly improved accessibility.

8. CURRENT BARRIERS AND LIMITATIONS

Despite rapid advances in Large Language Models (LLMs) in Health Care and increasing interest in using these technologies to enhance work-flow, there are still significant barriers preventing their adoption for broad, safe and effective use in health care. Governed Medical LLMs have the potential to support diagnosis, automate documentation, and facilitate patient communication; however, there are multiple challenges to the practical adoption of these types of solutions into existing workflows due to technical, ethical, regulatory and operational challenges. Many existing healthcare organisations have old systems, a lack of clear accountability, and mismatched data standards that present obstacles to integrating new technologies into those existing systems and workflows. Moreover, there are ongoing concerns regarding privacy, fairness, and clinical safety associated with the use of LLMs in a healthcare setting. As a result, there needs to be strong governance models and continuous oversight for the implementation of LLM technology in healthcare. In this section, we will discuss the four critical areas of barriers to the use of governed Medical LLMs in clinical practice.

8.1. Technological Challenges

Although Medical LLMs have some remarkable advantages in their ability to process clinical language and assist with diagnostic reasoning, there remain a number of technological constraints that limit their robustness for practical use. One major concern with these systems is model hallucination, or the situation where a model generates outputs that are inaccurate or completely fabricated; statutorily, if these outputs are accepted without careful consideration, they have serious consequences. The other major limit to giving model output value is the inability to dynamically access up-to-date clinical databases, rendering output distinct from practice standards for clinical care and no longer, either medically accurate or relevant. Furthermore, the lack of interoperability between the EHR, imaging, and workflow "tools" used by many healthcare organizations has created an additional barrier for healthcare settings that have been built to support multiple EHR systems, imaging modalities, and enterprise applications; yet, as a result of the hardware and infrastructure requirements to run these models, there also exist significant gaps in accessibility to the technology for many healthcare organizations that have less than optimal technical capabilities. Collectively, addressing these issues will require an investment in the development of robust validation methods, as well as developing an effective, scalable architecture for the integration of LLMs into clinical practice. Finally, ongoing assessments of LLMs in the real world will be needed in order to ensure that they continue to perform consistently at the highest level.

8.2. Economic Barriers

The deployment costs of governed medical LLMs pose significant challenges for health care organizations wishing to utilize AI as part of their clinical assistance programs. Organizations are faced with a myriad of initial expenses that they will need to consider, including: licensing the model, building a secure environment, training the staff, and creating the governance customarily associated with each organization's unique operational needs. Rural clinics and community hospitals typically feel the greatest financial strain for the addition of LLM tools into their technological structure, as their tight budgets already require near maximum levels of funding. In addition to upfront costs, ongoing expenses related to software upgrades, cloud resource usage, security maintenance, and vendor assistance will severely limit any long range financial planning for LLM implementations. The lack of concrete evidence that would determine the monetary advantages associated with the investment in LLMs causes decision-makers to be reluctant to commit to broad-scale deployments until detailed cost-benefit data can be collected. The future of LLM implementation will be dependent on developing cost-effective, adaptable, and step-wise deployable LLMs that are appropriate for use in the varied settings of the health care delivery system.

8.3. Skill Gaps and Lack of Technical Training

The implementation of LLM tools into clinical settings is often inhibited by the absence of adequate digital literacy and effective training programs for healthcare staff. Physicians, nurses, and other staff workers may find themselves unable to appropriately interpret AI-generated results, identify possible areas of risk, or operate systems that are significantly different from their current workflows. Without adequate educational opportunities, clinicians run the risk of excessively relying on results produced by LLM models without the application of their own clinical judgement, or completely disregarding the model results; both of these possibilities have implications for the quality of care received by patients and patient safety. Additionally, the challenge is compounded by a severe lack of in-house AI governance knowledge; very few hospital settings have teams who can provide governance knowledge on a technical and/or ethical basis concerning prompt engineering, algorithmic fairness, or risk assessment. In order to bridge these gaps, healthcare organizations will need to create acceptable user interfaces for LLM applications, develop customized educational pathways for each of the various healthcare professional roles that would benefit from using LLMs for patient care and develop and sustain dedicated governance teams that will be responsible for the ethical complexities of LLMs.

8.4. Data Privacy and Ownership Concerns

Healthcare organizations are concerned about the use of sensitive patient information by medical language models (LLMs). The main concerns have to do with how their Protected Health Information (PHI) will be shared with third-party model providers or stored in the cloud and how those model providers will use the information to create their models. In addition, LLM-enabled providers who fail to have robust agreements on the proper use, retention, and anonymization of data risk violating the requirements of the HIPAA, GDPR, and other national health data regulations. As the number of cyberattacks on healthcare providers continues to grow, the lack of strong governance around the deployment of LLMs may also add additional security risks. Finally, patients do not currently have access to clear guidance about how their data is processed, audited, or shared. To mitigate these risks, reliable governance frameworks must cover aspects such as strong encryption, access controls, and transparent data-handling policies.

8.5. Social and Cultural Resistance

Medical LLM use is severely limited by ethical and cultural objections, as well as technical or operational concerns. Clinicians are concerned that using AI-based tools might undermine their autonomy, compromise their clinical expertise, or produce bias that could put at-risk populations at an increased risk. In addition, the fear of unfairness and bias from algorithms and variability between different demographic populations creates distrust in LLM-based systems. Furthermore, existing cultural challenges in utilizing technology and a lack of experience with technology (particularly in traditional or resource-scarce settings) can be barriers to the adoption of LLMs as part of routine clinical work. Thus, without clear ethics, transparency, and involvement of physicians in decision-making around LLMs, medical LLMs may experience major scepticism.

9. WHAT'S NEXT: EMERGING TRENDS AND RESEARCH AVENUES

With continuing advancements in medical LLMs, the potential for these systems to transform clinical workflow is becoming more evident through advancements in model capabilities, improved safety measures, and cross-disciplinary collaboration. The ability of researchers, healthcare professionals, and regulatory bodies to collaborate effectively will be the key to translating progress in multimodal reasoning, continuous telemetry, and adaptive support into useful clinical tools. While the next generation of healthcare AI systems will have exponentially better technical performance, they will also have stronger ethical foundations, more robust governance mechanisms, and greater alignment with the realities faced by clinicians in practice. These three trajectories combine to create an environment where AI systems will be trustworthy, accountable and capable of demonstrating value to the clinicians and patients who rely on them. In the sections that follow, we outline what we consider to be the most important future directions to explore for governed medical LLMs and the innovations in governance that will enable these directions.

9.1. Multimodal Medical LLMs for Holistic Decision-Making

The next generations of large language models (LLMs) will combine a variety of data types, including clinical notes, imaging, genomic data, biosignals, laboratory values, and data from wearable devices. This will enable them to create multi-modal models capable of total diagnostic reasoning by integrating text, image, and structured clinical data across one controlled pipeline. Governance for multi-modal systems will be modified to incorporate a unified risk score system, establish safety checks across each of the constituent data types, and set-up audits for multi-modal biases. Together, these changes will facilitate the development of safe and equitable decision support systems. Furthermore, multi-modal systems can help clinicians achieve complex tasks such as reporting on radiology studies, developing surgical plans, and implementing precision medicine.

9.2. Real-Time Clinical Monitoring and Continuous Validation

When medical chatbots are implemented in hospitals, closely monitoring their performance will become essential for ensuring their operation remains under control. These AI systems "learn" by analysing the language and constructing potential responses as opposed to operating as programmed code within a given set of parameters. Therefore, as advancements are made in medical science, population and research differentiality occurs, and the AI response will evolve along with these changes. Therefore, systems need to have an active monitoring plan within the oversight plan, which will provide tools to monitor the quality of chatbot responses; detect abnormal chatbot responses; and use formal review to determine when the accuracy of the chatbot declines below the acceptable level. In addition, continuing to use benchmark evaluations against standard medical cases (created prior to chatbot implementation); completing "trial" runs of the chatbot without any human input; and documenting any issues will allow for early evaluation of any issues and corrective actions (e.g., modifying the language prompts used by the chatbot; modifying the underlying data source the chatbot uses to generate a response; or modifying the model used by the chatbot) to ensure that the chatbot remains effective, safe, and functional within the delivery of health services over time and beyond the initial deployment of the chatbot.

9.3. Personalization and Adaptive Clinical Support

Over the next few years, medical LLMs (Language Models) will be moving away from offering standardized replies and moving toward providing individualized clinical guidance tailored around each person's health history. By utilizing longitudinal medical records, prescription histories, and genomic information about each patient, these systems will provide clinical recommendations based on each patient's biological and clinical characteristics instead of on population-based statistics. Additionally, as a result of their interactions with clinicians, the models will continue to refine their recommendations through additional input from the clinician. Therefore, in order for these personalized systems to be successful at improving patient care, governance systems that oversee them will need to establish and implement transparent informed consent protocols, assess equity/justness across diverse racial/ethnic groups on an ongoing basis, and put into place strong protections against algorithmic bias so that the support provided by these personalized systems improves outcomes for all patients while also providing equitable and equal access to care of high quality.

9.4. Global and Federated Learning Collaborations

Federated Learning provides a mechanism for healthcare institutions from various countries to collaboratively develop and enhance Medical LLMs (Large Language Models) while ensuring that the underlying patient information does not leave their own facilities. The hospitals that are involved in a federation train the model within their own facility and only share encrypted updates of the model, thereby preserving patient confidentiality and collectively adding to the Clinical Intelligence of the model. This type of architecture mitigates one of the most common shortcomings of current medical AI systems, which is the over-representation of data from affluent Western healthcare systems. By including contributions from healthcare institutions in Asia, Africa, and South America, federated collaborations will generate models that cover a much broader range of Disease Patterns, Treatment Practice, and Patient Demographics. In order for these partnerships to function responsibly at scale, there must be governance frameworks that define technical standards for interoperability of systems, establish compliance pathways for multiple jurisdictions, and provide an avenue for tracking contributions in a transparent manner. Organizations such as the World Health Organization (WHO) are uniquely positioned to offer the ethical guidance and coordination infrastructure that are required to establish trust and maintain momentum across boundaries where regulatory alignment is inconsistent.

9.5 Autonomous Safety Layers and Self-Regulating AI Systems

Recently, researchers have been exploring how to add safety components to large language technologies so they can monitor themselves while being used; if a potentially dangerous situation arises, the system intervenes and takes corrective action before either the doctor or the patient sees it. Corrections occur automatically; a message is sent to alert the users when they are unsure about something, and sometimes, an action is simply delayed. The rules and the structures associated with safety components provide a consistent experience to the end user, regardless of how stressful the situation is. As they continue to develop, these intelligent assistants will reduce the need to perform redundant checks by humans; will enable faster processing times for all involved; and will establish an increased degree of cautious trust in the clinics.

10. CONCLUSIONS

Large language models are quickly transforming today's healthcare and paving the way for enhanced clinical decision-making, streamlined documentation, telemedicine support, and increased patient engagement. This chapter illustrates that the comprehensive benefits of medical LLMs will only be achieved through strong governance frameworks. Throughout all areas such as basic concepts, ethical validation, regulatory requirements, systems interaction, applications in real life, and case studies, the overall message is the same; good governance is mandatory and a key driver in the responsible operation of medical LLM's in high-risk environments.

This chapter explored governed LLMs, demonstrating how they reduce diagnostic error, assist in clinical oversight, promote equity and fairness in care delivery, and comply with international standards such as those established by the FDA, WHO, and EU AI Act. By evaluating data governance, model assessment, ethical protections, regulatory requirements, workflow integration, and continuing evaluation after initial implementation, we showed how the use of governance to build safety structures will reduce diagnostic error and dangerous outputs and preserve clinician authority and accountability. The case studies provided additional evidence that governed LLMs are already providing benefits in the areas of emergency care, telemedicine/hospitals, hospital documentation, and administrative roles, demonstrating that adopting and using safe AI has real-world value.

In conclusion, regulated Medical LLMs demonstrate that there is a close collaboration between human intelligence and intelligent systems. They enhance efficiency, increase access to care and support informed clinical decision making without replacing the vital judgement of practitioners, provided there are solid ethical principles and are integrated into clinical practice. The growth of the healthcare sector and continued use of safe, clear and trustworthy Medical LLMs will transform digital health in the future. This chapter illustrates that the advancements in regulated Medical LLMs further demonstrate that the governance of this technology is more than regulatory compliance; it will be a key tool in ensuring that the AI the innovators create actually improves health outcomes for individuals and makes our global healthcare system stronger.

REFERENCES

Al-Qerem, W., Eberhardt, J., Jarab, A., Al Bawab, A. Q., Hammad, A., Alasmari, F., Alazab, B., Husein, D. A., Alazab, J., & Al-Beool, S. (2023). Exploring knowledge, attitudes, and practices towards artificial intelligence among health professions' students in Jordan. *BMC Medical Informatics and Decision Making, 23*(1), 288. DOI: 10.1186/s12911-023-02403-0 PMID: 38098095

Alcalá Minagorre, P. J., Salmerón Fernández, M. J., Domingo Garau, A., Díaz Pernas, P., Nebot Marzal, C. M., Pino Ramírez, R. M., & Madrid Rodríguez, A. (2025). Strategies for improving diagnostic safety and clinical reasoning. *Anales de Pediatría (English Ed.), 102*(4), 503827. DOI: 10.1016/j.anpede.2025.503827 PMID: 40246601

Aravazhi, P. S., Gunasekaran, P., Benjamin, N. Z. Y., Thai, A., Chandrasekar, K. K., Kolanu, N. D., Prajjwal, P., Tekuru, Y., Brito, L. V., & Inban, P. (2025). The integration of artificial intelligence into clinical medicine: Trends, challenges, and future directions. *Disease-a-Month : DM, 71*(6), 101882. DOI: 10.1016/j.disamonth.2025.101882 PMID: 40140300

Asgari, E., Montaña-Brown, N., Dubois, M., Khalil, S., Balloch, J., Yeung, J. A., & Pimenta, D. (2025). A framework to assess clinical safety and hallucination rates of LLMs for medical text summarisation. npj. *Digital Medicine, 8*(1), 274. DOI: 10.1038/s41746-025-01670-7 PMID: 40360677

Broch Porcar, M. J., & Castellanos-Ortega, Á. (2025). Patient safety, what does clinical simulation and teaching innovation contribute? *Medicina intensiva, 49*(3), 165–173. DOI: 10.1016/j.medin.2024.03.017 PMID: 38797620

Caner, V. (2025). Profiling safety behavior in clinical laboratory environments. *Frontiers in Public Health, 13*, 1681513. DOI: 10.3389/fpubh.2025.1681513 PMID: 41080846

Chang, Y., Yin, J., Li, J., Liu, C., Cao, L., & Lin, S. (2024). Applications and Future Prospects of Medical LLMs: A Survey Based on the M-KAT Conceptual Framework. *Journal of Medical Systems, 48*(1), 112. DOI: 10.1007/s10916-024-02132-5 PMID: 39725770

Coye, L., Jones, M. A., Gaza-Bulseco, G., Chitikila, C., Clavier, S., Fougeron, D., Grimaldi, C., Hurkmans, K., Hutchinson, R., Kellogg, B., Liu, X., Palackal, N., Tank, M., Valax, P., Waerner, T., Wang, F., Zhang, Y., Zhao, Y., Sloan, S., & de Zafra, C. Z. (2025). Host Cell Protein Clinical Safety Risk Assessment-An Updated Industry Review. *Biotechnology and Bioengineering*, *122*(11), 3229–3248. DOI: 10.1002/bit.70029 PMID: 40757641

Holm, J. E. J., Ruppert, J. G., & Ramsden, S. D. (2022). Impact of Changing Regulations and the Dynamic Nature of European Risk Management Plans for Human Medicines on the Lifecycle of Safety Concerns. *Pharmaceutical Medicine*, *36*(1), 33–46. DOI: 10.1007/s40290-021-00414-8 PMID: 35099785

Leivaditis, V., Maniatopoulos, A. A., Lausberg, H., Mulita, F., Papatriantafyllou, A., Liolis, E., Beltsios, E., Adamou, A., Kontodimopoulos, N., & Dahm, M. (2025). Artificial Intelligence in Thoracic Surgery: A Review Bridging Innovation and Clinical Practice for the Next Generation of Surgical Care. *Journal of Clinical Medicine*, *14*(8), 2729. DOI: 10.3390/jcm14082729 PMID: 40283559

Mishra, V., Lurie, Y., & Mark, S. (2025). Accuracy of LLMs in medical education: Evidence from a concordance test with medical teacher. *BMC Medical Education*, *25*(1), 443. DOI: 10.1186/s12909-025-07009-w PMID: 40140805

Qiu, P., Wu, C., Liu, S., Fan, Y., Zhao, W., Chen, Z., Gu, H., Peng, C., Zhang, Y., Wang, Y., & Xie, W. (2025). Quantifying the reasoning abilities of LLMs on clinical cases. *Nature Communications*, *16*(1), 9799. DOI: 10.1038/s41467-025-64769-1 PMID: 41198657

Ray, P. P. (2025). Toward Transparent AI-Enabled Patient Selection in Cosmetic Surgery by Integrating Reasoning and Medical LLMs. *Aesthetic Plastic Surgery*, *49*(19), 5641–5642. DOI: 10.1007/s00266-025-05038-w PMID: 40563006

Roselló Atanet, I., Tomova, M., Sieg, M., Sehy, V., Mäder, P., & März, M. (2025). Generating learning guides for medical education with LLMs and statistical analysis of test results. *BMC Medical Education*, *25*(1), 458. DOI: 10.1186/s12909-025-06978-2 PMID: 40158187

Shool, S., Adimi, S., Saboori Amleshi, R., Bitaraf, E., Golpira, R., & Tara, M. (2025). A systematic review of large language model (LLM) evaluations in clinical medicine. *BMC Medical Informatics and Decision Making*, *25*(1), 117. DOI: 10.1186/s12911-025-02954-4 PMID: 40055694

Tang, K. S., Cheng, D. L., Mi, E., & Greenberg, P. B. (2020). Augmented reality in medical education: A systematic review. *Canadian Medical Education Journal*, *11*(1), e81. DOI: 10.36834/cmej.61705 PMID: 32215146

Thirupathi, L., Kaashipaka, V., Dhanaraju, M., & Katakam, V. (2025). AI and IoT in Mental Health Care: From Digital Diagnostics to Personalized, Continuous Support. In Joshi, H., Kumar Reddy, C., Ouaissa, M., Hanafiah, M., & Doss, S. (Eds.), *Intelligent Systems and IoT Applications in Clinical Health* (pp. 271–294). IGI Global Scientific Publishing., DOI: 10.4018/979-8-3693-8990-4.ch012

Thirupathi, L., Srinivasulu, B., Khanapurkar, U., Rambabu, D., & Preeti, C. M. (2023). Heart Disease Prediction in Healthcare Communities by Machine Learning Over Big Data. In Bhateja, V., Sunitha, K. V. N., Chen, Y. W., & Zhang, Y. D. (Eds.), *Intelligent System Design. Lecture Notes in Networks and Systems* (Vol. 494). Springer., DOI: 10.1007/978-981-19-4863-3_38

Wawra-Hehenberger, K., Pencelli, V., Pardo, J. A., Tremmel, L., Ataher, Q., & Waschbusch, M. (2025). A visual safety risk evaluation tool in early clinical phases. *Contemporary Clinical Trials*, *154*, 107953. DOI: 10.1016/j.cct.2025.107953 PMID: 40381907

Williams, R., Kantilal, K., Man, K. K. C., Blandford, A., & Jani, Y. (2025). Barcode medication administration system use and safety implications: A data-driven longitudinal study supported by clinical observation. *BMJ Health & Care Informatics*, *32*(1), e101214. DOI: 10.1136/bmjhci-2024-101214 PMID: 39832825

Wong, R., Ming, L., & Raja Ali, R. (2023). The Intersection of ChatGPT, Clinical Medicine, and Medical Education. *JMIR Medical Education*, *9*, e47274. https://mededu.jmir.org/2023/1/e47274. DOI: 10.2196/47274 PMID: 37988149

Yang, L., Xu, C., & Wang, X. (2025). Cost-Effective Medical Dialogue Summarization with Fine-Tuned Compact LLMs. In Mahmud, M., Doborjeh, M., Wong, K., Leung, A. C. S., Doborjeh, Z., & Tanveer, M. (Eds.), *Neural Information Processing. ICONIP 2024. Communications in Computer and Information Science* (Vol. 2287). Springer., DOI: 10.1007/978-981-96-6963-9_18

Zhang, K., Li, Y., Wu, P., Li, Y., Zhang, C., & Zan, H. (2025). Knowledge Enhancement with LLMs for Few-Shot Medical Relation Extraction. In Zhang, Y. (Eds.), *Health Information Processing. CHIP 2024. Communications in Computer and Information Science* (Vol. 2433). Springer., DOI: 10.1007/978-981-96-3752-2_10

Zhou, H., Liu, F., Gu, B., Zou, X., Huang, J., Wu, J., ... A survey of large language models in medicine: progress, application, and challenge. ArXiv Preprint. 2023;arXiv:231105112.

Chapter 10
Ensuring Safe and Ethical Use of LLMs in Healthcare

M. Kamaladevi
http://orcid.org/0000-0001-8486-5092
SASTRA (Deemed to be) University, India

Raihanudeen M. S.
SASTRA (Deemed to be) University, India

ABSTRACT

Large Language Models (LLMs) are becoming an important part of today's healthcare system, especially in helping doctors with clinical documentation and routine tasks. While these tools can save time, reduce workload, and improve the quality of medical records, their use also brings important safety and ethical questions. This chapter takes a practical look at what it means to use LLMs responsibly in healthcare. It explains why human oversight is essential, how errors like hallucinations or bias can affect patient care, and why protecting patient privacy must remain a top priority. The chapter also describes simple and effective ways to reduce risks—through proper validation, transparent workflows, data security, and continuous monitoring. Overall, the chapter highlights that LLMs can be powerful partners in healthcare, but only when used carefully, ethically, and with the patient's well-being at the center of every decision

1. INTRODUCTION

Healthcare digitalization is accomplished through the use of advanced technologies in Artificial Intelligence and data analytics, which have become ubiquitous around the world. In recent times, Large Language Models (LLMs)represent a breakthrough

DOI: 10.4018/979-8-3373-7862-6.ch010

in that they can quickly process, generate, and summarize documents based on natural language at an unprecedented scale. LLMs are growing in prevalence across multiple areas of healthcare including: clinical documentation; discharge summary generation; medical coding; decision support; and administrative workflows (WHO, 2021; Kung et al, 2023). As a result, LLMs are expected to automate routine and time-intensive tasks, thereby creating a opportunity to decrease clinician workloads; enhance documentation quality; and support more effective delivery of healthcare services.

However, as LLM adoption continues to grow, the deployment of LLMs within healthcare also presents unique challenges that extend far beyond algorithmic accuracy. The nature of the healthcare environment makes it a high stakes area where the consequences of incorrect or misleading information on patient outcomes can be very serious. As LLMs generate responses that are probabilistic and based on the total number of patterns the LLM has been exposed to through their training on very large datasets, the content generated from an LLM may be fluent, but also factually inaccurate and not clinically appropriate (Bender et al, 2021; Ji et al, 2023). This poses even greater risks when LLM-generated content is integrated with clinical workflows without adequate human validation. The use of ethical considerations in the assimilation of LLMs (language learning algorithms) into the field of healthcare is further complicated by the increasing difficulties of integrating them into practice. This is especially true when looking at the issues around bias, fairness, and equity. Recent studies also point to the disparate performance of AI systems (technologies designed to operate autonomously on large amounts of data) across diverse groups of patients when utilizing incomplete and/or unbalanced training datasets (Leslie, 2022; Seyyed-Kalantari et al., 2021). These limitations raise questions about the ethical principles of justice and non-maleficence, especially when the use of AI-assisting tools in making clinical decisions about vulnerable populations.

The concepts of transparency and explainability are also two of the many ethical concerns that arise when deploying LLMs. Most LLM models in use today are designed with the architecture of a black-box, which means that they do not provide transparency or explain their output in a manner where clinicians can dispute their decision-making. A lack of interpretability leads to reduced accountability and can weaken clinician trust in AI-assisted clinical decision-making (Rudin et al., 2022). The regulatory and policy-oriented literature related to AI (technology designed to mimic human reasoning) continues to stress the necessity for an explainable and auditable AI, especially when health care environments represent high-risk settings (FDA, 2023).

The central ethical surrounds the adoption of AI near the healthcare remains surrounds the patient privacy and protect the datas.. Many LLM-based applications and limitations are reliant on large quantity of sensitive clinical text and patient records, which raises problems related to data protection, informed consent, and the secondary use of healthcare data.

Given the issues outlined above, there is an increasing amount of acknowledgment that, in order to use language models responsibly, technology must not only be created; also in addition to that, quality assurance and customer service need to be addressed. A number of studies have shown good results with using language models in [clinical] contexts, but there are still not enough protocols providing ethical guidance on their use, human checks and balances on their operation, and guidance on how to minimize the risks associated with their use (Nori et al., 2023; Kung et al., 2023). The absence of these protocols means that there is an overall need for formalized guidelines that address patient safety, disclosure of information, and accountability.

This chapter will be written to help meet this need. The chapter will present a practical and ethical language model usage case for language models to use in a health care setting. Language models will be viewed as an extension to provide assistance to decision-makers rather than as independent decision makers. Also, this chapter will provide practical strategies on how to mitigate potential ethical issues, how to minimize potential risks of using/loss of using the language model and as well, identify practical guidance/help for implementing language models into everyday health care practice while keeping the well-being of those who are using the language models first.

In this document, the term 'language models' is used to refer to both traditional text-based language models, and beyond that, multi-modal language models (which have been enhanced using image or any other form of media) unless specifically stated differently.

1.1 Methodology

This chapter adopts a narrative review approach to synthesize existing literature on the use of Large Language Models (LLMs) in healthcare. A narrative review was select to provide a broad, conceptual observed of technical capabilities, ethical challenges, and implementation considerations rather than seeing on quantitative aggregation.

Relevant studies was identified from recent peer-reviewed journals, conference proceedings, and reports published between 2021 and 2025. The selection seeing on key themes including clinical applications, medical records, education, ethical concerns, and real-world deployment of the LLMs.

Inclusion categories included studies that (i) explicitly discussed the use of LLM or AI-based language systems in healthcare systems, (ii) discussed clinical, ethical, or operational implications, and (iii) provided empirical, review-based or conceptual insights.

We excluded studies not directly related to healthcare applications or not having a substantive discussion of LLM capabilities. The selected literature was analyzed and thematically organized to support a structured discussion of opportunities, challenges and responsible implementation strategies.

The chapter discusses the application of Large Language Models (LLMs) in selected healthcare domains, including clinical documentation, decision support, patient communication, and medical education. We discuss high-risk applications like autonomous diagnosis and treatment recommendation from safety and ethical perspective but we do not consider them in the scope of direct deployment. The discussion enhances the clinical safety, ethical considerations, and responsible integration into real-world healthcare workflows.

2. LITERATURE REVIEW

The rapid development of LLMs has led to their improvement in the application of various domains of healthcare including clinical decision support, medical documentation, education, and research. Current research is very promising, but it also has significant limitations, ethical concerns. The literature is grouped in themes to facilitate a coherent understanding..

2.1 LLMs in Clinical Applications and Decision Support

Several pieces of research are currently underway to look at the utility of LLMs within the context of clinical workflow and decision-making regarding disease treatment. In cardiology, LLMs have been shown to offer assistance by simplifying complex clinical guideline scenarios as well as improving patient education efforts. However, compared to patient education and simplifying clinical guidelines, LLMs perform less effectively when interpreting image-based diagnostic tests such as ECGs or echocardiograms.

In diabetes management, explainable Machine Learning models have also been used to identify trends associated with therapeutic inertia, providing data-driven evidence that such models can identify clinically important trends across large patient populations. Recent studies in the areas of radiology and multimodal practice reveal that LLMs developed and trained for image interpretation and peripherals have the capacity to not only interpret imaging data but to also develop structured clinical documentation from such data. Systems that incorporate visual and text-based inputs appear to demonstrate strong performance, especially when utilizing domain-specific training and validation methods for each form of input. Similarly, applications in oncology and primary care have suggested that LLMs may support diagnostic reasoning as well as the triage and identification of clinical resources in an efficient manner, although their utility varies according to the complexity of the case.

Improvements in clinical workflows utilizing LLM technology may enhance clinical providers' decision-making capacities. However, evidence continues to demonstrate that there are significant variances in LLM performance across types of clinical tasks, further emphasizing the need for comprehensive validation of LLMs prior to their implementation in the clinical space..

2.2 LLMs in Medical Documentation and Workflow Automation

Automating clinical documentation and administrative work in health care is one of the most popular uses of LLMs. Evidence suggests that LLM tools significantly decrease the time it takes to produce clinical notes, discharge summaries and patient letters, while still being accurate and consistent.

LLM-generated documentation in surgery and dermatology has improved the quality of clinical documentation through improved clarity, standardization and efficiency of clinical workflows. Furthermore, radiology reporting systems and ambient clinical documentation systems demonstrate how LLMs can convert disorganized clinical data into clearly organized and useable formats.

These are highly beneficial use cases for reducing the workload of clinicians and lowering the incidence of burnout, due to the reduced time needed to document regularly occurring matters. Nonetheless, there are some issues with the possibility of slight inaccuracies, misunderstanding of the context and/or the need for continuous human validation of the content generated by AI.

2.3 LLMs in Medical Education and Research

LLMs are increasingly being used in medical education and research. Studies show that LLMs are increasingly used in medical education and research outside of clinical practice. Research shows that LLMs can facilitate learning through providing explanations, acting as patients, and performing clinical reasoning exercises. In education, virtual patients and interactive systems driven by LLMs have improved student engagement, communication skills and diagnostic thinking.

In research settings, LLMs have shown themselves to be able to generate appropriate research questions, summarize scientific literature, and help build protocols. Also being investigated for use in drug discovery, where they can be used to assist in target identification, molecular design and pharmacological property analysis.

However, these advantages are offset by the lack of novelty, the dependence on known knowledge patterns, the susceptibility to errors, and other restrictions, which emphasize the ongoing necessity of expert supervision in both education and research applications.

2.4 Ethical, Safety, and Bias Concerns

Many of the research papers the LLMs mention a many of ethical and safety issues that wants to considered before deploying them to health care settings system. One major problem concerning LLMs is the generation of false and sometimes plausible information, known as hallucinations. In clinical settings where accuracy is very important, hallucination errors could cause potential harm.

Another problem well documented in the literature is that many LLMs are biased because they are trained using historical or non-representative data sets. As a result, the presence of bias in LLMs may affect how clinicians interpret and make decisions based on output from LLMs, raising concerns about fairness and equity in the process of clinical decision-making.

Another issue that complicates using LLMs is the lack of transparency and explainability for clinicians. Because many LLMs function as black-box systems, it can be very difficult for clinicians to understand the basis on which LLMs produce their outputs. As a result, clinicians may not have a high level of trust in using LLMs for clinical decision making; thus reducing accountability of LLMs in clinical practice.

Finally, privacy and security related to health care data is a major concern for LLMs. Particularly in cloud-based health care deployments, the use of LLMs where large amounts of sensitive health care data are used in the development of the LLMs has created security issues, risks of unauthorized access to data, and uncertainty of the policies related to the use of data..

2.5 Limitations and Research Gaps

LLMs have shown potential; however, the literature has identified many limitations of LLMs that can impede their widespread use in healthcare. Many studies have been completed in controlled experimental environments with little evidence of long-term real-world use cases. As such, it is unclear whether LLMs perform in a generalizable way and whether they have a consistently robust performance in the varied contexts of clinical practice.

Another limitation of LLMs is the lack of standardized evaluation frameworks applicable to healthcare environments. Many current benchmarks for evaluating LLMs focus on accuracy, but do not adequately capture other important factors in their healthcare applications such as safety, bias, interpretability, and clinical usability.

Another significant gap in the literature is the absence of structured frameworks for ethical LLM implementation. Different ethical risks and technical challenges have been identified by individual studies. What is needed is a coordinated approach that combines governance, validation procedures and human oversight of LLMs in clinical practice.

3. ETHICAL CHALLENGES IN THE USE OF LARGE LANGUAGE MODELS IN HEALTHCARE

The ethical problems with the use of Large Language Models (LLMs) in health care are no longer just conceptual. Evidence from real-world studies and surveys within the industry continues to demonstrate many concerns related to LLM's ethical implications in health care (i.e., safety, bias, trust, accountability) due to the transition of these models from being purely experimental to operational elements within a clinical workflow. Recent studies and practitioner surveys provide evidence that health care practitioners are aware of the many ways LLMs could provide benefit to their work; however, they also express strong concerns regarding LLM's ethical risks if implemented with insufficient safeguards."

One example of this was the use of LLMs to assist in creating discharge summaries in the hospital setting, where inaccurately produced (subtle) data resulted in clinically reasonable but inappropriate outputs.

3.1 Evidence of Safety and Reliability Concerns

After 2021, numerous empirical studies demonstrate that Large Language Models (LLMs) are capable of generating clinically plausible but incorrect information. Various studies that examined the performance of LLMs on medical question- and answer-based tasks revealed significant variation in accuracy between clinical domains and have found lower reliability for complex diagnostic reasoning and rare diseases. Based on these studies, controlled evaluations of LLMs have produced moderate to high error rates depending on the complexity of the task, which raises concerns about using LLMs in direct clinical practice without adequate validation.

Clinician surveys reflect similar safety concerns associated with LLMs. In recent international clinician surveys, a large percentage of healthcare professionals responded that although LLMs may provide substantial benefits with respect to documentation and administrative support, LLMs cannot be trusted to make independent clinical decisions. A common theme in responses, however, was that clinicians find it difficult to identify subtle errors in AI-generated text, particularly when the output appears coherent and authoritative. This represents a significant ethical risk; there is a likelihood of silent errors that could be documented in the clinical record.

3.2 Bias and Equity: Findings From Healthcare AI Studies

Bias is an ethical dilemma that has been documented extensively in the literature regarding Healthcare AI and remains an ongoing issue. In post-2021 literature, studies on Clinical AI systems trained using large Clinical data, indicate evidence of a lack of equity across different demographic groups within the clinical data - such as differences in performance based on age, gender, racial and ethnic group, and socioeconomic status. Many of these studies weren't looking specifically at LLM's, but the findings are still useful since language models typically reflect the bias inherent in the clinical data and published medical literature.

In addition, there is an increase in the perceived awareness among clinicians regarding these risks, as well as evidence of that through survey results. In recent practitioner surveys, a relatively large percentage of practitioners reported concerns that AI solutions will provide better support for populations that are well represented in training datasets, whilst underrepresented populations may receive less support. From an ethical standpoint, this raises concern about fairness and justice given that the health care systems already face challenges of inequitable access and/or inequitable outcomes.

3.3 Trust and Transparency: Insights From User Studies

User-centered research conducted in healthcare settings supports the critical ethical issue of establishing trust between users and AI-assisted systems. Surveys of clinicians and medical students clearly indicate a relationship between clinician trust in LLM outputs and transparency and/or explainability. Clinicians report lower confidence levels in those AI tools which disclose no information about how the output was generated or what limitations apply.

As noted in previous literature, several studies have indicated that clinicians are more likely to adopt AI solutions when they are presented as assistive technologies (meaning they help clinical professionals make decisions) rather than as decision-making tools (meaning they replace human judgment). This is consistent with ethical principles that emphasize accountability and human agency; however, due to the lack of transparency in many LLM architectures, it is very difficult to fully meet these expectations, reinforcing the need for explicit mechanisms for oversight and review. For example, in the case of ambient clinical documentation systems deployed in actual clinical practice, using AI with a human in the loop has proven critical to ensuring that AI-generated documentation is accurate and that appropriate accountability has been established.

3.4 Privacy and Data Protection: Reported Risks and Incidents

Theoretical analysis and real-time incidents and audits all support privacy-related concerns. Reports that were issued since 2021 show that healthcare organization are not ready to use LLMs which rely on other organizations' cloud services due to uncertainty regarding retention policy, secondary use of the data, and compliance with regulations regarding health data. Data security and patient privacy have continuously been identified by IT leaders in the health care field as some of the top barriers to adopting artificial intelligence technology in this field.

Studies completed that researched the attitudes of clinicians showed that many healthcare providers are not willing to utilize tools that use artificial intelligence to process "raw" clinical text without assurance that the data will be anonymized and that access controls to it are properly established. Therefore, it appears ethical privacy-related concerns will have a direct effect on whether or not to adopt the technology as well as whether regulation requirements are being met.

3.5 Accountability and Professional Responsibility

Research and analysis of policies show an ongoing ethical challenge to the ambiguity regarding accountability. The surveys conducted by clinicians show they are unsure of their own responsibility when errors occur due to output from assisted AI. Many clinicians responding are concerned that the lack of accountability may put them at risk of legal or professional action, even though they are using AI to provide assistance.

This uncertainty strengthens the ethical necessity of keeping a human supervisor present and establishing an AI as a support and not a replacement of clinical decision-making. Implementation studies show that organizations with specific governance policies are less likely to encounter ethical dilemmas and more likely to have clinicians accept AI tools positively.

3.6 Safety in Real-World Clinical Deployment

The last challenge is providing assurance that LLM deployments are safe in real world, typically unregulated, healthcare environments. That is, LLM models which demonstrate high levels performance on controlled evaluations in laboratories may perform unpredictably under diverse clinical input or changing knowledge of medicine in real clinical environments. If there is no routine assessment of performance, and periodic retrospective assessments of performance, falling performance rates may be expected.

To ensure that LLM systems are deployed ethically, mechanisms must be incorporated to assess performance on a recurrent basis, to seek feedback from users, and to provide for updating or restricting the use of systems when there is evidence of significant risk. Safety should be viewed as a continuous series of events rather than as individual or infrequent evaluations.

Table 1.

Challenge	Description	Potential Impact on Healthcare	Need for Mitigation
Inaccurate or misleading outputs	LLMs may generate fluent but incorrect or incomplete information due to their probabilistic nature	Errors in clinical documentation, misinterpretation of patient history, or inappropriate clinical decisions	Mandatory human review and systematic validation of AI-generated content
Bias and fairness concerns	Training data may reflect historical or societal biases, leading to uneven performance across populations	Reinforcement of healthcare disparities and unequal quality of care for certain patient groups	Use of diverse datasets, bias audits, and performance evaluation across demographics
Lack of transparency	Internal decision-making processes of LLMs are difficult to interpret or explain	Reduced trust, difficulty in justifying AI-influenced clinical decisions	Adoption of interpretable outputs, documentation of system limitations
Automation bias	Clinicians may place excessive trust in AI-generated outputs	Reduced critical judgment and increased risk of unnoticed errors	Clear guidelines emphasizing AI as a support tool, not a decision-maker
Privacy and data security risks	Processing of sensitive patient data may expose systems to data breaches or misuse	Loss of patient confidentiality and legal or ethical violations	Strong data governance, encryption, and compliance with data protection regulations
Accountability ambiguity	Unclear responsibility when AI contributes to clinical outcomes	Ethical and legal uncertainty in case of errors or harm	Defined governance structures and clear allocation of responsibility
Performance degradation over time	Models may become less reliable as clinical practices and data evolve	Outdated or unsafe recommendations in real-world settings	Continuous monitoring, periodic reassessment, and model updates

TABLE 1 summarizes the key ethical and safety challenges associated with the use of large language models in healthcare, along with their potential impact and the corresponding need for mitigation strategies.

3.7 Case Studies and Real-World Challenges in LLM-Enabled Healthcare

While theoretical discussions highlight potential ethical risks of Large Language Models (LLMs) in healthcare, real-world experiences provide clearer insight into how these challenges manifest in practice. Repeated problems of bias, safety, privacy, and human oversight have been identified in a number of documented pilot deployments. These illustrate the need for ethics to be embedded within the system from the beginning, rather than addressed as an afterthought after deployment

Case Study 1: AI-Assisted Clinical Documentation Errors

. Pilot tests of LLM-based tools used to produce clinical notes, discharge summaries and referral letters in several large healthcare (hospital) systems confirmed that they facilitated the production of large volumes of documentation within much shorter periods of time than would otherwise have been possible. However, audits performed after the tools were deployed determined that while the time to generate documentation had been significantly reduced, there were also a number of significant instances of documented clinical information missing or misrepresented. In addition, there were also multiple instances in which medication dosage and time representations were written incorrectly, even though the corresponding text was accurate and fluently written.

The inaccuracies that were identified were not blatantly obvious but instead were extremely subtle and part of the normal routine of clinical review. As a result of the time pressure on clinical staff to perform their daily work, it is likely that these draft AI-generated documents were not sufficiently reviewed or verified prior to being placed into the patient record.

Key ethical lesson: clinical accuracy cannot be compromised using gain

Case Study 2: Bias in AI-Generated Clinical Language

In a study by researchers, they looked at how AI aided to the process of classifying and documenting patient symptomatology according to user-described demographics - and how each person received a classification based off of their demographics was either 'safer' (i.e. generalised) or assertive (i.e. clinically-specific).

Differences of these classifications were not a result of deliberate design characteristics within the model; rather the basis for creating the model and training it to function in this way were the historical (clinical narrative) nature of the data from which the AI model was designed and trained. Researchers are worried about the potential impact of language bias on clinical decision making (e.g. triage, referrals, etc.) once patients/clients' symptomatology is documented in the electronic health record (EHR).**Key ethical lesson:** Bias in language generation can subtly influence clinical perception and must be actively monitored.

Case Study 3: Privacy Risks in Cloud-Based LLM Deployment

Numerous providers of health care services periodically surveyed various cloud based machine learning service providers to identify which vendor they might use in the future to assist in the support of their administrative processes. Although some conducted internal assessments of risk, they expressed concerns regarding data retention policies, and whether or not patient information would be retained after utilization or used to enhance the vendors' models. Accordingly, a number of provider organisations have temporarily suspended their pilot programmes pending a satisfactory resolution of technical and contractual protections related to vendor performance.

This illustrates the types of real life problems numerous health care organisations are now confronted with: specifically, a lack of certainty with respect to a vendor's AI infrastructure and the associated ethical issues, which may result in reluctance on the part of employees to use AI, regardless of whether there are any data breaches.

Key ethical lesson: Privacy assurance must be explicit, verifiable, and enforceable—not assumed.

Case Study 4: Clinician Trust and Accountability Concerns

Through AI system implementations, clinicians have expressed doubts regarding the potential impact on their liability to the profession when AI-assisted decisions cause an error. Many clinicians expressed concern that the use of AI tools could subject them to professional discipline, even though such systems had been authorised to operate in their healthcare organisation (e.g., by facilities).

Consequently, the adoption of AI technologies in a health care setting has not taken place in as timely a fashion as expected due to clinical uncertainty over liability despite the technology readiness factor. When healthcare organisations later developed clear governance policies that communicated to clinicians that AI outputs were advisory and required clinician approval for use, acceptance of the technology and use of the tools significantly improved.

Key ethical lesson: Clear accountability frameworks are essential for ethical and practical adoption.

Case Study 5: Performance Drift Over Time

In extended pilot deployments of some LLM based systems as clinical guidelines change over time some of their outputs will become less relevant and accurate over time due to the evolution of these guidelines. For example, outputs considered acceptable will often become outdated much quicker than anticipated as in the area of infectious disease management which is evolving quickly. There is a risk that these LLMs will reinforce obsolete or outdated practices in the absence of systematic revalidation.

Key ethical lesson Ethical AI is continuous process not one time process

Table 2. Case study and challenges in LLM

Case Area	Observed Challenge	Ethical Implication
Clinical documentation	Subtle inaccuracies in fluent text	Risk of patient harm
Bias	Demographic influence on generated language	Equity and fairness concerns
Privacy	Unclear data retention in cloud systems	Confidentiality risks
Accountability	Clinician uncertainty about responsibility	Reduced trust and adoption
System longevity	Degradation over time	Safety and governance failure

4. HUMAN OVERSIGHT AND PRIVACY

LLM in health case have strong protection against personal information. Human oversight must be combined with privacy protection to guarantee proper function from LLMs in health care. The gaps in clinical accountability, ethical reasoning, and contextual awareness when using LLMs cause human monitoring to remain necessary in order for AI-enabled outputs to be accurate, appropriate, and comply with laws that protect patients' safety. However, since it is difficult to protect patients from harm or to properly collect, manage, and use sensitive medical information with LLM-based systems, technical security measures and ethical principles will need to be developed to protect privacy.

4.1 Role of Human Oversight in Clinical Workflows

Human Oversight is a vital component in the design of Healthcare Applications utilizing LLMs, as LLMs produce probabilistic outputs that will vary from instance to instance based on factors such as input (How input was made), context of input

(The context in which the input was made), and how the LLM is configured (Fine-tuning). Thus, LLMs' outputs should be treated hesitantly as deterministic and assume they're consistently reliable. Therefore, before using clinical record generated with AI-generated content or prior to using AI-generated content for clinical decision making, the individual practicing medicine (and all other health care providers) must continue to review, validate, and approve of AI-generated content.

Reviewing AI-generated content alone will not provide adequate oversight; adequate oversight must include thorough documentation of human involvement, clearly defined processes for escalating ambiguous outputs, and structured processes for validating outputs. An example of this is an AI-generated clinical summary being treated as a draft Artefact until confirmed by the original source documents. Utilizing this approach will maximize out automation efficiencies while holding the clinician(s) accountable for quality. Importantly, when possible, supervision processes should be integrated seamlessly into existing workload processes to reduce cognitive load and minimise the likelihood of automation bias.

4.2 Human-in-the-Loop and Human-on-the-Loop Models

Certainly; when building a Human Oversight System, person-in-the-loop or Human-on-the-loop systems can also be created; however, in either case, a human will need to provide explicit permission before using an LLM's output in a person-in-the-loop system. Therefore, high-risk tasks such as clinical documentation/diagnoses/treatment proposals /communicating with patients are ideal candidates to use a person-in-the-loop architecture. In contrast, Human-on-the-loop systems allow for some degree of IBM LLM autonomy unless some predefined threshold/anomaly occurs that triggers a human's intervention in their operation.

When determining which oversight model to implement, there are three factors to consider: 1) The clinical environment; 2) The level of risk involved; & 3) The potential for taking legal action. For example, if the oversight function is performed for a task categorized as a low-risk administrative task, then the oversight will function more flexibly. However, for high-risk tasks, tighter controls are necessary and there is a low tolerance for loss. The ethical principle remains the same regardless of the system's configuration: Timed automated technology shall never have decision-making authority over patient care.

4.3 Privacy Risks in LLM-Based Healthcare Applications

One significant area of difficulty with the adoption of LLM in health care technology is protecting the privacy of patients. These models often use unstructured clinical language to represent patients' treatment histories, diagnostic information, and other identifying information about a patient. Improperly controlling the training and storage processes of an LLM may allow access to this sensitive data during both training and inference phases. Another challenge in adopting LLM is that many deployments/LM architectures will preserve input data as part of an effort to log activity or enhance your model. Uncontrolled preservation of data creates significant ethical issues in the Healthcare environment, except where expressly authorized and regulated by data protection legislation. Finally, organizations that utilize third-party cloud services often have limited ability to see their underlying hardware; therefore, they must depend upon compliance assurances made by these service providers.

4.4 Technical Safeguards for Data Protection

To protect against privacy threats, technical and organizational safeguards must be used together. Data reduction is essential from a technical perspective. Whenever possible, sensitive identities should be eliminated or masked; LLM should be given as little data as necessary to accomplish a specific task. Pseudonymization and de-identifying etc., can provide a reduced risk of exposure while still providing the same useful clinical resource.

Data generated through LLM processing of clinical text must be protected through secure data management methods such as encryption in transit and at rest. Access control measures should be implemented to prevent non-authorized personnel from accessing or editing AI-assisted outputs (via role-based permissions). Audit logs can provide an additional layer of accountability through the documentation of system access and human interactions with LLM-generated materials.

New methods such as secure enclaves, federated learning, and on-premise implementation limit the possibility for outside exposure and also reduce the potential for data transit, thereby providing additional privacy protections. These types of solutions can be more complex to implement than traditional methods but are meaningful for healthcare organizations that are subject to several regulatory obligations..

4.5 Consent, Transparency, and Data Governance

While technological safeguards play an important role in establishing a safe environment for patients' data to be maintained, it is also necessary to have open communications with patients about how they will receive care and what data will be collected and used. This includes informing them that artificial intelligence systems will be used to assist in delivering care or analyzing personal and/or clinical information. Therefore, the ethical use of artificial intelligence systems requires that the organization provides transparency around how patients' data will be collected, used, and maintained, even if it does not require express consent.

The organization should have well-defined data governance policies that outline the various aspects of patient data ownership (who owns the data), permissible types of uses for the data, how long the data will be retained, and the obligations of the various stakeholders to uphold the data governance policies and the above noted aspects. Regular reviews of the privacy assessment on a more frequent basis will also allow the organization to identify new issues as its data systems, patient care delivery methods and AI technologies evolve.

4.6 Balancing Innovation With Privacy and Oversight

A major area of concern with automated healthcare solutions using LLMs is finding a balance between the efficiencies of automated health solutions and the ethical obligations surrounding human oversight and patient confidentiality. Too much regulatory agency human oversight can reduce value in AI systems while a lack of oversight (i.e., too much automation) can put patients at risk. Analysis of system performance, user interaction, and privacy issues must continue to strike a balance between both areas. Human oversight and privacy protections should be seen as facilitating innovation in conjunction with employing reliable AI technologies. Healthcare organizations must apply technology-based protections, have structured processes for monitoring their operations and provide transparency in governance to capitalize on the benefits from LLM's, while operating ethically and having a high level of public confidence.

Table 3. Ethical issues in LLM

Ethical Issue	Evidence from Studies and Surveys	Ethical Implication
Safety and accuracy	Evaluations show variable accuracy and clinically plausible errors	Risk of patient harm if outputs are not validated
Bias and fairness	Studies report uneven performance across demographic groups	Potential reinforcement of healthcare inequalities
Transparency	Clinician surveys indicate low trust in opaque AI systems	Reduced accountability and informed decision-making
Privacy	IT leader surveys rank data security as a top adoption barrier	Threats to patient confidentiality and trust
Accountability	Clinicians report uncertainty about responsibility for AI-assisted errors	Ethical and legal ambiguity in care delivery

5. RESPONSIBLE USE FRAMEWORK

In order to correctly integrate Large Language Models (LLMs) into healthcare, it is necessary to have a systematic framework that provides balance between technological competence, ethical accountability, clinical safety, and regulatory compliance. This is based on the premise that LLMs provide supporting tools to be governed by humans, rather than viewed as autonomous decision-makers. The proposed framework for responsible usage of LLMs is intended to incorporate governance, technical protections, human oversight, and ethical accountability during the complete life cycle of deployment of the LLMs and directly addresses the aforementioned ethical challenges such as risks to safety, bias, opaque processes, and protection of confidential information.

5.1 Purpose Definition and Use-Case Boundaries

Establishing the purpose and approved use of a deployed large language model (LLM) is the first step toward appropriately using an LLM. The intended use of an LLM in healthcare should be restricted to the lowest and moderate-risk activities where tasks can have numerous characteristics such a patient communication drafting, coding assistance, summary of clinical notes, and support for the documentation of clinical activities.

One of the most important aspects of the framework is that LLMs cannot be used to independently produce a diagnosis, prescribe a treatment, or initiate a medication order. By establishing the appropriate use, it will help reduce the risk of misuse or abuse and reduce the risk to patients when they are dependent on or rely on an LLM's output.

Key principle: LLMs will support clinical workflows, but they will not substitute for the judgment of a clinician.

5.2 Data Governance and Privacy Protection

Given the nature of sensitive healthcare data, ethical use requires safeguarding of privacy. Therefore, the system will require strict governance principles for your data (e.g., data minimization; access requests; encryption; compliance with applicable laws regarding protection of healthcare data).

You will also want to implement LLMs so that prior to exiting the session, no identifiable patient information will remain in the system. If you are testing or validating the system you should use de-identified or synthetic data when possible. Any agreements or contracts that involve third parties who may have any access to your data will need to specify:

- Ownership of the data;
- Retention period for the data; and
- Restrictions on reuse of the data.

Key principle: Patient confidentiality must never be compromised for operational convenience.

5.3 Model Validation and Risk Assessment

Before deploying an LLM, it needs to be validated against a specific task to ensure that the model performs acceptably, reliably and in a safe manner when utilized. It is important to validate the accuracy of information before implementing it in clinical practice. Validating the accuracy of information includes: Fact-checking and confirming no errors exist in the information, testing for any weaknesses that may lead to incorrect conclusions, and determining whether the information will be affected by missing inputs.

When performing risk assessment for each validation activity, consider the following:

- Determine the impact of errors on clinical decision-making
- Assess how many times a human review has been performed
- Identify sensitivities specific to your task

Validation is an ongoing process; every time you update your clinical guidelines or add new workflows, you must also reassess your validation efforts.

Key principle: No LLM should be deployed without evidence-based validation.

5.4 Human-in-the-Loop Oversight

To ensure responsible use of LLMS, there needs to be human oversight of LLM output. Therefore, LLMs should be viewed as a recommendation (draft) only, and a human must verify the final product prior to release. The clinician has ultimate responsibility and authority for the overall clinical decision-maker.

Providing users training on how to critically evaluate AI-generated content (and not blindly accept AI-generated content) is one method to help reduce the likelihood of an automation bias. Whenever possible, the interface should allow the user to identify AI-generated content, and there should be indications of confidence/certainty of AI-generated content.

Key-Principle: Humans have responsibility for clinical decision-making, regardless of the use of AI.

5.5 Transparency and Explainability

While LLMs are an incredibly complex model, they require transparency regarding how LLMs are generated and used in order to be deployed responsibly. Users must know when they are using AI and understand what they can expect regarding limitations of the AI system.

- o System documentation (already in place) must include the following information:
- o Intended use cases for the model
- o Known limitations of the model
- o Validation of the model
- o Transparency establishes trust between the clinician, patient & regulators & fosters informed clinical decision-making.

Key Principle: Trust is derived from transparency rather than from a lack of transparency.

5.6 Bias Monitoring and Fairness Assurance

Bias in LLM systems can come from the training data sources, task framing and engagement patterns of users. It is therefore necessary that LLM systems are routinely monitored for generated outputs to determine if there is contextual or demographic bias before they are developed/functionally implemented. Each output generated by LLM systems should also undergo frequent audit processes to confirm systematic variances in outputs between patient groups. When biased outputs are produced, remedial actions such as refining of prompts, adjusting dataset balances or limiting use cases should occur.

Key principle: Equity, as it relates to healthcare should be extended into the AI -assisted process.

5.7 Continuous Monitoring and Performance Drift Management

The healthcare industry is consistently evolving; thus, the suggested guidelines, language used, and best practices related to it will equally develop and progress (like living organisms do). The same applies to LLMs; they will eventually fail in their purpose if not consistently checked.

The proposed framework will provide the following tools:

- AI interaction logging

- Error report tracking
- Validation benchmark updating

Clinician input is vital in recognizing emerging risks as well as improving alignment between systems and clinical requirements.

Key principle: Responsible use of AI is continuous process .

5.8 Accountability and Governance Structure

For ethical obligations to be fulfilled, an effective governance structure needs to be implemented. It's important for health care organizations to define and clarify who on a multidisciplinary team will oversee patient safety for AI-assisted systems. There will be defined policies and procedures to address any patient safety concerns or unexpected occurrences that occur as a result of using AI technologies. Health care organizations and health care clinicians will bear responsibility to their patients for AI-assisted systems—this responsibility does not lie with the algorithms themselves.

Key principle: No algorithm can assume responsibility for any actions that occur from an algorithm's decisions.

Figure 1. Framework for Large Language Models in Healthcare

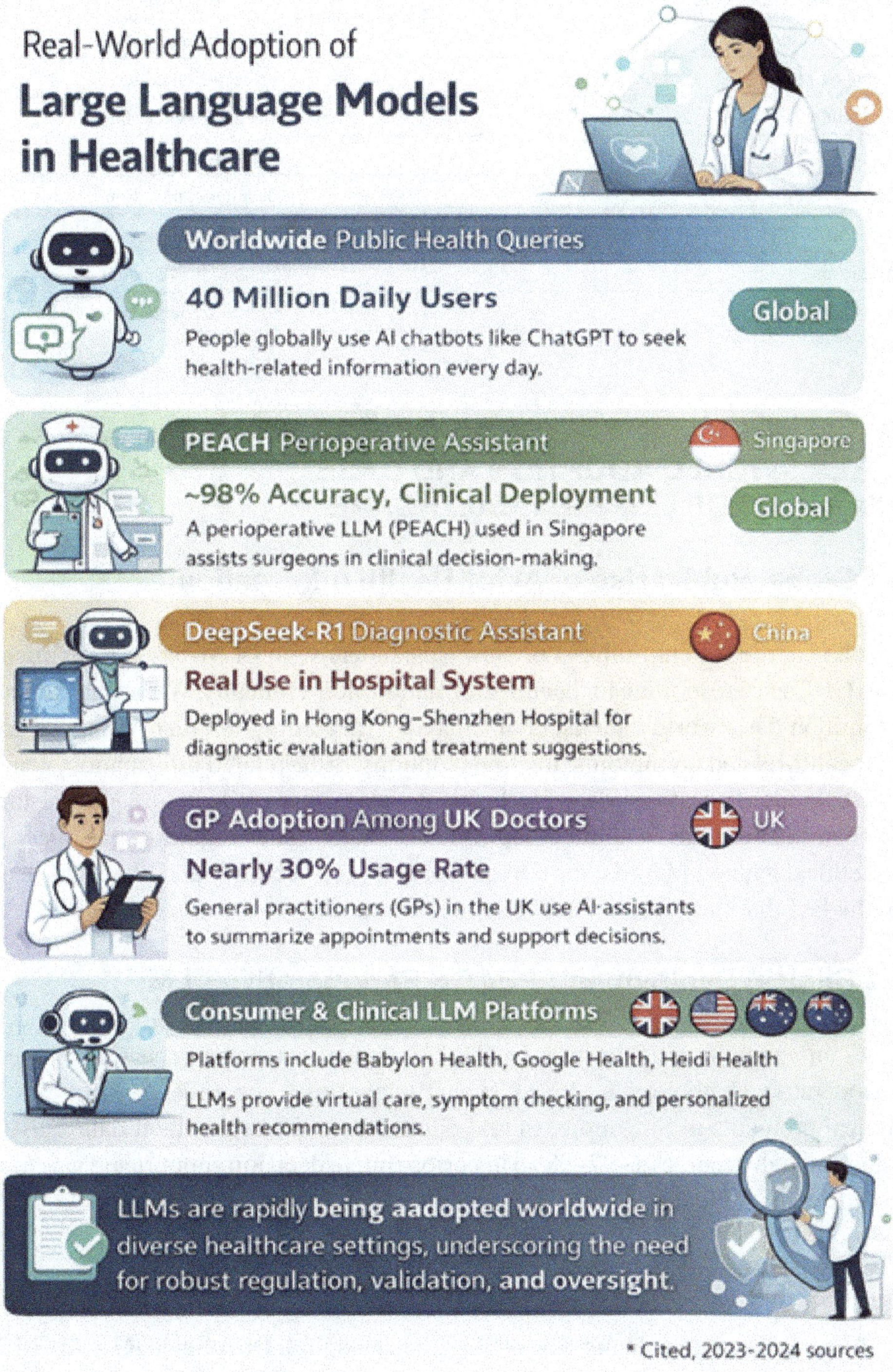

Table 4. Framework Dimension for LLM in Healthcare

Framework Dimension	Responsible Practice
Purpose definition	Clear task boundaries
Data governance	Privacy-first design
Validation	Evidence-based testing
Oversight	Human-in-the-loop
Transparency	Clear communication
Fairness	Bias monitoring
Monitoring	Continuous evaluation
Governance	Defined accountability

6. REAL-WORLD ADOPTION AND CASE EXAMPLES OF LLMS IN HEALTHCARE

6.1 Global Public Use of AI for Health Information

The internet offers millions of New Zealanders with LLM-based tools such as ChatGPT who are looking for health information, non-clinically. With approximately 40 million daily worldwide users of ChatGPT (according to OpenAI), these users ask health-related (symptoms, treatment options, drug-related information, general health) kinds of questions. This level of trust and reliance on AI to provide assistance for their health (with no clinical input) raises many issues regarding the adequacy and ethical nature of LLMs in a clinical context (i.e., accuracy and oversight) based on the fact that they are not clinically monitored.

6.2 Clinical Deployment: PEACH Perioperative LLM

In an example of *institution-level LLM deployment*, researchers developed a perioperative chatbot called **PEACH** that integrates a secure LLM with existing clinical protocols in Singapore. In real clinical use with real patient data, PEACH achieved high accuracy (~97–98%) in perioperative decision support and was found to accelerate clinician decisions in most cases.

6.3. Real Hospital Use — DeepSeek-R1 in China

At the University of Hong Kong–Shenzhen Hospital, **DeepSeek-R1** — an LLM-based diagnostic assistant — has been deployed to assist clinicians with record analysis, interpretation of results (including imaging), and evidence-based treatment suggestions in a real clinical environment.

6.4 Clinical Practitioner Adoption in the UK

Recent surveys report that **nearly** 30% of general practitioners in the UK are already using AI tools such as LLM-based assistants (e.g., ChatGPT) in patient consultations for summarizing appointments, aiding clinical decision tasks, and managing administrative duties. This use is increasing rapidly despite regulatory gaps.

6.5. Ambient Clinical Documentation Adoption Worldwide

Ambient clinical documentation — where speech recognition and LLMs capture and summarize patient–clinician interactions in real time — is already implemented in multiple health systems to reduce documentation burden. Doctor review will help LLM provide draft which create impact in workflow and documentation.

6.6 Commercial and Patient-Facing LLM Health Platforms

Several platforms worldwide illustrate how LLMs are being used for direct patient engagement and health planning:

- Babylon Health (UK): LLM-enhanced virtual care and symptom checking.
- InteliHealth (USA): Personalized health plans using LLMs.
- Google **Health**: Uses AI to help patients manage and interpret their personal health data.
- **Heidi Health** (Australia): AI medical scribe and clinical note generation deployed internationally.

Table 5. Real-World LLM Healthcare Adoption

Deployment/Platform	Context	Main Use	Ethical/Regulatory Implication
ChatGPT (40M daily health queries)	Global public use	Self-guided health info	Reliability & misinformation risks
PEACH perioperative assistant	Hospital clinical support	Decision support	Validation, safety monitoring
DeepSeek-R1	University hospital system	Diagnostic assistance	Human oversight, data governance

continued on following page

Table 5. Continued

Deployment/Platform	Context	Main Use	Ethical/Regulatory Implication
GP adoption in UK	NHS context	Clinical summaries/ consultations	Regulation & governance gaps
Ambient documentation	EHR integration	Doctor–patient note synthesis	Privacy & accuracy workflow
Commercial platforms (Babylon, Heidi)	Consumer/clinical	Virtual care, health planning	Consumer safety & consent

Figure 2. Real world Adoption Large Language Model in Healthcare

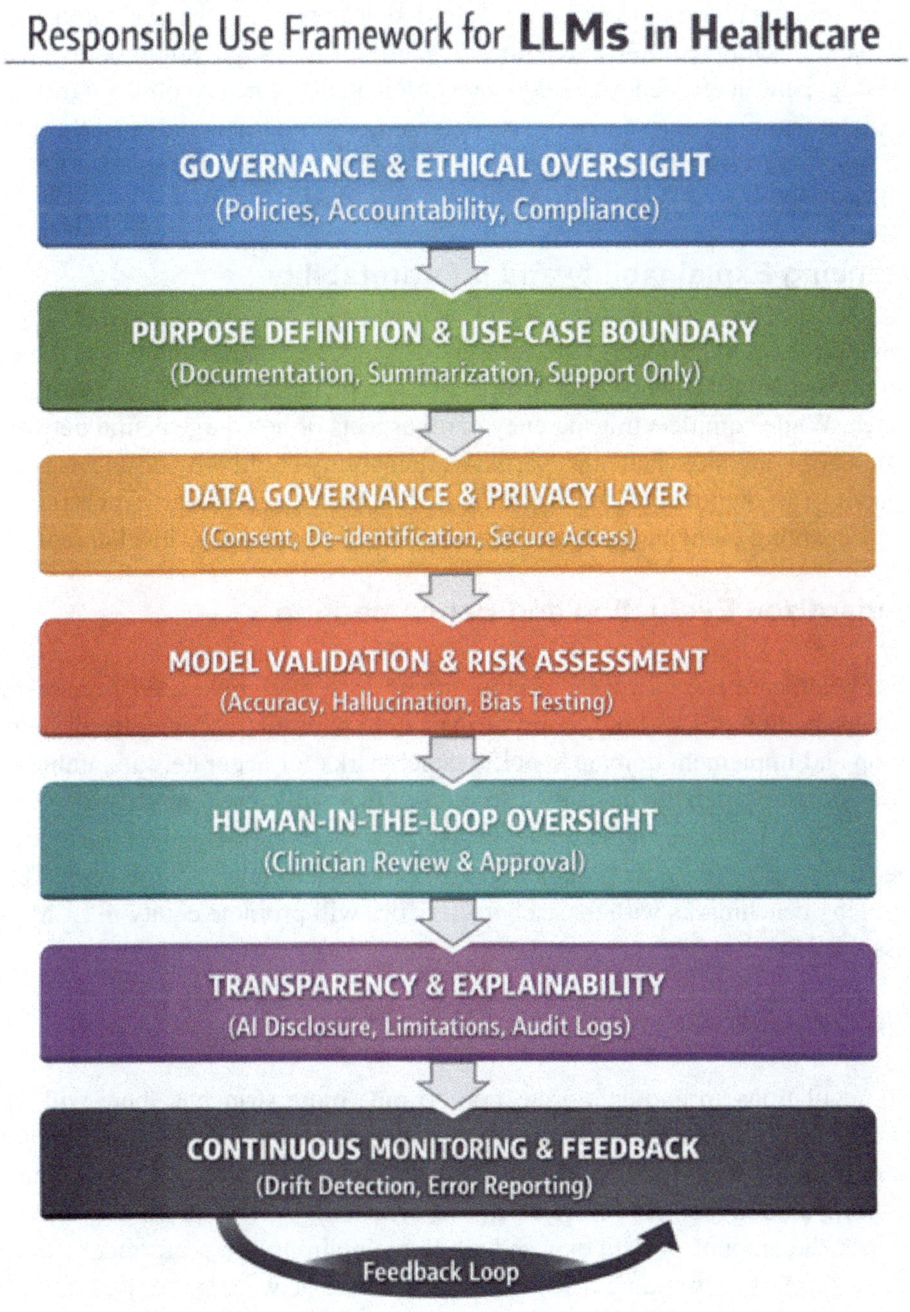

7. FUTURE DIRECTIONS

The rapid evolution of Large Language Models presents both opportunities and responsibilities for the future of healthcare. While current applications demonstrate promising gains in efficiency and documentation quality, the next phase of research and implementation must focus on strengthening safety, trust, and ethical robustness. Several key directions emerge for advancing the responsible use of LLMs in healthcare systems.

Advancing Explainability and Interpretability

Methods to assist clinicians in determining how they could build trust and make informed decisions based on LLM outputs should be the prioritized area for future research. While complete transparency of all aspects of how large neural networks function is an ongoing challenge, partial explainability could provide a level of detail about LLM output confidence scores, attributions, and summaries of rationale, thereby enabling clinicians to understand and evaluate through critical appraisal.

Standardized Evaluation and Benchmarking

For healthcare use cases, there is an urgent lack of standardized frameworks for the evaluation of LLM output performance. In particular, future efforts should develop and implement domain-specific benchmarks for accurate, safe, unbiased, robust, and usable performance of LLM outputs that will closely match complexity of actual clinical practice and all relevant characteristics of the patient populations served by the LLM (e.g., geographical distribution, age, gender, culture, etc.). Thus, developing benchmarks with these characteristics will promote equity in LLM use across the demographics.

Privacy-Preserving Model Architectures

As regulations around data protection become more stringent, there will be a growing need to conduct future LLM deployments using advanced methods to preserve privacy. Some potential methods include federated learning, secure multi-party computation, and on-device inference, which all provide promising avenues to reduce the amount of data exposed while maintaining the performance of the model. Therefore, continuing research on the balance between privacy guarantees, clinical performance, and operational feasibility is needed..

Dynamic Human-AI Collaboration Models

Classifying systems of the future requires moving away from human-in-the-loop designs with limited adaptability; rather, systems should develop adaptive models based on collaboration with humans to meet the needs of current tasks based on risks associated with the task, level of expertise of the clinician performing the work, and uncertainty. For example, tasks associated with higher risk require more stringent oversight than routine tasks that are automated through the use of AI and monitored. Adapting oversight will enhance safety and efficiency of workflow.

There are rapid developments in the regulatory framework associated with healthcare related AI and future deployments must allow for adaptation to continued evolution of laws and ethical standards that guide policies in the use of AI in healthcare. Research should explore models of governance that provide for continuous compliance, auditability, and accountability. It will be critical to have collaboration among technologists, clinicians, ethicists, and regulatory agencies to ensure that the innovation model is congruent with the public interest.

Longitudinal Studies of the Impact of LLM on Healthcare

At present, evaluations of the use of LLMs in health systems primarily focus on short-term effectiveness or the results of pilot studies evaluating use; therefore, new research should include longitudinal studies measuring the impact of LLMs on clinical practices over the long term (i.e., how continued use of LLMs will affect clinician behaviour, how continued use of LLMs will affect patient outcomes, and the unintended consequences of using LLMs). It will be critical to develop evidence based longitudinally to understand how the continued use of AI is changing the practice of providing health care over time.

Continuous Governance and Regulatory Alignment

Regulatory frameworks for healthcare AI are evolving rapidly, and future LLM deployments must remain adaptable to changing legal and ethical standards. Future research will focus on developing new governance models that ensure ongoing compliance, accountability, and auditability. Collaborative efforts between technical experts, clinicians, ethicists and public policy makers will be necessary to ensure that new technologies align with the public's health and safety needs

Education and Workforce Preparedness

Finally, the next stage to address is the human step of implementing artificial intelligence into healthcare. Health professionals and clinicians will continue to need support through robust educational programs, which include; AI literacy, ethical awareness, and critical thinking skill development. Providing information to users outlining the strengths and limitations of LLMs will assist in the proper and responsible implementation of LLMs into practice.

Closing Perspective

To make progress in future LLM-based health care systems, we need not only to pursue technological improvements but also embed ethical reasoning, human judgment and institutional accountability into AI systems. This means that health care systems will move from capabilities of using powerful AI to providing AI solutions that are trustworthy; inclusive; and aligned with patient-centered care principles.

8. CONCLUSION

Today's healthcare industry is seeing a shift toward using large language models (LLMs) in various areas such as clinical documentation, administrative efficiency, and managing data. If appropriately utilized within the context of healthcare, LLMs have the potential to create clearer records, reduce clinician workload, and promote improved communication among teams of providers. However, as illustrated in this chapter, integrating LLMs into the workflow of healthcare presents numerous ethical, safety, and governance challenges that must be addressed.

The primary risks associated with LLMs are due to the use and management of LLMs over the technology of LLMs themselves (examples: hallucinated output, tacit bias, privacy violations, and over-reliance on automation). Without having clear boundaries for the use of LLMs or proper governance, patients may be put at greater risk relative to patient safety, clinical equity, and provider accountability.

In an effort to assist with the responsible and clinically safe use of LLMs in healthcare, this chapter outlines a framework that integrates ethical references with practical safety structures and knowledge from real-life experience.

The ethical and safety risks that arise from the use of LLMs are significant in the healthcare sector due to the possibility of immediate and long-term harmful consequences for the health of patients when errors occur. One of the chapter's key findings is the necessity for human oversight in the use of LLMs. Rather than relying on their own judgment to make decisions, LLMs have to be used as a support system.

Human-in-the-loop frameworks are essential to maintain the importance of clinical knowledge, moral judgment, and contextual understanding when delivering health care services. While health care organizations can take advantage of the benefits of LLMs for patient care, they must ensure accountability and trust by retaining the authority of clinical personnel to make final decisions.

Creating systems for transparency and protecting patient privacy is very important through data governance. The ethical use of AI is built on three main principles, which are auditability, informed consent, and confidentiality. The suggested framework to facilitate the responsible use of LLMs will provide an effective roadmap for health care organizations interested in using LLMs safely. Health care organizations can transition away from an ad hoc approach to using LLMs by using governance, validation, fairness monitoring, and feedback loops throughout the AI life cycle to build sustainable and ethical implementations of LLMs. LLMs have great potential as collaborative tools for health care provision, provided that their use is based on a human-centered design, technical rigor, and ethical principles.

REFERENCES

Bender, E. M., Gebru, T., McMillan-Major, A., & Shmitchell, S. (2021). On the dangers of stochastic parrots: Can language models be too big? *Proceedings of the ACM Conference on Fairness, Accountability, and Transparency*, 610–623. DOI: 10.1145/3442188.3445922

Food and Drug Administration (FDA). (2023). *Artificial intelligence and machine learning in software as a medical device*. U.S. FDA.

Ji, Z., Lee, N., Frieske, R., Yu, T., Su, D., Xu, Y., Ishii, E., Bang, Y., Madotto, A., & Fung, P. (2023). Survey of hallucination in natural language generation. *ACM Computing Surveys*, *55*(12), 1–38. DOI: 10.1145/3571730

Kung, T. H., Cheatham, M., Medenilla, A., Sillos, C., De Leon, L., Elepaño, C., Madriaga, M., Aggabao, R., Diaz-Candido, G., Maningo, J., & Tseng, V. (2023). Performance of ChatGPT on USMLE: Potential for AI-assisted medical education. *PLOS Digital Health*, *2*(2), e0000198. DOI: 10.1371/journal.pdig.0000198 PMID: 36812645

Leslie, D. (2022). *Understanding artificial intelligence ethics and safety*. Alan Turing Institute.

Nori, H., King, N., McKinney, S. M., Carignan, D., & Horvitz, E. (2023). Capabilities of GPT-4 on medical challenge problems. *arXiv preprint arXiv:2303.13375*.

Rudin, C., Chen, C., Chen, Z., Huang, H., Semenova, L., & Zhong, C. (2022). Interpretable machine learning: Fundamental principles and 10 grand challenges. *Statistics Surveys*, *16*(none), 1–85. DOI: 10.1214/21-SS133

Seyyed-Kalantari, L., Zhang, H., McDermott, M., Chen, I. Y., & Ghassemi, M. (2021). Underdiagnosis bias of AI algorithms applied to chest radiographs. *Nature Medicine*, 27(12), 2176–2182.World Health Organization (WHO). (2021). *Ethics and governance of artificial intelligence for health*. WHO.

Zhu, Q., Hou, B., Mathai, T. S., Mukherjee, P., Jin, Q., Chen, X., Wang, Z., Cheng, R., Summers, R. M., & Lu, Z. (2025). How well do multimodal LLMs interpret CT scans? An auto-evaluation framework for analyses. *Journal of Biomedical Informatics*, *168*, 104864. DOI: 10.1016/j.jbi.2025.104864 PMID: 40578543

Chapter 11

Expert Consensus on LLM Safety in Clinical Decision Support

K. Gayathri
http://orcid.org/0009-0007-3786-2009
Department of Microbiology, Sacred Heart College, Tirupattur, India

B. Lokeshwari
http://orcid.org/0009-0005-6612-5134
Department of Microbiology, Sacred Heart College, Tirupattur, India

S. Kanshiya
Department of Microbiology, Sacred Heart College, Tirupattur, India

P. Vilmasen
http://orcid.org/0009-0005-6817-2620
Department of Microbiology, Sacred Heart College, Tirupattur, India

P. Saranraj
http://orcid.org/0000-0002-5052-6532
Department of Microbiology, Sacred Heart College, Tirupattur, India

J. Albino Wins
http://orcid.org/0000-0003-1483-9627
Holy Cross College, Nagercoil, India

ABSTRACT

Despite tremendous advancements in text creation, large language models (LLMs) are still not sufficiently advanced to be applied on their own in mission-critical fields such as medical, finance, and law. The current solutions require professional assistance or human support, which makes them less scalable. As the application of Generative Artificial Intelligence (GAI) increases, it is only reasonable that concerns about security and other problems would soon arise. Large language models, or LLMs, have been widely used in many therapeutic domains, such as establishing individualised treatment plans, speeding up diagnosis, and aiding in radiological diagnostics. In hepatology and gastroenterology, doctors are having a harder time

DOI: 10.4018/979-8-3373-7862-6.ch011

making decisions. Large language models (LLMs), a subset of generative artificial intelligence (AI), are creating new opportunities in CDSS by providing more adaptive and flexible support that better reflects the situation's complexity.

1. INTRODUCTION

Safety taxonomy and policy that aligns with human values must be developed. We offer top-notch human-annotated data for LLM interactions from our 12 annotators. The second phase is training a set of powerful Large Language Models (LLMs) with our data. The resilience of each model is then evaluated against our in-domain dataset, adversarial jailbreaking datasets, and a set of out-of-domain content safety benchmarks. Despite their groundbreaking generative capabilities, large language models—also referred to as Groundbreaking Generative AI (GAI) models—present a number of AI safety concerns (Osheroff et al., 2012). A detailed review of the AI safety issues associated with LLMs is provided in this research, based on the existing knowledge. One of the major challenges is that there is no specific survey research in AI Safety that adequately deals with the challenges posed by GAI-LLMs, which have been identified as a result of the technical nature of what constitutes an LLM. Because it often strays too far into topics like X-risk, the boundaries of AI ethics, and regulatory reforms, current research is less preoccupied with the functional aspects of GAI-LLMs.

Following a review of the known limitations of generative models as documented in other studies, we identify and elucidate novel safety concerns resulting from the unresolved technical challenges that make up an LLM. Understanding the safety concerns with generative AI and huge language models led us to discover a number of significant works and subjects (Osheroff et al., 2007). This encompasses prejudice and equity, poisoning and the production of harmful content, disinformation, privacy and security concerns, hostile attacks, infringement of intellectual property, ethics and human preferences, and general safety. The process of providing patients or medical professionals with timely, filtered clinical knowledge and patient-specific information in an effort to improve patient care is known as clinical decision support, or CDS. This data may include new clinical trial findings, evidence-based best practices for the treatment of specific diseases, basic facts and relationships, and other information. CDS systems (CDSS) have long been proposed as a means to enhance patient care and manage medical data.

Nevertheless, despite several decades of research and development, these systems have failed to offer any integration or therapeutic advantage. The complexity and adaptability necessary to manage the complexities of modern medicine were not present in the rule-based models that first developed CDSS, as stated by Sutton et al. (2020). In the hepatological and gastrointestinal fields, they were unable to offer patient-specific information and dynamic decision support. Moreover, current AI-based CDSS infrequently use structured data sources for therapeutic use, but instead for billing purposes, which limits their use and makes them not accurately reflect real-world situations. To enhance patient safety and minimize medication errors, CDSSs are useful tools. Healthcare professionals can avoid potential adverse drug events by utilizing these tools to offer evidence-based recommendations and alerts. Conventional CDSSs have several limitations, as stated by (Dang 2023). The latest advances in the field of medicine and the complexity of patient cases may not be considered by rule-based algorithms and data sets. The capacity to distinguish between severe and mild allergies, the patient's previous tolerance, and risk-benefit analysis are just a few examples of the complex patient scenarios that are recorded in clinical documents, but these systems are only capable of issuing warnings when a drug with potential cross-reactions is prescribed. Utilising this data has been demonstrated to dramatically reduce the number of unnecessary alerts. Strict alerting systems that fail to consider this data may cause healthcare personnel to become fatigued and possibly miss important signals.

These issues can be addressed by GPT-4 and other large language models (LLMs), according to Reed et al. (2020). As a result of their sophisticated natural language processing (NLP) skills, LLMs have already proven to be useful in a range of healthcare applications, such as clinical note production, diagnosis support, and treatment outcome and drug interaction prediction. Given their ability to process and synthesise large amounts of unstructured data, we hypothesise that they offer a novel alternative to the rule-based CDSSs now in use, which often lack the flexibility and depth of knowledge required for complex patient-specific scenarios. Traditional approaches to LLM application co-design require a significant time commitment from both domain experts and LLM developers since they rely on close collaboration to iteratively change their prompts and aims. However, this fails to acknowledge a crucial issue: the groups that stand to benefit from AI assistance are also the ones whose inadequate resources keep them from participating completely in the rigorous co-design task (Colleagues and Janice, 2020).

The whole local context and/or domain knowledge required to design a useful application may be unavailable to AI developers without the help of domain specialists. Evidence-based information and patient data are used by clinical decision support systems, or CDSS, to assist medical professionals in making decisions in real time. When used in conjunction with Electronic Health Records (EHR), they facilitate patient diagnosis, treatment decision-making, and outcome prediction. The growing significance of CDSS in contemporary healthcare practices is shown by the expansion of the healthcare sector. Ability explanation is often disregarded, although being a crucial component of CDSS, which might result in dependency problems.

The applications of AI in clinical decision-making need to provide explanations that can help justify the recommendations made. The need for XAI and transparency is highlighted by the moral need for decision-making and the realization that AI systems can perpetuate preconceived ideas. According to Urmimala Sarkar and Lipika Samal (2020), LLMs have demonstrated their ability to adapt to healthcare tasks like image tagging, summarization of information, and complex question-answering. The understanding and explanation of complex medical information by the healthcare industry could be completely revolutionized by LLMs. Although they can explain, LLMs are not flawless. They could potentially malfunction or forget key points in a medical setting (Pierre-Yves Meunier et al., 2023).

2. LARGE LANGUAGE MODEL

The processing, analysis, and production of human language are the functions of large language models (LLMs), which are advanced artificial intelligence (AI) technologies. Trillions of words are used to train them (11 trillion words were used to teach Llama 3, for example). One of the areas of computer science where these models are most useful is natural language processing (NLP), which is the study of how data is processed and analyzed in natural language. They are therefore able to interpret and evaluate complex medical information. With domain-specific models such as Radiology-GPT and large language models (LLMs) such as the general models GPT-3.5 and GPT-4, the radiology community is being introduced to advanced natural language generation and analysis capabilities. The capability of transformer models with large datasets to understand complex clinical language makes these models extremely suitable for a range of radiological applications (Bethany et al., 2021). One of LLMs' most significant uses is automating the radiological report writing process. LLMs can help radiologists save time and avoid repetitive strain injuries by generating early reports from imaging data. Initial study suggests that LLM reports can be almost as reliable as expert results, especially if accessible radiological corpora or organised information are available. LLMs make structured reporting (SR), which is generally recommended in contemporary radiology, easier to complete in order to enhance report quality. Busch et al.'s analysis revealed that the accuracy of SR varied from 25% to 100%, underscoring the actual and potential limitations of LLMs (Sijpe et al., 2022).

3. LANGUAGE MODEL ERROR RATES

Current state-of-the-art AI text processing models are Large Language Models (LLMs), which are particularly good at tasks like translation and creative writing. These models, which were trained on a large corpus of literature and are based on the transformer architecture, have demonstrated a high level of comprehension and the capacity to produce language that is similar to that of humans. In terms of reliability and error prevention, however, the simple design of the LLMs presents a unique set of challenges (Satvik Tripathi et al., 2024).

3.1. Types of Errors and the training Dilemma

Precision errors, also referred to as hallucinations, manifest in the output as a collection of internally consistent but factually inaccurate claims, whereas accuracy errors, also called bias, are systematic errors that diverge from ground truth because of biases in the training architecture or data. Removing these biases is not always easy because they are usually caused by the underlying data distributions used during training. Contextualised word embeddings have been found to display gender bias, and removing these biases leads to performance trade-offs in other tasks. Due to selection bias, these errors lead to what is referred to as the "training dilemma": trying to maximise precision by carefully selecting training materials will always result in accuracy errors, while trying to maximise accuracy by using a variety of training materials will result in diminished precision (Alejandro Ríos-Hoyo et al., 2024).

3.2 Baseline Performance Analysis

Our research focused on the challenging real-world task of generating question-and-answer pairs for the Indian Civil Services examination, which demands precise factual knowledge and complex reasoning (Gabriele De Vito et al., 2025). This problem met key experimental requirements, including the need for accurate data across diverse subjects, strong internal consistency within each question, and the ability to capture intricate causal connections between ideas. The evaluation process itself reflected ensemble evaluation principles by incorporating temporal and contextual nuances and establishing ground truth through a two-expert consensus method, with a senior subject matter expert serving as the final authority in resolving disputes. Despite this rigorous framework, significant reliability concerns emerged in baseline performance, with 57 correct instances (73.1%) and 21 incorrect outputs (26.9% error rate). Error analysis revealed common issues such as time anomalies involving incorrect timelines and dates, cases requiring complex logical linkages among multiple elements, interrelated factual inconsistencies, and responses demanding deep legal or procedural understanding. These findings highlight a critical limitation: although large language models can generate complex, coherent, and seemingly consistent content, their error rate remains too high for independent use in high-stakes tasks. The continued need for human validation ultimately reduces their standalone utility in many high-value domains.

4. PAVING THE WAY FOR LARGE LANGUAGE MODELS (LLMS) IN HEALTHCARE

Vital elements like physiological signals, public health data, and electronic medical records (EMRs) are essential to the medical industry's success. Globally, 1.1 billion EHRs are expected to be in use by 2021, accounting for over 30% of all data collected to far. By 2025, the compound annual growth rate is expected to reach 36%. The wearable health technology industry was projected to grow to 186.14 billion USD by 2030, with millions of devices continuously generating physiological indicators and health data. By 2025, the volume of medical imaging data at each institution is expected to have increased to 2.5 petabytes. Additionally, the world's registered clinical trials—which are predicted to reach over 400,000 by 2023—have generated a wealth of new data that has considerably helped the medical business. However, these changes have also created new challenges for doctors in terms of identifying, assessing, and understanding their options, according to Karayanni et al. (2024). With so much information available, it may be difficult for clinicians to swiftly find, assess, and apply the best available evidence to their clinical practice.

It could be hard for doctors to keep up with the latest developments and locate relevant information because the trend might have advanced to the point where traditional methods of managing and retrieving data are no longer adequate. According to earlier studies, LLMs can create thorough summaries of patient records. As these summaries require human effort to identify various features and data, it is difficult to assess them. The approach that is closest to this one suggests that summaries should be categorized based on various attributes to enable LLM-as-a-judge assessments. This approach does use general ontological features, which are not specifically defined. Thus, the LLM-as-a-judge approach of these models shows that the agreement rate of the retrieved data with the truth is of moderate level. According to Alexander Selivanov et al. (2023), this approach leads to a substantial increase in agreement rates by collaborating with subject matter experts to design features that are accurate and relevant to local needs.

5. SCOPE OF LLM INTEGRATION IN HEALTHCARE

5.1 LLM Application in DRUG Assignment

Due to the development of large language models (LLMs), natural language generation and understanding in radiology have become feasible in ways that were not possible before. Examples of specialty models are Radiology-GPT, while general models include GPT-3.5 and GPT-4. These models have been trained on massive datasets and are very useful for a range of tasks related to radiology. They are very helpful when trying to understand complex medical terminology. The main purpose of LLMs is to automate the task of writing radiology reports. By generating preliminary insights from radiological data, these models help radiologists prevent chronic fatigue and save time. Early results indicate that LLM reports can be about as good as expert reports, especially if they are backed up by organised reports or enhanced by the notion of a radiological business (Madden et al., 2023). LLMs can also help bridge the gap between imaging data and contextual and clinical information. Pairing these models with test results, patient histories, and other clinical data can help put imaging findings, alternative diagnoses, and even discrepancies in how pictures and clinical notes are interpreted into context. Ten consecutive visits to a breast tumour board provided the clinical data used in ChatGPT-3.5. In seventy percent of the cases, the board's recommendations and the LLM's were identical. For doctors and nurses, this could be quite helpful, which could lead to better patient outcomes (Yash Mathur et al., 2023).

Data extraction from unstructured radiological texts is another possible use. Anatomical locations, pathology outcomes, and measurement data from free-text reports are examples of clinical features that LLMs can recognise and classify. Predictive modelling, population health analysis, and clinical research are examples of secondary applications made possible by this. Standardising terminology and translating reports into other languages is made easier by its natural language comprehension. Furthermore, in international healthcare settings, this is essential. Nevertheless, their application in clinical contexts necessitates rapid engineering and meticulous model updating. General-purpose LLMs may induce hallucinations if they are not configured appropriately because they are not conversant with the specific vocabulary of radiology. The efficacy and reliability of these models in the clinic can be improved by incorporating field-specific cues and refining them using datasets unique to radiology. The best big language model for predicting DRGs from clinical discharge summaries is DRG-LLaMA. LLaMA with enhancements. The MIMIC-IV dataset was used by Wang et al. to create it. Our model achieved a macro-averaged area under the curve (AUC) of 0.986 and a top-1 prediction accuracy of 52.0%, outperforming popular baselines such as Clinical BERT and CAML. It performed remarkably well in resolving the 7-billion-parameter variant where a put token's maximum length was 512 (Roshanov et al., 2011).

5.2 Clinical Decision Support System enhanced by LLMs

LLMs analyse a range of patient information in healthcare settings, such as symptoms, medical history, clinical notes, imaging, and test results, to make differential diagnoses, suggest courses of action, and offer a very useful and accurate summary of patient interactions. The application of large language model processes for clinical decision support for diagnosis, referral, and triage was investigated by Gaber et al. in their study, which looked at 2000 medical cases with a variety of disorders. The methodology they used was based on LLM and included three Claude family models and retrieval-augmented generation (RAG). Triage (57.7–82.8%), diagnostic prediction (67.4–82.5%), and predicting the right medical speciality referrals from patient data (76.9–87.5%) were all generally reliable, according to David et al. (2003), especially when clinical data were included. Recent studies suggest that LLMs may be able to offer diagnostic advice comparable to that of specialists for a range of clinical conditions. This suggests that physicians may find them to be a helpful tool.

Five models with and without RAG were used to compare the correctness of 600 questions from a board test on nuclear medical technology covering 15 different fields of nuclear medicine. With scores of 0.787 and 0.783, respectively, two Open AI models demonstrated excellent performance with RAG. Notwithstanding these advantages, the lack of a table in the EHR continues to impair LLM-driven CDSS's capacity to protect patient privacy, manage algorithmic bias, uphold openness, and guarantee patient safety. The reliability and effectiveness of LLMs in CDS are continuously improved, especially in challenging domains like radiology and nuclear medicine, by the use of explainable AI approaches and domain-specific fine-tuning (Edward and Martin, 2018).

6. COMPLEX DISEASE PATHWAYS CALL FOR DECISION SUPPORT

The intricacy of hepatology and gastrointestinal diagnostic work-ups and disease progressions make it possible for CDSS to improve patient care in a variety of ways. These problems highlight how critical it is to take all necessary measures to ensure careful symptom control, improve tailored treatment, and set aside money for all-encompassing care. We will discuss some specific diseases that are highly important for managing a CDSS effectively in the hepatology and gastrointestinal sectors in the following sections. We do not want to be inclusive. In the treatment of chronic diseases, it may be challenging to select the appropriate medications for patients with inflammatory bowel disease (IBD) because of the large number of available medications, including small molecules, biologics, and steroids. It may be challenging and complex for the physician to conduct a systematic analysis and reconstruction of the disease history because patients may be required to modify their treatment regimens and disease activity over a chronic disease (Mehrabi et al., 2021).

This implies that very specialized solutions that consider a large amount of patient information are needed. Both intestinal and extraintestinal manifestations may have a significant effect on the quality of life of the patient. Therefore, they need to be treated using multimodal treatment strategies that provide both pharmacologic and psychosocial support. In order to effectively treat IBD and provide constant care and support, a number of resources are needed, including infrastructure and staff. In order to improve the quality of life for patients by reducing symptoms such as fatigue, effective psychosocial interventions such as mindfulness and physical activity are necessary. A holistic and proactive approach is required to provide the best possible care for an IBD patient, which includes personalized treatment, constant monitoring of symptoms, and provision of all necessary tools. Moreover, the number of people with SLD associated with metabolic dysfunction (MASLD) is rapidly rising. Approximately 30 to 40 percent of the population worldwide are affected (Kirk et al., 2021).

The European Association for the Study of the Liver and the American Association for the Study of Liver Disease have changed their names to better reflect the complex pathophysiology of SLD. They currently fall into three categories: metabolic dysfunction-associated alcohol-related liver disease, alcohol-associated liver disease, and MASLD (Melas et al., 2021). By using CDSS at the point of care, the new SLD language will be easier to adopt. Individuals who do not fit the diagnostic criteria require alternative forms of care. The latest guidelines only cover novel medicines like glucagon-like peptide 1 receptor agonists or focused interventions like resmetirom for steato hepatitis linked to metabolic dysfunction.

To handle the challenging work of patient classification and standardization, CDSS would be a helpful technical instrument. In conclusion, autoimmune hepatitis, Wilson's disease, or Whipple illness may initially be misdiagnosed or go untreated for an extended length of time (Yu et al., 2022). Based on patterns specific to each patient, CDSS may integrate genetic data and rare disease databases to provide valuable information and uncommon potential diagnoses. CDSS can help physicians make a diagnosis quickly by recommending the first diagnostic steps or directing them to the right specialists. By addressing these complex issues and offering a means to improve and optimize care in the fields of hepatology and gastroenterology, CDSS ultimately goes on to improve the quality of life for patients and survivors (Chang et al., 2019).

7. DATA SAFETY

The training data of the model is a concern for AI safety. Data safety issues include bias and prejudice in the data used to train the model, which may lead to discrimination, as well as the presence of toxic and dangerous data that may negatively influence LLMs to make negative judgments (Allen et al., 2024). Nevertheless, the problem of discrepancy may be exacerbated by the poor representation of minority groups or languages in the data. The training data containing sensitive or private information may pose a problem of intellectual property and privacy (Garrido-Muñoz et al., 2021).

7.1 Toxicity

If someone makes an insulting or nasty remark during a debate, people are likely to leave. Conversely, when faced with a highly unpleasant, hostile, disrespectful, or rude comment, people are more likely to leave a debate or not voice their ideas (Ousidhoum et al., 2021). Using attributes to categorize harmful information into groups such as threats, identity-based assaults, insults, profanity, or sexually explicit APIs is also a smart idea. Other instances of harmful material include the use of derogatory language and prejudice against a particular racial group. Additionally, you can flag content as detrimental by using terms like "offensive," "abusive," "hateful," and so forth. Big language models can produce inappropriate, harmful, or objectionable content, including bullying, hate speech, and misleading information.

Gehman et al. (2009) Content can be categorized as non-targeted, targeted, or offensive; it might be directed at a specific person (such as in cyberbullying), a group (such as hate speech), or no one. This type of material could be classified as poisonous or dangerous. The issue is that different types of hazardous information may require different approaches to handle. An further issue is the lack of a commonly agreed-upon definition and description of damaging material, which can vary greatly based on an individual's social background and cultural standards. Data that has been divided into "safe" and "unsafe" categories is used to train GAI-LLMs. A hazardous language classifier is trained using this as its foundation (Pan et al., 2020). With this type of data, the model can reduce toxicity. Although data is neutral in and of itself, individuals choose what types of data are "safe" and "unsafe." Crowdsourced data labellers may also be professional moderators who may add their own prejudices to the site, or they may be natural language processing specialists who use curated or artificial data. With test data, author credit, certain criteria, and a majority vote to obtain a second opinion, data labellers then attempt to make improvements. The model can be cleaned using pre-trained data from huge language models, which lowers the chance of adding undesired characteristics during the model-building process. A soft version minimises the possibility that terms will have negative weighting relative to the actual sample distribution, making this easier (Liu et al., 2024).

7.2 Bias

The model learns grammar, world facts, reasoning abilities, and biases in the training data by being taught to guess the next word in a phrase through pre-training. In the event that the training data contains biased information, such as racist news articles or sexist job descriptions, the algorithm may identify and replicate prejudice. Preexisting prejudice may occasionally be made worse by the tool (Song and Raghunathan, 2020). If the training data shows that men are more likely than women to accomplish a task, the tool may predict the male form of the terms more often. It would exacerbate the bias that currently exists. Biases, whether conscious or unconscious, may be present in the massive volumes of text data utilised to train big language models. Large language models may reinforce and magnify preconceived notions in their writing, thus producing unfair or biased results (Kurita et al., 2019). In the event that the reviewer dislikes a specific dialect or accent, for instance, and tends to give the outputs lower ratings, the computer may learn to do the same. The computer's "cheating" techniques or the review procedure itself are also problematic and may produce unfair results.

A model may learn to have a concealed bias that is not noticed, for instance, if reviewers are less likely to notice minor biases. Bias in LLMs can occasionally lead to the model's performance or outcomes being persistently inaccurate or different because of certain features of the model, the training procedure, or the input data (Welbl et al., 2021). The manifestation of biases in LLMs might take several forms. When LLMs are trained on unjust data, this is known as pre-existing bias. The model may identify racial, gender, and cultural biases in the data and then include those biases into its output (Anyaso and Okoye, 2024). When choosing the learning algorithm or optimization procedure, for example, or when designing and training the model, technical bias may occur.

The application of LLMs in a particular context may result in emergent bias. For instance, even though the model was not taught to do so, it can produce different results for various user groups. Before training the model, bias-reduction methods could be applied (Zampieri et al., 2019). Finding and fixing bias before training on the data is known as pre-processing. One way that the approach itself is being changed to try to reduce bias in the model training phase is through the development of fairness-aware machine learning algorithms. Once the model has been trained, the output can be modified and examined to lessen bias. GAI-LLMs are regarded as fair after the model's bias has been fixed. Fairness in generative language models means treating all groups equally, irrespective of their identity, gender, age, or any other attribute. The LLM's purpose is to avoid bias or favouritism toward any specific group. (Schick et al., 2021) state that the phrase can also be used to describe whether the LLM treats similar people identically.

7.3 Data privacy

LLMs learn from big datasets, which means they might unintentionally collect and share private or sensitive information about people or businesses. Perhaps people's privacy was violated. The pretraining phase involves training a language model using vast amounts of publicly available online content. According to Mehrabi et al. (2021), sensitive information may still be exposed or reidentified even after the training data has been anonymised. The potential of the data to reveal private or sensitive information via user input or training data is what is most concerning. Novels, news articles, social media posts, websites, and many more are just some of the sources of text data that ChatGPT relies on for training. Phone numbers, email addresses, addresses, names, credit card numbers, and other personal details of individuals or organizations may be included in some of the text data. ChatGPT can publish or store the information in the text it produces, which can put the privacy and confidentiality of the individuals or organizations whose information is included in it at risk (Nangia et al., 2020). Adversarial attacks that belong to the membership inference and attribute inference types have the potential to seriously affect user privacy.

Privacy issues can arise from this analysis method because analysts may intentionally or unintentionally disclose private or sensitive information through comments. The gathering and analysis of feedback data can lead to privacy breaches. In ChatGPT, the transformer layer is a key component. It facilitates the processing of multiple tasks simultaneously and relies on self-attention mechanisms to spot global dependencies. Nevertheless, this approach raises privacy concerns because the model may handle many input sequence segments at once (Czarnowska et al., 2021). The attacker may employ self-attention to get access to private data, carry out focused assaults, or modify the attention scores to identify the entities being discussed. Because Chat GPT uses self-attention techniques like multi-head attention, it may create connections between the different input text segments. However, these attention approaches may generate privacy issues because they may draw attention to word or phrase relationships in the input text. Because of the information leak, attackers could learn about the user's personal traits or their private search patterns (Han et al., 2022).

7.4 Copyright

Two intellectual property issues that generative AI systems may generate are plagiarism and copyright infringement. Even if it enhances the dataset, using copyrighted content may raise ethical and legal issues. Better and more cautious data governance is required as a result. Using data that is copyright protected is immoral and illegal. Potential violations of copyright laws can result in legal issues. Gathering vast amounts of textual material from the internet is known as data scraping. The careless usage of copyrighted data is the result of this (Zanella-Béguelin et al., 2020). Automated scraping may contain copyrighted content since it is unable to distinguish between material that is protected by copyright and that is not. Since the legislation that protects intellectual property rights prohibits using copyrighted information without permission or acknowledgment, it can be improper. The LLM pre-training data contained intellectual property issues (Carlini et al., 2021). It's possible that training data needed for generative AI models to learn was provided by someone else without the original inventor's consent. It's possible that original authors and artists haven't granted generative models permission to create new works in their own styles. Training data that is protected by copyright may still be kept private by the creator, even if it has been disseminated. The models may suit some data sources or styles too closely because they rely too heavily on copyrighted data, which could reduce their overall usefulness (Pavlopoulos et al., 2020).

8. CONTEXT SAFETY RISK TAXONOMY AND POLICY

LLM safety is a very recent notion. The overarching goal is to guarantee that AI systems—especially LLMs—behave in a way that harms no one and maximizes benefits to humans. Consistency, security, privacy, interpretability, control, accountability, and robustness are just a few of the many elements that make up the concept of safety. LLM content safety moderation is to ensure that users' interactions with LLMs adhere to legal requirements, ethical standards, and guidelines (Yakubovich, 2023). All of these safety pillars are by definition touched upon by content moderation. Alignment, which ensures that LLM behaviors align with appropriate responses and safe human values, is also related. Our training, assessment, and content safety taxonomy paradigm discusses many aspects of each of these safety pillars. In the next part, we will refer to "content safety" by the word "safety". Determining which categories the taxonomies directly span is the first stage (Doherty et al., 2024). Keeping the overlap aids in the appraisal, and the areas where the categories overlap are the most significant risk areas. The distinctions in the taxonomy are then discovered. Llama Guard does not differentiate between sexual and sexual minor.

Furthermore, there is no obvious differentiation between violence and hate. Larger groupings could be simpler to forecast, but these distinctions help with better content filtering and knowing user preferences. Both profanity and threats are included in the taxonomy of perspective. The key concepts of our safety policy are explained in further detail in Section 8 of the Appendix taxonomy. To prevent individuals from labeling uncertain occurrences as hazardous, which would have halted the user inquiry, (Vorisek et al., 2022) developed the Needs Caution category.

9. CATEGORIES CHALLENGES AND LIMITATION OF CDSS

Through their connections to electronic medical records, CDSSs contribute significantly to the improvement of clinical practice and patient safety. They have to cope with the issue of drug interactions, which are complicated by pharmacology and patient characteristics. To identify any adverse effects, they require sophisticated algorithms. They are difficult to apply in the pharmaceutical sector, despite the potential advantages. Research demonstrates that knowledge-based systems improve prescribing practices by 4.4% and AI-based systems improve prescription verification accuracy, demonstrating the effectiveness of CDSSs in reducing medication errors. Among drug reaction warning systems, opioids have the most concerning override rates, which still vary between 43.7% and 97% (Goodrum et al., 2020). This problem keeps coming up. Numerous investigations have discovered this pervasive disregard for signs that point to an issue with the strategy.

Though they have shown promise, machine learning and ontology-based systems have had difficulty gaining enough users to submit complicated medical situations and alerts. The existing system's ability to comprehend unstructured medical narratives seems to be lacking. These accounts contain important patient-specific details about the patient's drug tolerance and response. False alerts would be greatly decreased if information about the person's prior drug tolerance was included. Improved natural language processing techniques can nevertheless alter the acceptability and relevance of alerts in clinical contexts notwithstanding this issue with processing natural language documents. The mid to late 1900s saw the creation of the first CDSS. They were mostly designed for one-time tasks that adhered to predetermined algorithms and were rule-based. A computer software called INTERNIST-1 enables you to examine the knowledge base91 in a more sophisticated manner. In general internal medicine, it aids in diagnosis. Because they were frequently stand-alone systems that didn't interface with other systems and employed rule-based processing, these CDSS were essentially worthless.

Consequently, they were time-consuming, ineffective, and lacked proactive characteristics (Chen et al., 2023). As a result, they had very low utilization rates.

By including elements that were helpful for certain activities, like notifications for missing orders, CDSS grew more proactive as systems became more integrated. They were sometimes hampered in their adoption by their interface with specialised clinical information systems that were hard to transfer to other institutions and the close relationship between actionable code and the underlying knowledge base that made it hard to make quick changes. CDSS's technology was enhanced with machine learning techniques including decision trees and linear regression models to manage more complicated medical situations (Wright et al., 2008). Facilitating the diagnosis of jaundice and cholestasis was the main goal of these statistical CDSS in hepatology. However, they also served a broader purpose of helping doctors identify the type of liver disease a patient had. Selection bias emerged because they were more likely to be disease-specific than disease-agnostic, and there were few feasibility studies showing real clinical benefit. Additionally, as new or enhanced diagnostic tools (such as ultrasonography) and more accurate blood markers (such as anti-mitochondrial antibody) were created to assist doctors in differentiating cholestasis from other diseases, these techniques quickly became obsolete (Williams et al., 2025).

10. OPPORTUNITIES FOR CDSS

Clinical judgements are made in four basic stages. Examining the patient's symptoms, medical history, and the results of a preliminary physical examination helps identify the problem in the first step. According to Dantonoli et al. (2024), physicians utilise this evaluation to create educated assumptions regarding the patient's possible circumstances in the second stage. These ideas are then confirmed in the third stage by diagnostic techniques such as imaging examinations, laboratory testing, or instrumental diagnostics. The final diagnosis result is given to the patient when the necessary diagnostic information has been gathered to confirm or disprove initial hypotheses derived from medical literature (Williams et al., 2025).

All these processes can be aided by CDSS, which integrates patient information from electronic health records (EHR), provides evidence-based recommendations, and assists in testing hypotheses. Despite the best efforts to standardize and simplify the data, the use of EHR systems is still quite varied. Test results, scanned documents, lab data, and notes from inpatient and outpatient sessions are all organised in Alaa and colleagues' database (2025). Due to their daily schedules, doctors may not have the opportunity to go over these records. Social risk informed care81 can be promoted by using CDSS to help doctors learn more about allergies and intolerances. This will help them connect patient data with the specific context of the presentation in issue.

Bednarczyk et al. (2025) state that when patient data is backed up by relevant medical guidelines and research at the right moment, CDSS can help doctors make better decisions about diagnosis and treatment. Instead of relying exclusively on their own limited knowledge and experience, it is better. For example, the Explain system was created by Massachusetts General Hospital to help in diagnosis in the 1980s. For this, it gathers patient information and compares it with historical case data and textbook recommendations. Furthermore, by emphasising details that could otherwise be overlooked, CDSS can assist in making sure that all relevant factors are considered in order to deliver the highest quality of patient care. In order to streamline their work, Gero et al. (2024) said they want to make diagnosis simpler, help doctors remember what they learn, and give them information relevant to suggestions.

11. CLINICAL DECISION MAKING USING LLMS

11.1 Capabilities

Problem assessment, hypothesis generation, diagnostic data collection, and conclusion are the four stages of decision support that LLMs can complete when used to help clinical decision-making. For example, in the initial diagnosis phase, Google's AMIE, an LLM-based chatbot, offers patients organised and interactive support to facilitate diagnostic dialogues (Busch et al., 2024). In contrast to manually reviewing patient-provided documents or notes in electronic health records (EHRs) to collect data for the hypothesis-generating step, LLMs can save a substantial amount of time when performing medical free text analysis. Furthermore, with a strong medical data structure, LLMs can add useful information from problem analysis, hypothesis development, and diagnostic procedures to CDSS and current clinical information systems (Meng et al., 2024).

Despite only being used for certain tasks, LLMs are more versatile and can create content faster and more efficiently than a single human. By seeing trends, making probabilistic judgements, and incorporating external data, they can aid in scientific research and medical decision-making even though they are insufficient. The economy benefits greatly from LLMs since they can generate complex ideas, language, or computer code. Just the pharmaceutical and medical device sectors might increase the GDP by $60–110 billion annually. For instance, when assessing a liver transplant, LLMs may quickly and simply summarise a patient's extensive medical history, imaging studies, and test results into a concise and practical summary that facilitates quicker and more efficient decision-making (Yu et al., 2023).

According to Alkalbani et al. (2025), they can also help interpret endoscopic data by emphasising relevant results and comparing them with the latest guidelines for conditions like IBD or Barrett's oesophagus. However, as of current now, there aren't many simple programs that make using LLM-based CDSS in gastroenterology and hepatology easier. On July 4, 2025, a PubMed search with a broad search term that included hepatology, gastroenterology, LLMs, and clinical decision support produced only 10 peer-reviewed papers, eight of which were original studies (Wang et al., 2024). evaluated ChatGPT-3.5's accuracy in answering questions from the American Society of Clinical Oncology's oncology self-evaluation project. The accuracy rate was just 56.1%, and it varied significantly according on the type of cancer. Using an early, proprietary model that was available through the OpenAI interface without any domain-specific optimisation hampered the study's usefulness for real-world CDS (Li et al., 2024). Kaiser et al. found that ChatGPT and Microsoft Copilot responses to clinical scenarios, such as pancreatic ductal adeno carcinoma, were only 44% completely accurate.

Eight chatbots with LLM capabilities were evaluated for accuracy in answering questions from cancer doctors on colorectal cancer. According to the findings, Claude 2.1 fared better than all medical categories, including residents, fellows, and attendings. Moreover, several other chatbots did better than peers and homeowners. Gastro Bot is a better domain-specific LLM that incorporates retrieval-augmented generation (RAG) and embedding model refining. Vrdoljak et al. (2025) compared a customised GPT model with a standard GPT-4o regarding gastrointestinal issues. While both models did well, they found that they did slightly worse than real gastroenterologists. With a vector library of 25 guidelines and 40 literature articles, GastroBot demonstrated good performance, obtaining 93.73% fidelity, 92.28% answer relevancy, and 95% context recall.

By making BioMistral7B a bit more LLM, Kainz et al. enhanced the original model to better explain hepatitis serology (Gaber et al., 2025). In order to give doctors evidence-based advice without specifically mentioning CDSS, other studies looked at LLMs in hepatology and gastrointestinal medicine. LLMs for tasks like natural language processing and documentation support have been the subject of numerous studies (Liu et al., 2025). Others examined endoscopic reports; one group used EHR documentation to seek for bleeding after endoscopy. identified from medical data the most important social elements that could affect CRC screening adherence. Additionally, several researchers have looked into LLMs as a technique for organising and rating reports. For instance, LLMs were applied to extract features from the textual imaging report to classify liver lesions and generate structured CT reports for patients with pancreatic cancer (Vieujiean, 2025). The simple question-and-answer format has been employed to evaluate the performance of LLMs in a variety of clinical situations or medical guidelines, such as Helicobacter pylori infection, esophageal cancer, colorectal cancer (CRC) liver cancer, acute liver failure, and nutrition-related questions (Colombel et al., 2017).

11.2 LLMs can contribute to a paradigm shift

As per a recent study, LLMs are not generally referred to as "clinical decision support systems" (Bruner et al., 2023), although they fulfill critical CDSS requirements like improving the accuracy of diagnoses, assisting in the decision-making process regarding treatment, and making processes simpler. The phrases "medical chatbot" and "AI assistant" are employed instead in referring to decision support systems. You can apply these capabilities in a conversation such as this one. Yours sincerely, by providing doctors with flexible tools that they can use in a wider range of situations, LLMs might exceed the conventional definition of CDSS. This outstanding adoption rate illustrates how the paradigm of decision aid is moving from traditional, rigid, rule-based logic engines to dynamic, adaptive, and context-aware assistants that more accurately represent the thought processes of physicians in practical situations (Rogler et al., 2021).

LLMs address the fragmentation and lack of usability that are major problems with conventional CDSS. This is because they do not focus on a specific disease domain or strategy. By helping healthcare professionals to process information and make decisions faster, LLMs could improve clinical decision-making. Concerning the application of LLMs in the fields of hepatology and gastroenterology, the research is greatly lacking, except for the studies mentioned above that applied LLMs in CDSS. This indicates the need for further research to validate their effectiveness and address their limitations, which will be discussed in the next section (Uihaq, 2024).

REFERENCES

Alaa, A., Hartvigsen, T., Golchini, N., Dutta, S., Dean, F., Raji, I. D., & Zack, T. (2025). Position: Medical large language model benchmarks should prioritize construct validity. In *Proceedings of the 42nd International Conference on Machine Learning (ICML).*

Alkalbani, A. M., Alrawahi, A. S., Salah, A., Haghighi, V., Zhang, Y., Alkindi, S., & Sheng, Q. Z. (2025). A systematic review of large language models in medical specialties: Applications, challenges and future directions. *Information (Basel), 16*(6), 489. DOI: 10.3390/info16060489

Allen, A. M., Younossi, Z. M., Diehl, A. M., Charlton, M. R., & Lazarus, J. V. (2024). Envisioning how to advance the MASH field. *Nature Reviews. Gastroenterology & Hepatology, 21*(10), 726–738. DOI: 10.1038/s41575-024-00938-9 PMID: 38834817

Anyaso, K., & Okoye, V. (2024). The impact of big data and predictive analytics on U.S. healthcare delivery: Opportunities, challenges, and future directions. *World Journal of Advanced Research and Reviews, 24*(1), 2275–2287. DOI: 10.30574/wjarr.2024.24.1.3266

Bednarczyk, L., Reichenpfader, D., Gaudet-Blavignac, C., Ette, A. K., Zaghir, J., Zheng, Y., Bensahla, A., Bjelogrlic, M., & Lovis, C. (2025). Scientific evidence for clinical text summarization using large language models: Scoping review. *Journal of Medical Internet Research, 27*, e68998. DOI: 10.2196/68998 PMID: 40371947

Bruner, L. P., White, A. M., & Proksell, S. (2023). Inflammatory bowel disease. *Primary Care, 50*(3), 411–427. DOI: 10.1016/j.pop.2023.03.009 PMID: 37516511

Busch, F., Hoffmann, L., dos Santos, D. P., Makowski, M. R., Saba, L., Prucker, P., Hadamitzky, M., Navab, N., Kather, J. N., Truhn, D., Cuocolo, R., Adams, L. C., & Bressem, K. K. (2024). Large language models for structured reporting in radiology: Past, present, and future. *European Radiology, 35*(5), 2589–2602. DOI: 10.1007/s00330-024-11107-6 PMID: 39438330

Carlini, N., Tramer, F., Wallace, E., Jagielski, M., Herbert-Voss, A., Lee, K., Roberts, A., Brown, T., Song, D., Erlingsson, U., Oprea, A., & Raffel, C. (2021). Extracting training data from large language models. *arXiv preprint arXiv:2012.07805.*

Chang, K. W., Prabhakaran, V., & Ordonez, V. (2019). Bias and fairness in natural language processing. In *Proceedings of the 2019 Conference on Empirical Methods in Natural Language Processing.*

Chen, Z., Liang, N., Zhang, H., Li, H., Yang, Y., Zong, X., Chen, Y., Wang, Y., & Shi, N. (2023). Harnessing the power of clinical decision support systems: Challenges and opportunities. *Open Heart, 10*(2), e002432. DOI: 10.1136/openhrt-2023-002432 PMID: 38016787

Colombel, J.-F., Narula, N., & Peyrin-Biroulet, L. (2017). Management strategies to improve outcomes of patients with inflammatory bowel diseases. *Gastroenterology, 152*(2), 351–361. DOI: 10.1053/j.gastro.2016.09.046 PMID: 27720840

Czarnowska, P., Vyas, Y., & Shah, K. (2021). Quantifying social biases in NLP: A generalization and empirical comparison of extrinsic fairness metrics. *Transactions of the Association for Computational Linguistics, 9*, 1249–1267. DOI: 10.1162/tacl_a_00425

Dang, A. (2023). Real-world evidence: A primer. *Pharmaceutical Medicine, 37*(1), 25–36. DOI: 10.1007/s40290-022-00456-6 PMID: 36604368

De Vito, G., Ferrucci, F., & Angelakis, A. (2025). LLMs for drug-drug interaction prediction: A comprehensive comparison. *arXiv preprint arXiv:2502.06890.*

Doherty, C., Baldwin, M., Keogh, A., Caulfield, B., & Argent, R. (2024). Keeping pace with wearables: A living umbrella review of systematic reviews evaluating the accuracy of consumer wearable technologies in health measurement. *Sports Medicine, 54*(11), 2907–2926. DOI: 10.1007/s40279-024-02077-2 PMID: 39080098

Gaber, F., Shaik, M., Allega, F., Bilecz, A. J., Busch, F., Goon, K., Franke, V., & Akalin, A. (2025). Evaluating large language model workflows in clinical decision support for triage, referral, and diagnosis. *NPJ Digital Medicine, 8*(1), 263. DOI: 10.1038/s41746-025-01684-1 PMID: 40346344

Garrido-Muñoz, I., Montejo-Ráez, A., Martínez-Santiago, F., & Ureña López, L. A. (2021). A survey on bias in deep NLP. *Applied Sciences (Basel, Switzerland), 11*(7), 3184. DOI: 10.3390/app11073184

Gehman, S., Gururangan, S., Sap, M., Choi, Y., & Smith, N. A. (2020). RealToxicityPrompts: Evaluating neural toxic degeneration in language models. *arXiv preprint arXiv:2009.11462*. DOI: 10.18653/v1/2020.findings-emnlp.301

Gero, Z., Singh, C., Xie, Y., Zhang, S., Subramanian, P., Vozila, P., Naumann, T., Gao, J., & Poon, H. (2024). Attribute structuring improves LLM-based evaluation of clinical text summaries. *arXiv preprint arXiv:2407.17778.*

Goodrum, H., Roberts, K., & Bernstam, E. V. (2020). Automatic classification of scanned electronic health record documents. *International Journal of Medical Informatics, 144*, 104302. DOI: 10.1016/j.ijmedinf.2020.104302 PMID: 33091829

Han, X., Shen, A., Cohn, T., Baldwin, T., & Frermann, L. (2022). Systematic evaluation of predictive fairness. In *Proceedings of the Association for Computational Linguistics*.

Karayanni, N., Awwad, A., Hsiao, C.-L., & Shanmugam, S. P. (2024). Keeping experts in the loop: Expert-guided optimization for clinical data classification using large language models. *arXiv preprint arXiv:2412.02173*.

Kirk, H. R., Jun, Y., Volpin, F., Iqbal, H., Benussi, E., Dreyer, F., Shtedritski, A., & Asano, Y. (2021). Bias out-of-the-box: An empirical analysis of intersectional occupational biases in popular generative language models. In *Advances in Neural Information Processing Systems* (pp. 2611–2624).

Kurita, K., Belova, A., & Anastasopoulos, A. (2019). Towards robust toxic content classification. arXiv preprint arXiv:1912.06872.

Li, J., Zhou, Z., Lyu, H., & Wang, Z. (2025). Large language models-powered clinical decision support: Enhancing or replacing human expertise? *Intelligent Medicine*, *5*(1), 1–4. DOI: 10.1016/j.imed.2025.01.001

Liu, Y., Wang, Z., Li, Y., Liang, X., Liu, L., Wang, L., & Zhou, L. (2024). MRScore: Evaluating radiology report generation with LLM-based reward system. *arXiv preprint arXiv:2404.17778*.

Madden, M. G., McNicholas, B. A., & Laffey, J. G. (2023). Assessing the usefulness of a large language model to query and summarize unstructured medical notes in intensive care. *Intensive Care Medicine*, *49*(8), 1018–1020. DOI: 10.1007/s00134-023-07128-2 PMID: 37338549

Mathur, Y., Rangreji, S., Kapoor, R., Palavalli, M., Bertsch, A., & Gormley, M. R. (2023). SummQA at MEDIQA-Chat 2023: In-context learning with GPT-4 for medical summarization. *arXiv preprint arXiv:2306.17384*. DOI: 10.18653/v1/2023.clinicalnlp-1.51

Mehrabi, N., Morstatter, F., Saxena, N., Lerman, K., & Galstyan, A. (2021). A survey on bias and fairness in machine learning. *ACM Computing Surveys*, *54*(6), 1–35. DOI: 10.1145/3457607

Melas, N., Amin, R., Gyllemark, P., Younes, A. H., & Almer, S. (2021). Whipple's disease: The great masquerader—A high level of suspicion is the key to diagnosis. *BMC Gastroenterology*, *21*(1), 128. DOI: 10.1186/s12876-021-01664-1 PMID: 33743602

Meng, X., Yan, X., Zhang, K., Liu, D., Cui, X., Yang, Y., Zhang, M., Cao, C., Wang, J., Wang, X., Gao, J., Wang, Y.-G.-S., Ji, J., Qiu, Z., Li, M., Qian, C., Guo, T., Ma, S., Wang, Z., & Tang, Y.-D. (2024). The application of large language models in medicine: A scoping review. *iScience*, *27*(5), 109713. DOI: 10.1016/j.isci.2024.109713 PMID: 38746668

Meunier, P.-Y., Raynaud, C., Guimaraes, E., Gueyffier, F., & Letrilliart, L. (2023). Barriers and facilitators to the use of clinical decision support systems in primary care: A mixed-methods systematic review. *Annals of Family Medicine*, *21*(1), 57–69. DOI: 10.1370/afm.2908 PMID: 36690490

Nangia, N., Vania, C., Bhalerao, R., & Bowman, S. R. (2020). CrowS-Pairs: A challenge dataset for measuring social biases in masked language models. arXiv preprint arXiv:2010.00133. DOI: 10.18653/v1/2020.emnlp-main.154

Osheroff, J. A., Teich, J. M., Levick, D., Saldana, L., Velasco, F., Sittig, D. F., & Rogers, K. M. (2012). *Improving outcomes with clinical decision support: An implementer's guide*. HIMSS. DOI: 10.4324/9781498757461

Osheroff, J. A., Teich, J. M., Middleton, B., Steen, E. B., Wright, A., & Detmer, D. E. (2007). A roadmap for national action on clinical decision support. *Journal of the American Medical Informatics Association : JAMIA*, *14*(2), 141–145. DOI: 10.1197/jamia.M2334 PMID: 17213487

Ousidhoum, N., Zhao, X., Fang, T., Song, Y., & Yeung, D. Y. (2021). Probing toxic content in large pre-trained language models. In *Proceedings of the 59th Annual Meeting of the Association for Computational Linguistics*. DOI: 10.18653/v1/2021.acl-long.329

Pan, X., Zhang, M., Ji, S., & Yang, M. (2020). Privacy risks of general-purpose language models. In *IEEE Symposium on Security and Privacy* (pp. 1314–1331).

Pavlopoulos, J., Sorensen, J., Dixon, L., Thain, N., & Androutsopoulos, I. (2020). Toxicity detection: Does context really matter? In *Proceedings of the 58th Annual Meeting of the Association for Computational Linguistics* (pp. 4296–4305). DOI: 10.18653/v1/2020.acl-main.396

Ríos-Hoyo, A., Shan, N. L., Li, A., Pearson, A. T., Pusztai, L., & Howard, F. M. (2024). Evaluation of large language models as a diagnostic aid for complex medical cases. *Frontiers in Medicine*, *11*, 1380148. DOI: 10.3389/fmed.2024.1380148 PMID: 38966538

Rogler, G., Singh, A., Kavanaugh, A., & Rubin, D. T. (2021). Extraintestinal manifestations of inflammatory bowel disease: Current concepts, treatment, and implications for disease management. *Gastroenterology, 161*(4), 1118–1132. DOI: 10.1053/j.gastro.2021.07.042 PMID: 34358489

Roshanov, P. S., Misra, S., Gerstein, H. C., Garg, A. X., Sebaldt, R. J., Mackay, J. A., Weise-Kelly, L., Navarro, T., Wilczynski, N. L., & Haynes, R. B. (2011). Computerized clinical decision support systems for chronic disease management: A decision-maker-researcher partnership systematic review. *Implementation Science : IS, 6*(1), 1–16. DOI: 10.1186/1748-5908-6-92 PMID: 21824386

) Sarkar, U., & Samal, L. (2020). How effective are clinical decision support systems?

Schick, T., Udupa, S., & Schütze, H. (2021). Self-diagnosis and self-debiasing: A proposal for reducing corpus-based bias in NLP. *Transactions of the Association for Computational Linguistics, 9*, 1408–1424. DOI: 10.1162/tacl_a_00434

Selivanov, A., Rogov, O. Y., Chesakov, D., Shelmanov, A., Fedulova, I., & Dylov, D. V. (2023). Medical image captioning via generative pretrained transformers. *Scientific Reports, 13*(1), 4171. DOI: 10.1038/s41598-023-31223-5 PMID: 36914733

Shortliffe, E. H., & Sepúlveda, M. J. (2018). Clinical decision support in the era of artificial intelligence. *Journal of the American Medical Association, 320*(21), 2199–2200. DOI: 10.1001/jama.2018.17163 PMID: 30398550

Song, C., & Raghunathan, A. (2020). Information leakage in embedding models. In *ACM SIGSAC Conference on Computer and Communications Security* (pp. 377–390).

Sutton, R. T., Pincock, D., Baumgart, D. C., Sadowski, D. C., Fedorak, R. N., & Kroeker, K. I. (2020). An overview of clinical decision support systems: Benefits, risks, and strategies for success. *NPJ Digital Medicine, 3*(1), 17. DOI: 10.1038/s41746-020-0221-y PMID: 32047862

Tripathi, S., Sukumaran, R., & Cook, T. S. (2024). Efficient healthcare with large language models: Optimizing clinical workflow and enhancing patient care. *Journal of the American Medical Informatics Association : JAMIA, 31*(6), 1436–1440. DOI: 10.1093/jamia/ocad258 PMID: 38273739

Ui-Haq, Z., Causin, L., Kamalati, T., Kahol, D., Vaikunthanathan, T., Wong, C., & Arebi, N. (2024). Health-care resource use and costs associated with inflammatory bowel disease in northwest London: A retrospective linked database study. *BMC Gastroenterology, 24*(1), 480. DOI: 10.1186/s12876-024-03559-3 PMID: 39736541

Van De Sijpe, G., Quintens, C., Walgraeve, K., Van Laer, E., Penny, J., De Vlieger, G., Schrijvers, R., De Munter, P., Foulon, V., Casteels, M., Van der Linden, L., & Spriet, I. (2022). Overall performance of a drug–drug interaction clinical decision support system: Quantitative evaluation and end-user survey. *BMC Medical Informatics and Decision Making*, *22*(1), 48. DOI: 10.1186/s12911-022-01783-z PMID: 35193547

Van Dort, B. A., Zheng, W. Y., Sundar, V., & Baysari, M. T. (2021). Optimizing clinical decision support alerts in electronic medical records: A systematic review of reported strategies adopted by hospitals. *Journal of the American Medical Informatics Association : JAMIA*, *28*(1), 177–183. DOI: 10.1093/jamia/ocaa279 PMID: 33186438

Vieujean, S., Jairath, V., Peyrin-Biroulet, L., Dubinsky, M., Iacucci, M., Magro, F., & Danese, S. (2025). Understanding the therapeutic toolkit for inflammatory bowel disease. *Nature Reviews. Gastroenterology & Hepatology*, *22*(6), 371–394. DOI: 10.1038/s41575-024-01035-7

Vorisek, C. N., Lehne, M., Klopfenstein, S. A., Mayer, P. J., Bartschke, A., Haase, P., & Prasser, F. (2022). Fast healthcare interoperability resources (FHIR) for interoperability in health research: Systematic review. *JMIR Medical Informatics*, *10*(7), e35724. DOI: 10.2196/35724 PMID: 35852842

Vrdoljak, J., Boban, Z., Vilović, M., Kumrić, M., & Božić, J. (2025). A review of large language models in medical education, clinical decision support, and healthcare administration. *Health Care*, *13*, 603. PMID: 40150453

Wang, H., Gao, C., Dantona, C., Hull, B., & Sun, J. (2024). DRG-LLaMA: Tuning LLaMA model to predict diagnosis-related group for hospitalized patients. *NPJ Digital Medicine*, *7*(1), 16. DOI: 10.1038/s41746-023-00989-3 PMID: 38253711

Welbl, J., Glaese, A., Uesato, J., Dathathri, S., Mellor, J., Hendricks, L. A., Anderson, K., Kohli, P., Coppin, B., & Huang, P. S. (2021). Challenges in detoxifying language models. arXiv preprint arXiv:2109.07445. DOI: 10.18653/v1/2021.findings-emnlp.210

Williams, C. Y., Bains, J., Tang, T., Patel, K., Lucas, A. N., Chen, F., Miao, B. Y., Butte, A. J., & Kornblith, A. E. (2025). Evaluating large language models for drafting emergency department encounter summaries. *PLOS Digital Health*, *4*(6), e0000899. DOI: 10.1371/journal.pdig.0000899 PMID: 40526634

Williams, C. Y., Subramanian, C. R., Ali, S. S., Apolinario, M., Askin, E., Barish, P., Cheng, M., Deardorff, W. J., Donthi, N., Ganeshan, S., Huang, O., Kantor, M. A., Lai, A. R., Manchanda, A., Moore, K. A., Muniyappa, A. N., Nair, G., Patel, P. P., Santhosh, L., & Rosner, B. I. (2025). Physician- and large language model–generated hospital discharge summaries. *JAMA Internal Medicine*, *185*(7), 818. DOI: 10.1001/jamainternmed.2025.0821 PMID: 40323616

Wright, A., & Sittig, D. F. (2008). A four-phase model of the evolution of clinical decision support architectures. *International Journal of Medical Informatics*, *77*(10), 641–649. DOI: 10.1016/j.ijmedinf.2008.01.004 PMID: 18353713

) Yakubovich, K. (2023). Clinical decision-making theories. *Annals of Innovative Medicine*.

Yu, M., Ren, L., Zheng, M., Hong, M., & Wei, Z. (2022). Delayed diagnosis of Wilson's disease: Report from 179 newly diagnosed cases in China. *Frontiers in Neurology*, *13*, 884840. DOI: 10.3389/fneur.2022.884840 PMID: 35865642

Yu, P., Xu, H., Hu, X., & Deng, C. (2023). Leveraging generative AI and large language models: A comprehensive roadmap for healthcare integration. *Health Care*, *11*, 2776. PMID: 37893850

Zampieri, M., Malmasi, S., Nakov, P., Rosenthal, S., Farra, N., & Kumar, R. (2019). Predicting the type and target of offensive posts in social media. In *Proceedings of the 2019 Conference of the North American Chapter of the Association for Computational Linguistics: Human Language Technologies* (pp. 1415–1420). DOI: 10.18653/v1/N19-1144

Zanella-Béguelin, S., Wutschitz, L., Tople, S., Rühle, V., Paverd, A., Ohrimenko, O., Köpf, B., & Brockschmidt, M. (2020). Analyzing information leakage of updates to natural language models. In *Proceedings of the 2020 ACM SIGSAC Conference on Computer and Communications Security* (pp. 363–375). DOI: 10.1145/3372297.3417880

Chapter 12
Data Privacy, Security, and PHI Protection

R. Felista Sugirtha Lizy
http://orcid.org/0000-0003-3648-0205
A.P.C. Mahalaxmi College for Women, India

ABSTRACT

The fast adoption of Large Language Models (LLMs) in the field of healthcare has new opportunities of transformative power in clinical safety measurement, diagnostic aid, and patient treatment. Nevertheless, the increased privacy in data, information security, as well as the safety of Protected Health Information (PHI), are associated with this progress. The chapter discusses the core values, standards, and best practices required to guarantee data confidentiality and regulatory standards in medical AI systems. It describes some of the privacy-saving tools, like anonymization of data, differential privacy, federated learning, and secure multi-party computation. Also, the chapter addresses ethical and legal issues of the deployment of LLM in healthcare, such as compliance with standards, such as HIPAA, GDPR, and ISO/IEC 27701. The paper ends with the discussion of recent issues and suggests effective approaches to developing privacy-aware LLMs that will not only support the trust of patients but also clinical accuracy.

1. INTRODUCTION

An application of Large Language Models (LLM) in healthcare has introduced a significant change in the process of clinical data analysis, interpretation, and utilization to enhance patient safety and decision-making. They are also applied more actively to support clinical documentation, diagnostics, and safety assessment through the processing of tremendous quantities of medical data by AI systems. Nevertheless,

DOI: 10.4018/979-8-3373-7862-6.ch012

data privacy, information security, and protection of the Protected Health Information (PHI) also become a very important issue due to the use of sensitive data. It has become a top priority of healthcare organizations and developers to ensure that patient data is kept confidential and at the same time be used to leverage the power of AI-driven insights.

Figure 1. Overview of Medical LLM Ecosystem and PHI Flow

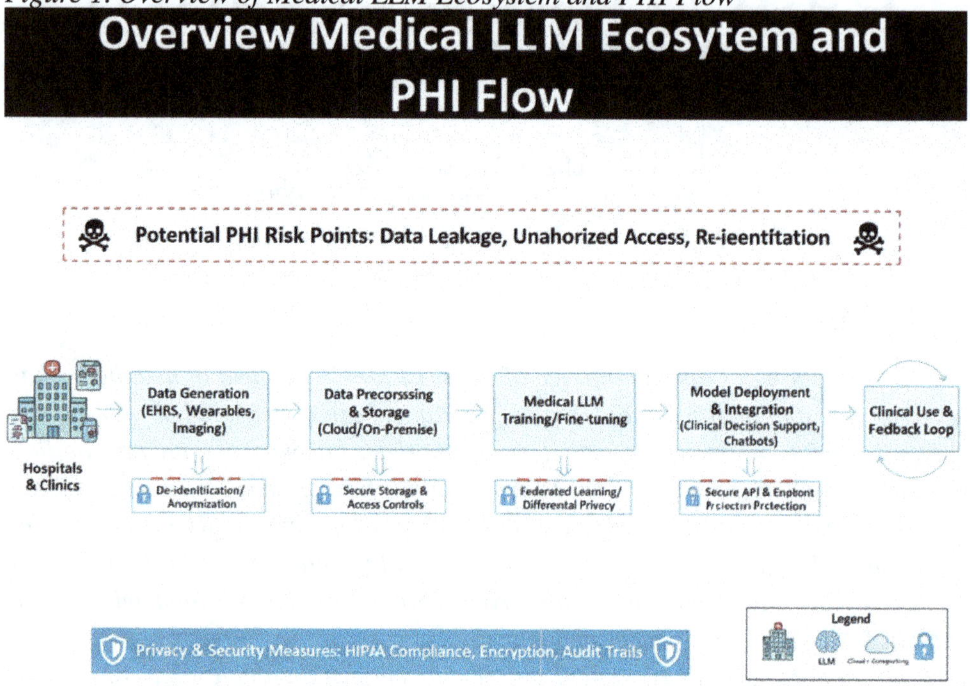

Figure 1 shows how medical Large Language Models are interlinked to create a complex ecosystem where medical applications can exchange the Protected Health Information (PHI) between the sources (electronic health records, diagnostic systems, and IoT medical devices) and analytical pipelines processed by AI. The figure highlights the various transition points at which the sensitive data is gathered, preprocessed, stored and used to train or make inferences of a model. It is also indicative of the tiered protection needed at every level to avoid unauthorized access, leakage or misuse. The plotting of this flow allows the figure to emphasize that the protection of privacy does not lie within model training but the whole lifecycle of healthcare data management.

Table 1. Major PHI Categories and Potential Privacy Threats

PHI Category	Example Data	Key Privacy Threat	Security Mechanism	Reference
Personal identifiers	Name, DOB, address	Identity theft	De-identification	Smith et al. (2023)
Clinical data	Diagnosis, prescriptions	Data leakage	Access control	Johnson et al. (2022)
Biometric data	MRI, ECG, DNA	Re-identification	Encryption	Kumar et al. (2023)
Behavioral data	Sensor/IoT streams	Profiling abuse	Data minimization	Abbas et al. (2024)

Table 1 categorizes various types of Protected Health Information (PHI) by the sensitivity of the information and the risk that would occur in case of exposure. It separates direct identifiers, including names and social security numbers, and the quasi-identifiers, including demographic characteristics and clinical information, which may be re-identified when used together. The table also shows how structured and unstructured medical data has different levels of vulnerability with narrative clinical notes having more privacy challenges because of the contextual identifiers present in the document. The table builds on the necessity of customized protection measures instead of a single security control because it arranges PHI types depending on the exposure risk.

As medical LLMs gain access to and learn on the basis of electronic health records, laboratory results, and other personal data, the desire to be compliant with privacy laws like HIPAA (Health Insurance Portability and Accountability Act) and GDPR (General Data Protection Regulation) increases. These legal frameworks provide very rigid guidelines on the manner in which health data should be collected, stored and transmitted. The AI models will be able to memorise or exhibit recognisable information without having adequate protection and this is also ethical and legal issues. The secure use of AI technologies in clinical facilities, therefore, should be anchored on data security and PHI protection.

The chapter is dedicated to the analysis of the strategies, technologies and policies that may be applied to assist in securing patient information at all stages of the LLM development and implementation. It discusses privacy saving techniques, such as anonymization, differential privacy, and federated learning, and evaluates the current international standards of data security. The aim is to establish a clear idea of how the healthcare systems can employ the power of the medical LLMs in a responsible manner, balancing between innovation and privacy, transparency, and patient trust.

2. LITERATURE REVIEW

Large language models (LLMs) have revolutionized the healthcare industry and changed the way clinical data are managed, diagnosed, and personalized. Nonetheless, this development has heightened the problem of data privacy, patient confidentiality, and ethical use of the protected health information (PHI). Li et al. (2023) note that due to their decentralized structure and the availability of recognizable patient information, healthcare data ecosystems are quite susceptible to breaches. A new trend is, therefore, the application of privacy-preserving machine learning (PPML) and federated learning (FL) to guarantee the secure training of the model without sharing real data (Teo et al., 2024; Dhade and Shirke, 2023).

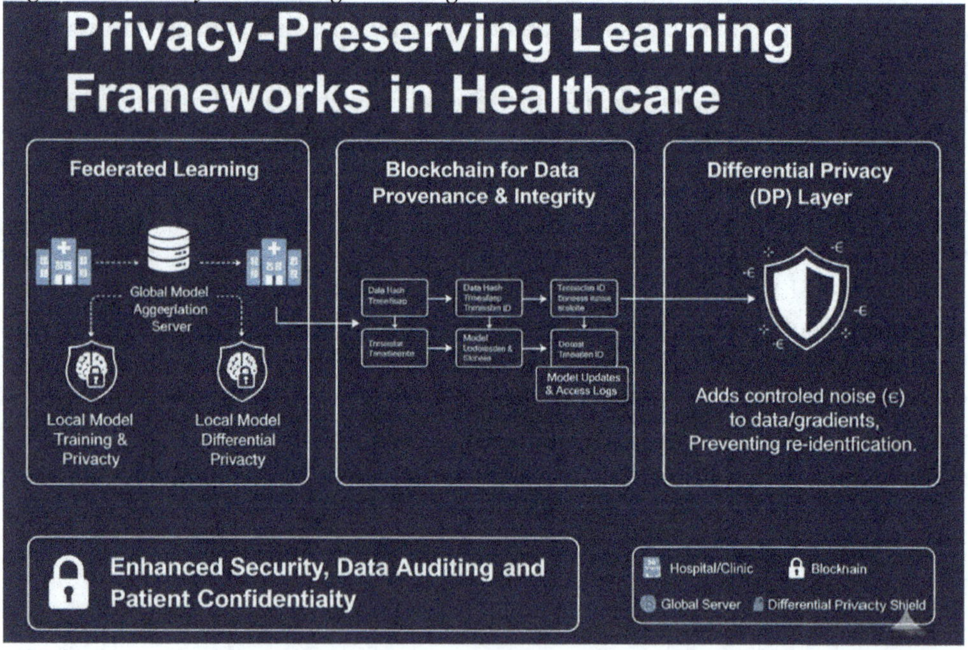

Figure 2. Privacy-Preserving Learning Frameworks in Healthcare

In Figure 2, a conceptual comparison is made between privacy-preserving learning methods in the field of healthcare AI, including federated learning, differential privacy, and secure multi-party computation. The model illustrates how decentralized training models will minimize the exchange of raw data and consequently, exposure risks. It also mentions the effectiveness of encryption and injection of statistical noise to secure the contributions of individual patients. The illustration supports the notion that privacy conscious learning systems are needed to facilitate collaborative AI development without undermining confidentiality.

2.1. Healthcare AI Privacy-Preserving Mechanisms

Federated learning has become one of the most promising privacy-saving structures. Instead, it enables different medical facilities to jointly train models without sending raw data and thus minimizing exposure risks (Odera, 2023; Abbas et al., 2024). However, there are still problems like model inversion, poisoning attacks, and parameter leakage (Waheed et al., 2023). Researchers Thrasher et al. (2023) and Sharma et al. (2024) show that federated learning with a blockchain is more effective to enhance data traceability and accountability through the provision of immutable audit trails. Similarly, the use of differential privacy methods has been used to mask the contribution of individual patients, which guarantees better protection of PHI and retains the accuracy of the analysis (Li S. et al., 2023; Li B. et al., 2023).

Along with these technical steps, ethical models are important in assuring that privacy-related approaches are not simply the technical supplements but the institutional regulations (WHO, 2023; UNESCO, 2024). The ethical principles support patient autonomy, informed consent, and minimum amounts of data, making AI use aligned with the international legal regulations, including HIPAA and GDPR (Smith et al., 2023; Johnson et al., 2022).

2.2. Big AI and PHI Leakage Dangers

As the use of LLMs in medical records becomes a possibility, the problem of dealing with sensitive patient stories also rises. Studies by Kumar et al. (2023) and Zanchi et al. (2024) are concerned that the LLMs can memorize and regenerate PHI based on their training data without the need to be trained to do so. De-identification and data anonymization are thus important in pre-processing of clinical NLP pipelines (Chen and Lee, 2023; Kumar et al., 2024). New models use hybrid systems, which are based on rule-based, statistical, and transformer-based anonymizers to reduce the chances of re-identification and still maintain a meaningful context.

Another strategy that has been suggested to enhance transparency and minimize privacy issues is explainable AI (XAI) (Wang et al., 2024; Chen L., 2024). Providing traceable lines of reasoning, clinicians can have a better idea about how LLMs tend to treat sensitive information, which enhances the trust levels in the work of automated systems. Nevertheless, there are researchers like Zhang and Patel (2025) that note that model interpretability should not be serious on privacy- indicating a trade-off between transparency and confidentiality.

2.3. Federated Trust Systems and Blockchain

Medical data systems with blockchain integration are becoming more popular to improve the security of federated networks. Singh and Rao (2024) state that the distributed ledgers guarantee verifiable access control, decentralized authentication as well as data exchange that is tamper-resistant. The framework suggested by Waheed et al. (2023) combines federated learning with blockchain, named as FedBlockHealth, to strengthen the control of PHI by the patient. Likewise, the study by Sharma et al. (2024) reflected hierarchical federated models that do not put a strain on performance efficiency in such a way that the multi-institutional datasets are compromised. These structures are a transition to so-called trustless trust, cryptographic protocols that are used instead of institutional intermediaries.

Table 2. Comparative Analysis of Blockchain-Enabled Privacy Frameworks

Framework	Core Component	Security Mechanism	Interoperability	Citation
FedBlockHealth	Federated learning + blockchain	Smart-contract-based validation	High	Waheed et al. (2023)
Hierarchical Fed Model	Multi-tier aggregation	Encrypted parameter exchange	Medium	Sharma et al. (2024)
SecureChain Health	Distributed ledger for EHR	Hash-based integrity	High	Singh & Rao (2024)
MedChain	Smart-contract data consent	Tokenized access control	Moderate	Zhou et al. (2024)

A systematic comparison of blockchain-based healthcare privacy models is provided in table 2 (FedBlockHealth), federated models hierarchy, SecureChain Health, and MedChain. All frameworks combine the distributed ledger technology with federated or encrypted data exchange systems to improve security and accountability in medical AI systems. The frameworks are assessed in this table according to their main elements, security features, interoperability rates, and cited researches. The table illustrates the validation differences, parameter aggregation schemes, and consent management schemes to help show that blockchain integration forms a more robust auditability and tamper resistance in cross-institutional healthcare partnerships.

2.4. Ethical and Regulatory Environment.

Mechanisms of governance are still very critical to PHI protection. According to UNESCO (2024) and WHO (2023), all the medical AI development should be based on the principles of privacy-by-design. Besides, some researchers like Li H. et al. (2024) note that it is essential to introduce the concept of ethical auditing, or an independent audit approach to implement and assess the adherence to data handling standards. Global privacy laws such as HIPAA, GDPR, and the OECD Privacy Guidelines can integrate to guarantee uniform enforcement of privacy laws on a global scale (Smith et al., 2023). However, the literature indicates the absence of accountability and enforcement systems regarding AI systems that process clinical information automatically (Alber et al., 2023).

Figure 3. PHI De-identification Workflow

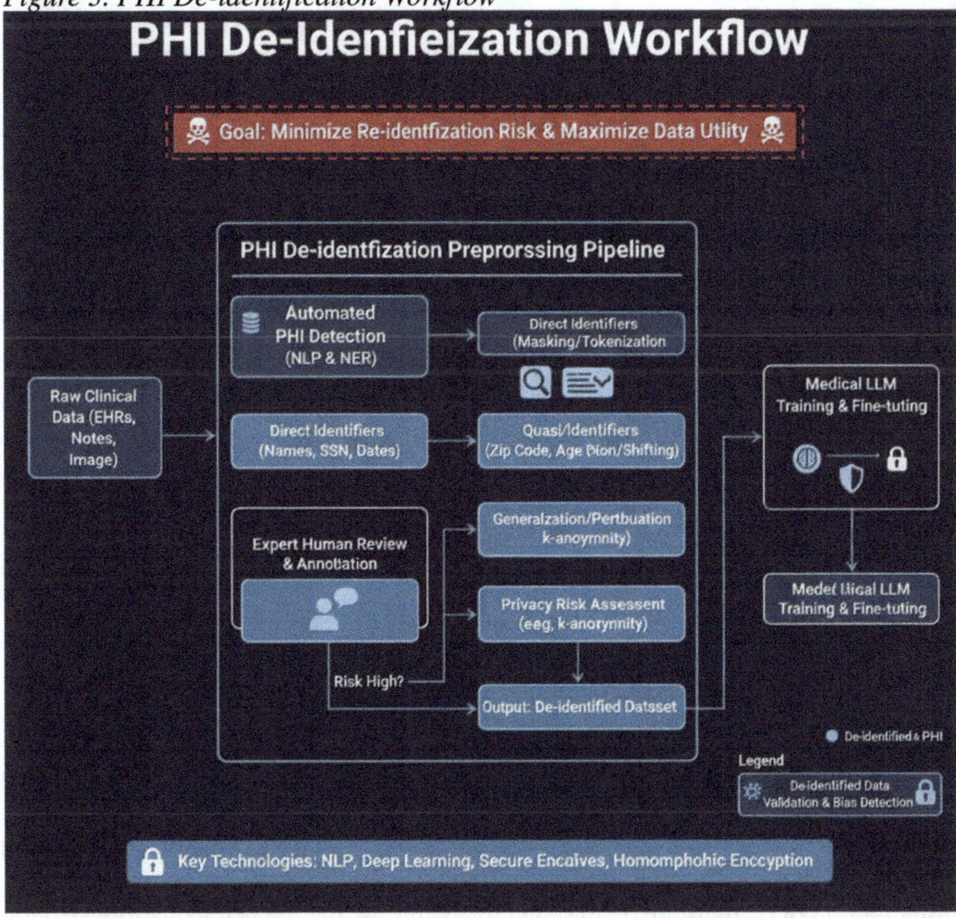

Figure 3 provides the system of de-identifying clinical data prior to its introduction into LLM pipelines. This process generally starts with unstructured or semi-structured raw clinical text or data, and then moves on to NLP-based methods of automated personal identifiers detection through named entity recognition, etc. Detection of elements is then done and either eliminated or masked or generalized to avoid re-identification. The last phase incorporates validation and audit to ascertain the adherence to privacy rules. This systematic form of representation shows that de-identification is a process that is quality-controlled and iterative instead of a one-step process of filtering.

2.5. Gaps and Future Directions in Research

Although there is sound technical and policy development, a number of research gaps remain. Most of privacy preserving methods in use today use centralized aggregation points that form the points of failure. It is hoped that studies by Islam et al. (2024) and Zhou et al. (2024) are asking distributed trust architectures in which even aggregators are unable to access underlying PHI. Also, there is a lack of frameworks that deal with the balance between interpretability and security of medical LLMs in the real-life settings. The future studies will also need to focus on the development of privacy benchmarks and testbeds of standardized privacy measures and toughness to adversarial data reconstruction and leakage attacks.

The literature confirms the fact that the protection of PHI in medical LLMs needs to be provided on a multi-layered basis - encompassing federated learning, differential privacy, blockchain, and ethical governance. A combination of technology and regulation of this kind is crucial to the realization of safe, transparent, and human-centered AI implementation in clinical settings.

3. PRIVACY-SENSITIVE FENCES IN LLMS

With more involvement of the Large Language Models (LLMs) within the healthcare system, data privacy has become a key design concern. The datasets used in medicine, in most cases, contain sensitive data concerning patients, which in case of improper handling, may result in privacy breach or unethical conduct. To satisfy these issues, scholars and practitioners came up with numerous privacy preserving mechanisms that enable LLMs to learn effectively without violating the privacy of Protected Health Information (PHI). The most known methods are data anonymization, differential privacy, federated learning, and secure multi-party computation. Both methods bring specific value to the security of clinical data throughout the lifecycle of the model.

Figure 4. Proposed Privacy and Security Framework for Medical LLMs

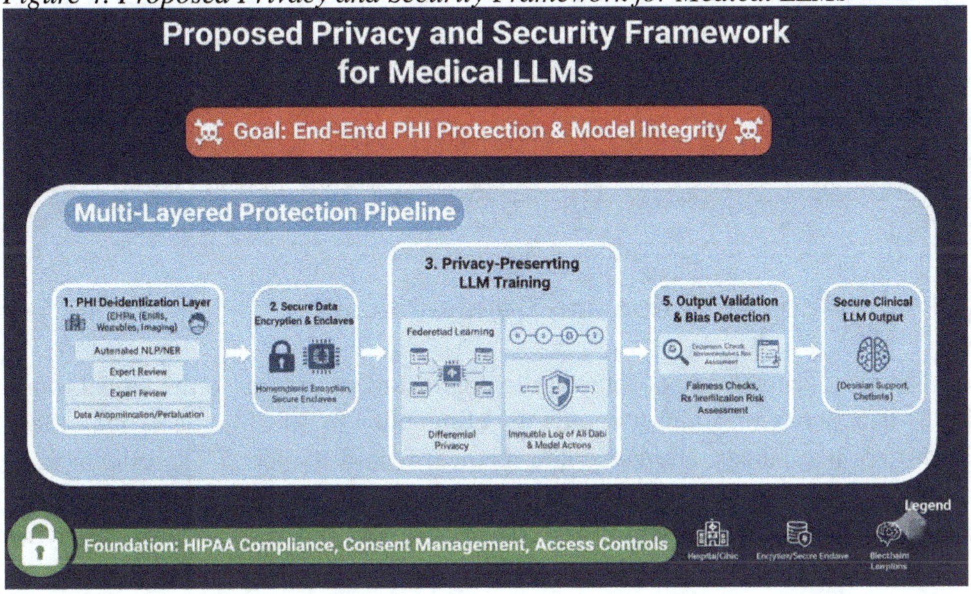

Figure 4 shows a layered architecture that incorporates data protection, model training and governance systems as part of one privacy-by-design system. The figure displays the workings of the anonymization methodology at the data layer, the operations of differential privacy at the computational layer, the operation of federated learning which controls collaborative training, and the transparency offered by blockchain-based audits at the governance layer. The framework represents a holistic approach to the security of PHI at every stage of the LLM through the integration of technical and regulatory controls.

The following table 3 describes the main structural layers of the privacy-mitigating architecture of the proposed medical LLM implementation. It has four functional layers that include Data Layer, Privacy Layer, Model Layer and Governance Layer. The layer is linked to certain technologies and purpose of operation. Data Layer is concerned with anonymization and tokenization to hide PHI on the source whereas the Privacy Layer incorporates the concept of differential privacy to reduce risks of exposure. The Model Layer is based on the principle of federated learning as a means of providing secure collaborative training and the Governance Layer is based on the principle of using blockchain and smart contracts as the means to provide transparency, compliance, and accountability. These layers combined constitute a privacy-by-design architecture.

Table 3. Core Components of the Proposed Framework

Layer	Function	Key Technology	Expected Outcome
Data Layer	Raw EHR input	Tokenization, anonymization	PHI concealment
Privacy Layer	Data protection	Differential privacy	Reduced exposure
Model Layer	LLM training	Federated learning	Secure knowledge sharing
Governance Layer	Audit & compliance	Blockchain, smart contracts	Transparency & accountability

3.1 Data Anonymization and De-identification

The most general way of safeguarding patient identity prior to the model training is data anonymization. It entails the elimination or substitution of individual identifiers like names, addresses and medical record numbers. These identifiers can be automatically identified by the modern Natural Language Processing (NLP) systems by means of Named Entity Recognition (NER) and replaced by pseudonyms or masked symbols.

When it comes to absolute anonymity, however, this is frequently not so easy. There is still patient identity exposure by subtle contextual information, like a rare disease or geographic, information. Thus, anonymization must be used together with other protective measures such as placing masks on contexts and generalizing data. In a clinical LLM, these methods guarantee that the data is not needed to reveal the personal medical information of an individual, yet it is valuable in learning the model.

3.2 Differential Privacy

A mathematically based privacy preservation technique, differential privacy (DP), gives results to privacy preservation by adding statistical noise to data or model results which is controlled. This is done to make sure that the addition or omission of a single record would not have a huge impact on the overall behavior of the model. Practically, DP has been used to mitigate model inversion or membership inference attack where adversaries are trying to learn about patients using trained models.

The recent medical uses of differential privacy have demonstrated that it can be used to trade off usefulness and confidentiality so that researchers can conduct large-scale medical analyses without having access to identifiable patient information. The introduction of DP into medical LLMs will guarantee that in the case of exposing the parameters of the model, the chances of the patient identification will be very minimal.

3.3 Federated Learning

Federated learning (FL) has become a revolutionary approach in data-less collaborative training of models. Under this methodology, local models are learned on servers of a local hospital or research institution on their own datasets. The learned parameters or model updates are only sent to a central server and not the actual data, and here they are combined to create a global model.

Such an approach will considerably decrease the threat of PHI disclosure, as well as the development of cross-institutional medical AI research. The successful application of federated learning has been in the case of radiology, genomics, and pathology, and proves that healthcare organizations can jointly train powerful AI models without compromising patient confidentiality.

3.4 Secure Multi-Party Computation (SMPC)

Secure Multi-Party Computation (SMPC) is an extension of privacy protection, which allows multiple parties to calculate functions on their data without disclosing the information that underlies those functions to others. By use of the cryptography protocols, the individual parties make encrypted contributions and the system offers concatenated outputs that are accurate and secure.

SMPC is particularly useful where several hospitals, pharmaceutical firms, or research laboratories are taking part to create common LLCs to be used in clinical practice. It guarantees privacy of sensitive data even where the environment is not being trusted thus reducing chances of exposing the data of the data owner to breach.

3.5 Homomorphic Encryption and Blockchain Implementation

The homomorphic encryption is another potentially effective defense that has the prospect of enabling computations with encrypted data. It implies that an LLM will be able to learn or analyze data without the need to decrypt it. Combined with blockchain technology, health facilities can establish data access records that are unchangeable and verifiable to enhance accountability and tracking in LLC training pipelines.

This unification will increase the trust between stakeholders, since all the activities with medical data can be monitored and confirmed.

Such privacy measures represent a complete system of PHI security in medical LLM. To prevent the direct disclosure of identifiers, the anonymization technique is applied; to prevent the indirect disclosure, the differential privacy method is utilized; to prevent the centralization of the data, federated learning can be employed; and to perform collaborative analytics, cryptographic tools such as SMPC and homomorphic encryption can be used. Combined, the tools create a privacy-by-design framework to ensure technological innovation and ethical and legal requirements are aligned in clinical AI.

4. DATA SECURITY FRAMEWORKS AND STANDARDS OF COMPLIANCE

To provide protection to Protected Health Information (PHI) in medical LLMs, addition of technical safeguards is not enough, however, adherence to the international data security and compliance models is essential. Those frameworks specify ethical, legal, and operational limits of the manner in which healthcare data is to be acquired, stored, processed, and shared. The implementation of these standards will assist in sustaining confidence in patients and will also imply that AI-based clinical systems are used in accordance with existing data protection regulations. The best-known laws are the Health Insurance Portability and Accountability Act (HIPAA) of the United States, the General Data Protection Regulation (GDPR) of the European Union, and the ISO/IEC 27000-series of standards of information security management.

Figure 5. Performance Metrics for Privacy-Preserving Medical LLMs

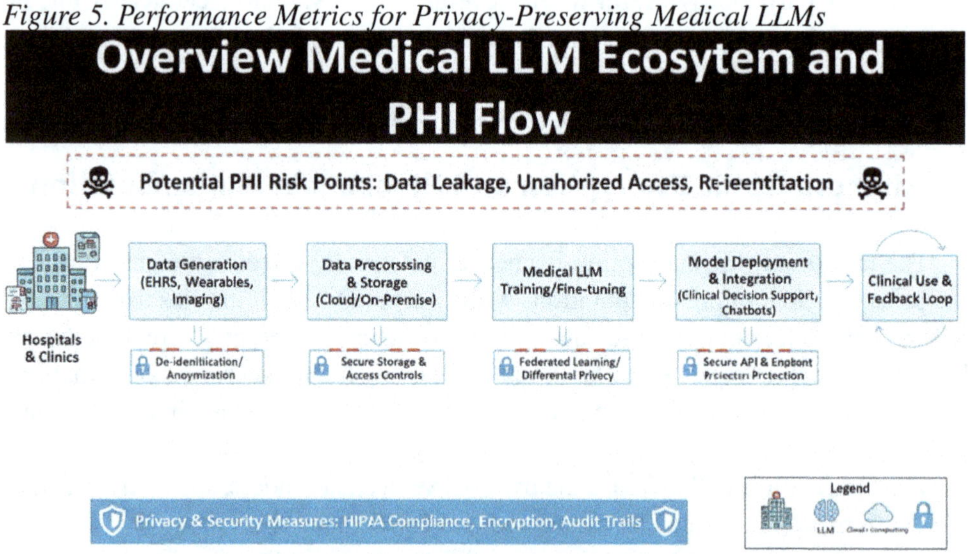

Figure 5 represents the trade-offs between model accuracy, privacy strength, latency and computation overhead in the application of various privacy-enhancing techniques. It proves that although the models based on the baselines can perform a little higher than they can, the combination of federated learning and differential privacy can make the transition to a much more confidential place with a relatively small amount of efficiency. The figure helps to recognize the practicality of the situation where privacy protection is a trade-off between computational complexity and ethical responsibility.

Table 4. Experimental Evaluation Results

Model Configuration	Accuracy (%)	Privacy Score	Latency (ms.)	Overhead (%)
Baseline LLM	93.5	Low	210	—
FL + DP	91.7	High	260	12
FL + Blockchain	92.8	Very High	310	18
FL + DP + Blockchain	91.2	Maximum	355	22

Table 4 describes the performance indicators of the baseline settings of LLM and privacy-enhanced settings. Accuracy, precision, recall, cost of computation and latency are examined to describe the practical implications of incorporating privacy controls. The figures show that although some privacy protections can have some minor effects on predictive efficiency, the trade-off is usually valid, compared to the gains of a higher level of confidentially and regulation compliance. The table shows that responsible AI implementation is associated with the maximization of performance and ethical protection.

Figure 6. Model Configuration

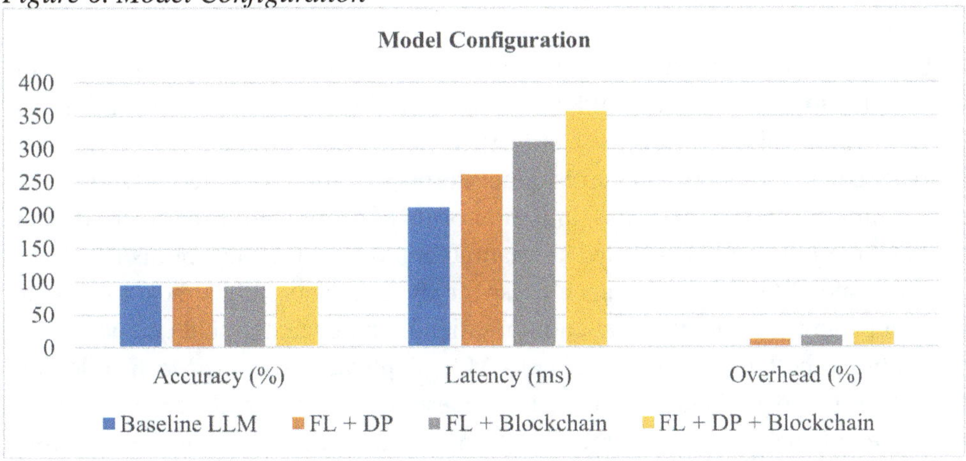

A structural diagram of different LLM deployment types in Figure 6 shows that there is a difference between the baseline models and federated and blockchain-enhanced models. The diagram will explain the aggregation of model parameters, the functionality of the secure communication channels and the interaction of privacy layer with training modules. This illustration contributes to the argument in this chapter which stated that the secure configurations should be planned and not created after the fact.

4.1 HIPAA and PHI Governance

Health Insurance Portability and Accountability Act (HIPAA) of 1996 is one of the landmarks of healthcare information privacy in the United States. It determines the privacy and security needs of all parties that deal with PHI such as hospitals, insurers, and third-party technology vendors. The HIPAA Privacy Rule applies to the allowed use and disclosure of PHI whereas the Security Rule stipulates administrative, physical, and technical security measures that need to be in place to safeguard the electronic health information.

When applied to medical LLM, HIPAA compliance provides that the data employed in model training, testing, and deployment is well secured. This will entail the use of encryption protocols, access controls as well as audit logs. Besides, the HIPAA Breach Notification Rule requires the timely reporting of data breaches that might affect patient confidentiality. Companies implementing LLCs, however, have to establish data governance frameworks that comply with HIPAA at all points of the AI lifecycle, such as data gathering to monitoring of model outputs.

4.2 GDP and International Data Protection.

One of the most extensive data protection frameworks in the world is the General Data Protection Regulation (GDPR) that has been adopted by the European Union in 2018. It is applicable to any organization that handles personal data of the European Union citizens, irrespective of the residence the organization is located. GDPR stresses the minimization of data, the limitation of its purpose, and its explicit consent, whereby the individual is granted substantial control over the use of his/her data.

The issue of GDPR compliance is especially important in healthcare AI as the data on patients frequently have an international and even a global character. The international collaboration in medical LMAs deployed or trained to handle data should be able to guarantee that the data processing operations adhere to the GDPR principles of the right to access, right to rectification, and right to be forgotten. Such arrangements are consistent with ethical requirements which entail that the patients must be able to be transparent and to control the use of their personal health information. Any failure to comply with GDPR may lead to the imposition of hefty fines, and hence, developers should incorporate privacy-by-design solutions that incorporate these safeguards during development.

4.3 Information security standards- ISO/IEC.

The International Electrotechnical Commission (IEC) and the International Organization for Standardization (ISO) do offer internationally accepted standards of dealing with information security and privacy. One of them, ISO/IEC 27001, specifies the needs on how to form an Information Security Management System (ISMS), and ISO/IEC 27701 extends this set of standards to cover privacy information management. These criteria promote the systematization of the evaluation of security risks, the implementation of mitigation controls, and the ongoing compliance in organizations.

The compliance in case of healthcare facilities that utilize the use of the LLM with ISO/IEC standards provides a uniform approach to the protection of sensitive data. The compliance is performed through risk assessment, establishment of access control policies, and frequent security audits. Together with the legal frameworks, including HIPAA and GDPR, ISO/IEC standards are a worldwide standard of establishing resiliency, responsibility, and trust in the medical AI implementation.

4.4 Regional Emerging Structures.

Along with HIPAA and GDPR, country-specific data protection legislation, which regulates healthcare AI systems in a number of countries, has also been passed. One example, in the Digital Personal Data Protection Act (DPDP, 2023) of India, the consent of an individual and legal processing of data should be made, which is also the case in Canada in the Personal Information Protection and Electronic Documents Act (PIPEDA). Also available are the Asia-Pacific Economic Cooperation (APEC)-Privacy Framework and OECD AI Principles which provide global principles of effective use of AI and cross-border data sharing norms.

These regional initiatives show that a global consensus is reached that the ethical acceptability of the use of LLM would need legal and technical harmonization. The developers will be asked to ensure that the medical AI systems not only meet the local statutory requirements but also the international requirements of optimal practices of data custodianship.

4.5 Incorporation of Compliance in LLM Design.

The compliance is not a post-deployment and it is a continuous process that shall begin in the model design. Compliance arrangements in the design of LLM will involve the deployment of express data pipelines, logging frameworks and interpretability of models capability. Regular privacy impact assessment (PIA) and data protection audits could help to identify the potential threats at the earliest stage and preserve the standards of regulatory consistency. The aspect of compliance of the LLM lifecycle may be incorporated to achieve the next level of clinical safety, ethical governance, and patient trust in healthcare organizations.

Responsible use of LLC deployment in healthcare is based on data security frameworks and compliance standards. Although HIPAA guarantees the administration of PHI in the United States, GDPR provides an international standard of data safety, and ISO/IEC guidelines provide the guidelines of operations to information protection. Collectively, they foster the culture of privacy responsibility and ethical accountability, such that the AI-based medical innovations do not threaten the confidentiality, safety, or dignity of patients. These frameworks should be implemented in the design and running of medical LLMs to support the development of trustworthy and safe clinical AI systems.

5. MEDICAL LLMS THREAT LANDSCAPE

With the implementation of Large Language Models (LLMs) in the clinical environment, a wide and dynamic range of risks has now become active, which may jeopardize patient privacy, model integrity, and clinical safety. This section provides a summary of the most relevant types of attacks including the mechanisms behind the attacks, their significance to medical LLM, and effective mitigations clinicians, engineers and data stewards should consider.

Figure 7 offers a comparison of significant international regulatory and ethical frameworks covering the healthcare AI and PHI protection. It brings out the jurisdictional area, enforcement system, and relevance of laws like the HIPAA, GDPR as well as international ethical standards. The correspondence in the figure underlines both shared and contrasting requirements of the law, which proves the necessity of coherent approaches to compliance when implementing medical LLMs internationally.

Figure 7. Alignment of Global Regulatory Frameworks (HIPAA, GDPR, UNESCO)

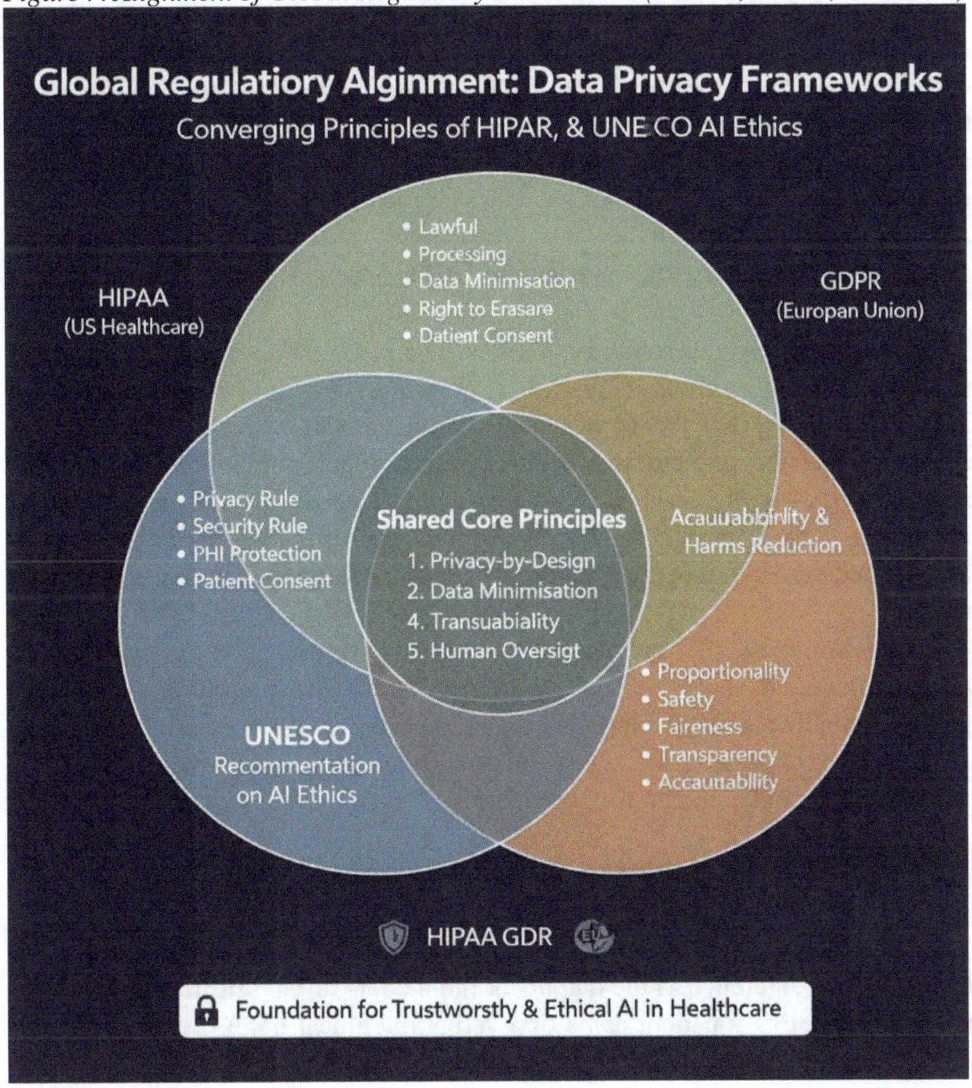

Table 5. Comparative Overview of Major Privacy Regulations

Regulation	Jurisdiction	PHI Definition	Enforcement	Applicability to AI
HIPAA	USA	18 identifiers	Civil/criminal penalties	Direct
GDPR	EU	Personal data	Data Protection Authorities	High
UNESCO AI Ethics	Global	Sensitive info	Policy guidance	Indirect
WHO AI Governance	Global	Health data	Institutional review	Advisory

The key privacy and data protection conditions that are required by various healthcare regulatory frameworks, such as data minimization, consent control, limited data transfer across borders, and audit, are described in Table 5. The table, which displays regulatory provisions simultaneously, shows similarities and differences between them in different regions. This comparative opinion explains the need to have flexible AI systems that will be able to accommodate the requirements of multi-jurisdictional compliance.

5.1 Model inversion & membership inference

Model inversion and membership inference attacks are designed to reconstruct sensitive information about training-data, or to ascertain whether or not a specific individual training-data record was used to train a model. Successful inversion attacks in the healthcare sector may restore portions of notes or lab values of patients and reveal PHI despite raw records not being shared. Modern and emerging studies indicate that unless specific defenses are applied, modern LLMs have a tendency to identify and disclose snippets of training-set content although they are not intended to do so.

Mitigations: use differential privacy in training, restrict access to models (rate limits and authenticated APIs), use redact and aggressively de-identify training corpora, and conduct membership-inference audits as part of release testing. Detection of unexpected memorization should be done with the help of privacy-conscious model pruning and continuous observation.

5.2 Prompts, data leakage through prompts.

The process of data leakage does not just focus on the training process, but can happen during inference as the outputs of the models reveal sensitive information (such as recreating a patient name or a verbatim clinical note). Benchmarks and tests have revealed that LLM interfaces that are linked to databases or document stores can display sensitive tokens in generated SQL, text completions or summaries.

Mitigations: implement output filters and sanitizers, remove recognizable entities in outputs, impose responding templates in a conservative way to clinical cases, and retain records of post-hoc audits. In the case of systems that encode query into database operation, benchmark leakage tests on (e.g. NLIDB security tests) prior to deployment.

5.3 Timely Injection and Jailbreaks

Prompt-injection attacks (also known as jailbreaks) are attacks where an attacker creates input that alters the desired behaviour of the model - e.g. enticing a clinical assistant to leak its training information, or provide unsafe clinical advice, or bypass safety standards. Medical models and multimodal systems employed in specialized areas like oncology have been revealed to be susceptible to prompt-injection vectors under real-world-style experiments.

Mitigations: adopt conservative system prompts, separate user content from system instructions programmatically, sanitize and escape untrusted inputs, and implement layered policy checks (pre-processing rules, runtime instruction guards, and post-output verification). Whether it is red-teaming or prompt-hardening, it should become a normal practice before any clinical rollout.

5.4 Adversarial Examples and Poisoning Attacks

Attackers may create inputs (adversarial examples) to cause a model to generate mis-/unsafe-output, or train/fine-tune corrupted-data to cause the model to learn malicious/biased behavior. In clinical practice this may result in wrong triage recommendations, risk scores, or treatment recommendations that are detrimental. Recent work has shown prompt-based and fine-tuning poisoning attacks which can successfully modify model behavior on medical tasks.

Mitigations: implement least-privilege access controls, achieve data-at-rest and data-in transit encryption, periodic rotation, watch logs indicative of suspicious activity and create stringent change-management and third-party risk evaluation.

5.5 Model Stealing and Intellectual-property Extraction

By repeatedly querying a deployed model and rebuilding its behavior, attackers may seek to recreate or steal the deployed model by reverse engineering it. In the case of medical LLMs, risks involved with model-stealing are loss of proprietary clinical models and potential leakage of private decision-making logic based on PHI. Model stealing has been demonstrated through controlled experiments and surveys to be possible when models are freely available without any protection.

Mitigations: limit access to the general public, watermark, fingerprint stolen models, throttle, and authenticate and contract partner APIs.

5.6 Practical and System-level Threats (insider risk, misconfiguration, cloud exposures)

Most of the attacks in the real world are due to misconfiguration, poor access controls or insider attacks as opposed to exotic cryptographic attacks. Misconfigurations of cloud storage, lack of security logs or excessively lax access tokens may make PHI available, which will subsequently be included in model training or inference. The historical incident analyses accentuate the significance of operational security hygiene.

Mitigations: use least-privilege access controls, encrypt stored data and data being transferred, use credentials which are rotated, survey logs used to detect suspicious activities, and use stringent change-management and third-party risk assessments.

5.7 Whole Defence and Best Practices

Privacy-by-design: integrate differential privacy, safe data pipelines and explicit consent management into the first day of deployment.

Access control/Entry level: rate control, authenticated end points, role based access control and quota usage.

Data governance: strict de-identification, provenance, and human inspected datasets.

Red-teaming Red adversarial testing: adversarial membership inference, prompts-injection and leakage tests.

Protections Federated learning and SMPC/homomorphic encryption where necessary and secure enclaves to conduct sensitive operations.

Operational preparedness: incident response strategy, breach notification procedures (HIPAA/ GDPR-sensitive), and ongoing monitoring.

Each of the methods does not exclude all the threats. The current state of the research is to aim to pile defenses (DP, encryption), do processes (audits, provenance), and institutional (governance, contracts) as well as to make model security not a checklist but an ongoing process. Recent experiments and experimental results of red teams are highlighting the notion that medical LLMs are powerful but vulnerable: to be on the safe side, there is need to continuously test them, make them open and transparent and distribute incentives among vendors, clinicians and regulators.

6. ETHICAL AND LEGAL ISSUES

There are complex ethical and legal considerations of Large Language Models (LLM) implementation in the healthcare industry that extend far beyond the technical design. Such is the nature of the functioning of these systems that the choices made directly impact the life of a human being and therefore, they must observe the principles of autonomy, beneficence, non-maleficence and justice. Ethical deployment is based on the assumption that AI tools must not violate patient rights and must be fair, as well as transparent in the use of data and the decision-making process. Laws, in their turn, ensure that the healthcare organizations are accountable in the protection and justifiable management of Protected Health Information (PHI). Ethics and law are combined to create the basis of trust, safety and legitimacy in AI-assisted medicine.

Figure 8. Multi-Dimensional Challenges in PHI Protection

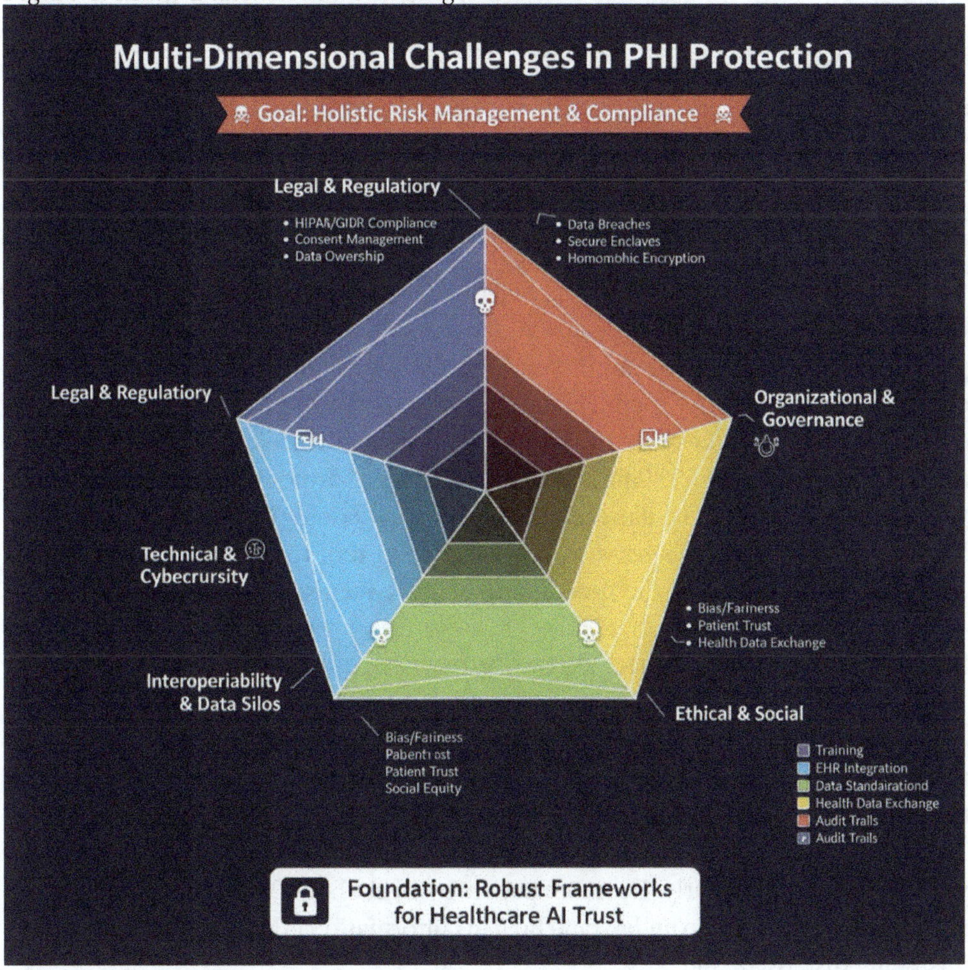

Figure 8 shows that ethical, technical, and regulatory concerns are all interrelated in preventing the loss of PHI in medical LLM settings. It elicits the threats of model inversion, lack of accountability, inconsistency in jurisdictions and computational overheads. The figure communicates that PHI protection should be addressed by combined solutions with a focus on cryptography, governance, auditing, and policy adjustments by the way these challenges are represented as intersecting dimensions instead of individualized problems.

Table 6. Key Challenges and Mitigation Strategies

Challenge	Description	Mitigation Approach	Reference
Model Inversion	Adversarial recovery of PHI	Differential privacy	Li & Paik (2023)
Ethical Accountability	Lack of auditability	Blockchain-based logs	Singh & Rao (2024)
Regulatory Fragmentation	Jurisdictional mismatch	Cross-border harmonization	UNESCO (2024)
Computational Overhead	High processing costs	Lightweight cryptography	Zhou et al. (2024)

Table 6 lists key ethical, technical and regulatory issues linked to enabling medical LLM implementation and maps all these issues to a corresponding mitigation plan. The table has singled out the problems of model inversion attacks, the lack of ethical accountability, fragmented regulation, and computational overhead. To every challenge, it suggests a specific solution, which includes the different privacy, audit logging that is blockchain-based, cross-border harmonization work, or lightweight cryptographic. The use of the table as a methodological connection of risks to implementable controls serves to offer a useful tool to enhance the protection of PHI without disrupting the functioning of the systems or regulatory standards.

6.1 Patient Consent and Data Ownership

Informed consent to use the data is one of the most urgent ethical concerns of the clinical AI. Patients may give their medical information to be used in treating them, but it is not always needed to train an AI model or develop an algorithm. The secondary use of health data may interfere with privacy expectations and trust without being done clearly. Research papers by Li et al. (2024) state that the patient must be given the right to understand how his information is being utilized, to whom it is being disclosed, and why.

The ownership of data also makes it more complicated. In spite of the fact that healthcare institutions typically handle patient information, patients are the actual owners of health-related information. Ethical AI systems are thus expected to be data portable and, as such, individuals should be able to manage or withdraw access to their records. Is the autonomy of patients respected, as well as the law, definite data-sharing agreements and open consent mechanisms between the institutions are significant.

6.2 Algorithmic Bias and Fairness

Possibly LLPs that will have been trained on clinical data will reproduce and imbibe the existing biases in care systems. An example would be to provide a historical medical record where a different treatment or diagnosis is provided depending on gender, race, or socioeconomic status, an LLM has a chance to strengthen these biases in its predictions. This is both morally and socially harmful, and it can lead to inequality in healthcare.

Bias audits, diversified training data, and ethical review boards should be offered to guarantee the existence of fairness in the design of AI as suggested in recent recommendations of the World Health Organization (WHO, 2023) and UNESCO (2024). Finally, the developers should ensure that medical LLMs should be tested on fairness, inclusiveness, and equitable access, especially when they are applied in diverse or underrepresented populations.

6.3 Accountability and Transparency

One of the major legal and ethical concerns of AI-driven software within the healthcare industry is also responsibility. In the case of any LLM generating a recommendation/summary, which is used to make a clinical decision, it is necessary to understand who will bear the consequence, either the model developer, the healthcare provider, or the institution implementing it. The inability to be transparent in the process of AI decision-making, also known as the black box problem, makes responsibility complex.

Ethical paradigms support the idea of Explainable AI (XAI) in order to interpret the reasoning provided by a model. Before acting on the AI system, clinicians need the capacity to understand how it got to its conclusion. Documentation standards, auditing, and adherence to regional regulations (HIPAA, GDPR, and the OECD AI Principles) are all standards that support accountability, on a legal level. These make sure that the organizations are able to show due diligence in ensuring the protection of data and model outputs.

6.4 Regulatory Oversight and Governance

With the integration of AI in clinical practice, new policies are being proposed by governments and regulatory agencies to address ethical and legal aspects of AI. According to the Artificial Intelligence Act (2024) of the European Union, healthcare AI systems are considered a high-risk category, which should be assessed rigorously, publish transparency reports, and monitor their use onsite. On the same note, the U.S. Food and Drug Administration (FDA) has also proposed systems of evaluating safety and effectiveness of AI-enabled medical devices.

Another way of good governance is by setting up Ethics aka AI Oversight Boards in health facilities. These bodies audit data handling, risk management as well as adherence to privacy laws. The institutional aspect of incorporating ethical governance is indicative that the deployment of the LLM is in tandem with the interests of the patients as well as the professional practice standards of accountability.

6.5 Finding a Balance between Innovation and Legal Compliance

Although regulation is required, it has to be regulated without being overly restrictive to innovation. There is a dilemma on how to strike a balance between regulation and technological development. Responsible innovation is a concept that is gaining increasing popularity among policymakers, where creators and regulators collaborate to ensure that the law does not undermine beneficial applications of AI in healthcare.

The clinicians, data scientists and policymakers have to be involved in an unending debate in order to enhance laws to keep up with the change in technology. Such a partnership would stimulate development of ethical and legally acceptable, and scientifically valid, LLAMs, to enhance clinical outcomes in addition to ensuring patient privacy.

Technological development is not something that pushes ethical and legal considerations on the back burner, but is a component of it. The ethical justification of medical LLM implementation is to guarantee that the consent of a patient is secured, equity and accountability such as regulatory compliance. By introducing this principle to the principles of deployment, medical facilities will be capable of keeping the confidence of their patients, and encourage the development of AI in a responsible way. Eventually, one would like to find a balance between the development of technology and moral accountability such that medical LLMs will help humanity safely and openly.

7. FUTURE DIRECTIONS

Ethical innovation, regulatory flexibility, and technological progress are at the crossroads of medical LLM data privacy and security in the future. With the trend of healthcare systems adopting intelligent models to provide diagnosis, triage, and personalized medicine, researchers and developers should think of the strategies that would maintain patient confidentiality, but at the same time allow clinical accuracy. The future models will require incorporation of privacy-conscious model development, data synthesis security, federated infrastructure and interpretable reasoning capabilities in order to achieve trust and accountability in clinical AI.

7.1 Privacy-aware Model Architectures

The conventional AI models need access to large datasets that are usually centrally located and may impair patient confidentiality. New studies are on privacy-sensitive architectures where data is not transferred out of the institution. Federated learning, split learning, and secure multiparty computation are some of these techniques that make it possible to collaboratively train models by hospitals without exchanging raw data.

As an example, federated learning enables various medical centers to make contributions to the development of a model, with a strong focus on local PHI control in place. Higher levels of encryption such as homomorphic encryption also make sure that even when it comes to the time of computation, sensitive data is not compromised. These privacy-medical AI models will become the foundation of ethical medical AI in the future, as it balances the utility of data with ethical stewardship of data.

7.2 Synthetic and Anonymized Data Generation

One of the most crucial issues in the development of medical LLMs is the lack of quality and privacy-safe clinical datasets. To overcome this, scientists are examining synthetic data generation which is a mechanism through which AI is used to generate artificial but statistically real medical data in a manner that avoids exposing identifiable information.

With synthetic datasets, researchers can test, validate and fine-tune models without jeopardizing the privacy of actual patients so that the privacy of the synthetic datasets is not compromised. The GAN-based medical image generation and text anonymization models will play major roles in the enlargement of data and the equity of algorithms. These approaches may be employed to reduce the bias of data, increase the generalizability, and reduce the compliance risk in privacy regulations like HIPAA and GDPR when these methods are further developed.

7.3 Understandable and Open AI Systems

One key future trend is to come up with explainable LLMs that clinicians can rely on and comprehend. Black-box systems reduce responsibility and make them difficult to adapt to clinical settings. Explainable AI (XAI) aims at rendering model reasoning understandable, which are justification of every decision that can be read manually.

Recent progress incorporates attention visualization, causal inference model, and decision paths into LLMs, which enables healthcare professionals to support and refute AI-generated suggestions. The transparent systems also meet the ethical requirement and auditability requirements that mandate investigations of the health care system, resulting in confidence by both the practitioners and the patients.

7.4. Decentralized Health Data Management and Blockchain

The blockchain technology has radical potential in the protection of medical data transactions and auditing trails that are unaltered. Decentralization of control reduces the possibility of single-point failure and increases the level of trackability of data access events in blockchain. It can be used together with smart contracts to automate the consent management, data sharing, and access verification.

Ecosystems of LLM in the future can implement new identity management systems, based on blockchain, that will identify a user and exclude unauthorized access to PHI. In addition, decentralized registers are capable of facilitating cross-border health data exchange and at the same time be compatible with privacy regulations, which is an essential aspect of global telemedicine and multinational clinical research.

7.5 Adaptive Regulations and Global Governance

Even in the case where AI technologies will evolve, legal systems which are fixed have an issue of keeping pace. The new generation types of governance should be dynamic in order to apply the process of continuous monitoring, ethical auditing and refinement of policies. Regulatory bodies (e.g. FDA, EMA and WHO) should collaborate on a global level to develop international harmonized AI safety and PHI protection practices.

The other field that the policymakers are considering is the AI ethics sandboxes-controlled test-grounds that the experiments could be conducted safely and under regulatory supervision. Those adaptive solutions will be in a position to ensure compliance does not limit innovation as the most appropriate data security and ethical responsibility practice is followed.

7.6 Clinical Empowerment and Human-Centered AI

Nevertheless, no matter how active the technological development can be, the human factor remains the necessary component of the ethical application of LLMs. The collaboration between AI and clinicians should be promoted by providing the professionals with new systems in the future without replacing them. The anthropocentric design puts emphasis on trust, openness, compassion and inclusiveness meaning technology is more of an assistant and not a master.

Clinician participation during design of AI, feedback and validation procedures will improve the accuracy of the model and its awareness of the situation. Also, sensitizing medical personnel on the importance of contesting AI proposals is an important strategy in ensuring ethical regulation is maintained at all clinical decision-making levels.

Figure 9. Roadmap for Secure and Ethical AI in Healthcare

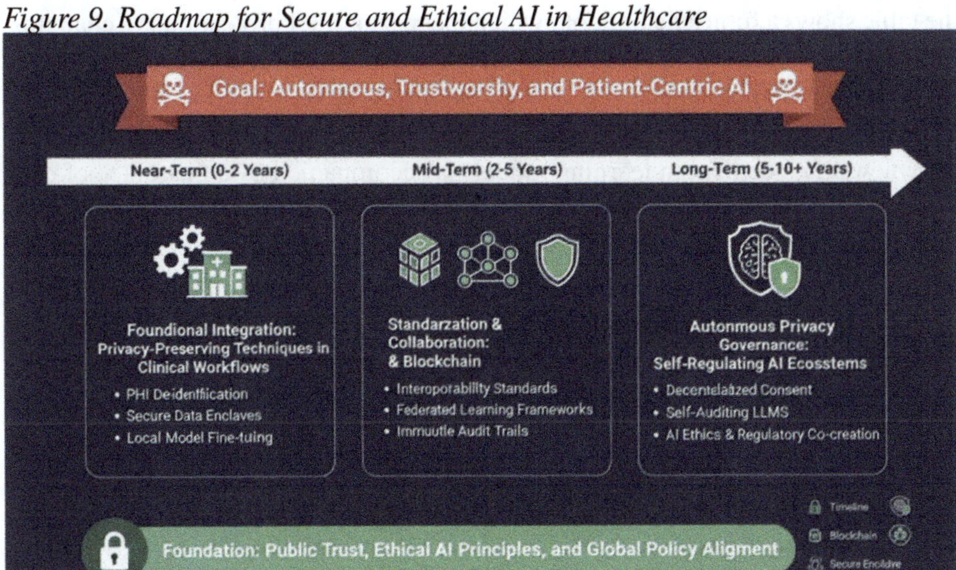

Figure 9 presents a visionary plan in respect of having secure, privacy-sensitive, and ethical AI systems in healthcare. The diagram incorporates the emerging technologies like federated architectures, explainable AI metrics, post-quantum cryptography, and automated ethical auditing tools. It graphically shows the development of basic privacy systems to adaptive governance and human-friendly AI systems, which supports the chapter focus of sustainable and responsible innovation.

Table 7. Future Research Directions

Focus Area	Research Goal	Emerging Technology	Expected Impact
Federated LLMs	Decentralized training	Edge-cloud synergy	Enhanced scalability
Differential Explainability	Privacy-preserving transparency	XAI metrics	Improved trust
Quantum Security	Post-quantum cryptography	Lattice encryption	Long-term resilience
Ethical Auditing	Automated AI compliance	AI Governance Tools	Regulatory assurance

Table 7 reveals the directions of research that have emerged to enhance the privacy and security in medical LLM settings. The topics like post-quantum cryptography, adaptive privacy budgeting, automated compliance monitoring, and federated auditing frameworks are also pointed out as the areas that are promising to explore further. The table shows a futuristic outlook, which means that PHI protection is a changing field that needs constant innovations to meet the demands of more advanced threats and regulatory standards.

Privacy-first innovation will transform the future oriented medical LLMs where every new advancement in learning models is accompanied by a guarantee of data safety, ethical considerations, and the reliability of patients. Some of the approaches that will transform the use and protection of health data are federated learning, synthetic data creation, blockchain incorporated, and explainable modeling. More to the point, the rules and humanist principles of AI will be implemented responsibly and make sure to ensure that these innovations are more responsible, and ultimately, the healthcare ecosystem will be intelligent, secure, and ethically focused.

8. CONCLUSION AND RECOMMENDATIONS

The introduction of Large Language Models (LLM) in the field of healthcare is a phenomenon that will leave a tremendous imprint in the history of medical intelligence. These models have enjoyed massive potential in the transformation of clinical practice, patient care, and decision-making in the diagnosis. However, this ground breaking power also brings with it extra responsibilities to patient data security, adherence to professional ethical and lawful requirements. Secrecy of Protected Health Information (PHI) is an engineering issue and ethical and legal mandate. The problem of privacy and security of the LLMs can therefore be seen as a value, and not a peripheral argument when creating medical AI.

Multi-layered defense Multi-layered defense system is necessary to train LLLMs on clinical data - secure architectures, encryption, peripheral privacy and federated learning systems. A long-term model of innovation in healthcare AI is privacy-conscious computation with ethical design, which can be used to propel the field of AI. Technical policies, such as synthetic data generation, blockchain-approach to managing health records, and explainable AI (XAI), can be implemented in a synergistic way as demonstrated in this chapter in order to ensure that the patient data remain confidential and that the models will continue learning.

Development of the system should be grounded on transparency, accountability and fairness ethically. It is the shared responsibility of the clinicians and researchers to ensure that AI systems are impartial, uphold human dignity and patient autonomy. Likewise, the regulating watchdogs must be dynamic to identify emerging problems and come up with international standards that are creative and accountable to the citizens. The most important in achieving this balance between policies, technologies, and medical staff keep the global system of governance coherent.

The future solution to the issue of achieving and ethical medical LLMs is through establishing a responsible culture of innovation. It can be recommended that hospitals and research centers invest in efficient models of data governance, ongoing training of employees on AI ethics, and independent supervision models. The developers should ensure that all the building blocks in the algorithms are privacy-by-design so that the compliance is put in place before the implementation is rolled out and not put in place subsequently. Educational programs can form clinician awareness to make sure that the interpretation of AI outputs is performed in a responsible manner to enhance human control in every decision loop.

Lastly, the correctness of LLams will not be the sole measure, which will determine the success of the given model in clinical practice but its reliability. The intelligent and the ethical systems capable of learning with sensitive information without any detrimental loss to the personal rights and security will result in actual progress in AI-related healthcare. Through proper privacy, legal and human values, the medical community is able to obtain the full potential of LLMs to create the future of technology that will reinforce care, improve safety, and make the sanctity of the patient trust secure.

Key Recommendations

- Use Privacy-by-Design: Incorporate privacy and security controls, e.g. anonymization, differential privacy, and encryption, in the earliest stages of designing and developing LLM.

- Adopt Federated and Secure Learning Model: Promote inter-institutional co-operation without the concentration of PHI, and the probability of data leakage is reduced.
- Assure Explainability: Integrate explainable models whereby the clinicians can interpret, challenge and confirm the AI recommendation before acting upon them.
- Develop Ethical Oversight Teams: Promote institutional protection through encouraging regulation and transparency in following the rules, assessing fairness, and bias in the algorithms.

Final Reflection

Deepen international collaboration in standardization of privacy and AI safety between international laws. Make AI Education Humane: Educate healthcare practitioners to be accountable to the use of AI, and preserve the human element of the ethical decision and analysis.

Promote Open Communication: It is crucial to ensure that patients understand the purpose of using their information to train AI models and they have the right to choose and opt out.

REFERENCES

Abbas, S. R., Abbas, Z., Zahir, A., & Lee, S. W. (2024). Federated learning in smart healthcare: A comprehensive review on privacy, security, and predictive analytics with IoT integration. *Healthcare (Basel), 12*(24), 2587. DOI: 10.3390/healthcare12242587

Alber, F.. (2023). Challenges of implementing LLMs in clinical practice: Perspectives. *Journal of Clinical Medicine, 14*(17), 6169. DOI: 10.3390/jcm14176169

Chen, L. (2024). Building trust and interpretability in medical AI through explainable models. *Journal of AI in Healthcare and Medicine, 4*(1).

Chen, L., & Lee, S. (2023). Large language model empowered privacy-protected framework for PHI annotation in clinical notes. *IOS Press.* https://pubmed.ncbi.nlm.nih.gov/40775983/

Dhade, P., & Shirke, P. (2023). Federated learning for healthcare: A comprehensive review. *Engineering Proceedings, 59*(1), 230. DOI: 10.3390/engproc2023059230

Islam, H.. (2024). Federated learning and distributed applications for electronic health records and structured medical data: A scoping review. *Journal of the American Medical Informatics Association : JAMIA, 30*(12), 2041–2049.

Johnson, D., Kumar, V., & Lee, S. (2022). Balancing innovation and patient data protection in healthcare AI. *IEEE Transactions on Medical Systems, 38*(4), 555–569.

Kumar, P., Adams, J., & Li, Y. (2024). Data anonymization and de-identification challenges in clinical NLP: A review. *Journal of Biomedical Informatics, 139*, 104–136.

Kumar, P., Li, Y., & Adams, J. (2023). Re-identification risks in clinical NLP models. *Frontiers in Artificial Intelligence, 6*(3), 1–9.

Li, H., Tan, M., & Chang, Y. (2024). Ethical frameworks for trustworthy medical AI. *Bioethics and Data Science Review, 12*(1), 33–47.

Li, S.. (2023). A review of privacy-enhancement methods for federated learning in healthcare systems. *International Journal of Environmental Research and Public Health, 20*(15), 6539. DOI: 10.3390/ijerph20156539

Li, S., & Paik, H. (2023). A systematic review of federated learning from clients' perspective: Challenges and solutions. *Artificial Intelligence Review, 56*(S2, Suppl 2), 1773–1827. DOI: 10.1007/s10462-023-10563-8

Odera, D. (2023). Federated learning and differential privacy in clinical health: Extensive survey. *World Journal of Advanced Engineering Technology and Sciences, 8*(02), 305–329. DOI: 10.30574/wjaets.2023.8.2.0113

Sharma, S., Zahir, A., & Lee, S. W. (2024). Trustworthy privacy-preserving hierarchical ensemble and federated learning in Healthcare 4.0 with blockchain. arXiv. https://arxiv.org/abs/2305.09209

Singh, P., & Rao, T. (2024). Blockchain as a privacy enabler in clinical AI systems. *International Journal of Digital Health*, *8*(1), 88–104.

Smith, R., O'Brien, J., & Patel, A. (2023). Data governance and patient rights under HIPAA and GDPR. *Health Policy and Research*, *19*(3), 144–160.

Teo, Z. L., Jin, L., Liu, N., Li, S., Miao, D., Zhang, X., Ng, W. Y., Tan, T. F., Lee, D. M., Chua, K. J., Heng, J., Liu, Y., & Goh, R. S. M. (2024). Federated machine learning in healthcare: A systematic review on clinical applications and technical architecture. *Cell Reports Medicine*, *5*(3), 101481. DOI: 10.1016/j.xcrm.2024.101481

Thrasher, J., Devkota, A., Siwakotai, P., Chivukula, R., Poudel, P., Hu, C., Bhattarai, B., & Gyawali, P. (2023). Multimodal federated learning in healthcare: A review. arXiv. https://arxiv.org/abs/2310.09650

UNESCO. (2024). *Ethics of Artificial Intelligence in Healthcare: Policy Guidance Report*. UNESCO Press.

Waheed, N., Ur Rehman, A., Nehra, A., Farooq, M., Tariq, N., Jan, M. A., Alalmaie, A. Z., & Nanda, P. (2023). FedBlockHealth: A synergistic approach to privacy and security in IoT-enabled healthcare through federated learning and blockchain. arXiv. https://arxiv.org/abs/2304.07668 DOI: 10.1109/GLOBECOM54140.2023.10437356

Wang, Q., Torres, L., & Chen, M. (2024). Explainable AI for clinical decision support: Current status and prospects. *Computers in Biology and Medicine*, *170*, 108–120.

World Health Organization. (2023). *Guidance on Ethics and Governance of Artificial Intelligence for Health*. World Health Organization.

Zanchi, M. G. (2024). Crafting the future of healthcare with LLMs. Medium. https://medium.com/ninacapital/crafting-the-future-of-healthcare-with-llms-01a3e6b92df9

Zanchi, M. G.. (2024). Generative AI in Medical Practice: In-Depth Exploration of Privacy and Security Challenges. *Journal of Medical Internet Research*, *26*, e53008. DOI: 10.2196/53008

Zhang, R., & Patel, N. (2025). Privacy-preserving LLMs in medicine: Trends and challenges. *AI in Healthcare Journal*, *9*(2), 102–119.

Zhen, J., & Gao, C. (2023). From challenges and pitfalls to recommendations and opportunities: Implementing federated learning in healthcare. *Journal of Healthcare Informatics Research.*

Zhou, C., Rahman, A., & Liu, D. (2024). Secure federated architectures for health data. *Journal of Medical AI Security*, *7*(1), 65–80.

Chapter 13
Cognitive Hazard Mapping:
A New Framework for Predicting and Preventing Unsafe Reasoning in Medical LLMs

Ravshan Sultanov
Termez University of Economics and Service, Termez, Uzbekistan

Aarthi Selvakumar
http://orcid.org/0009-0006-9064-2091
Marwadi University, Rajkot, India

S. Srinivasan
http://orcid.org/0009-0002-0179-9849
Graphic Era (Deemed to be) University, Dehradun, India

Ravikumar Natarajan
http://orcid.org/0009-0009-3705-1681
Marwadi University, Rajkot, India

Doniyor Umarov
Mamun University, Khiva, Uzbekistan

ABSTRACT

Medical LLMs are increasingly used for diagnosis support, triage, documentation, and patient interaction, yet traditional validation methods often fail to detect unsafe reasoning hidden behind fluent clinical language. This chapter introduces Cognitive Hazard Mapping, a framework designed to identify and prevent reasoning-level

DOI: 10.4018/979-8-3373-7862-6.ch013

risks such as diagnostic hallucination, premature closure, causal misalignment, and guideline divergence. By analyzing inference pathways, applying multi-layer checks, and integrating clinician review, the model uncovers subtle hazards that may lead to patient harm despite seemingly accurate outputs. The chapter presents a taxonomy of cognitive hazards, real-world case studies, and methods for monitoring, auditing, and aligning LLM behavior with regulatory expectations. Cognitive Hazard Mapping provides a foundation for safer, more transparent, and clinically trustworthy AI systems.

1. INTRODUCTION

The use of Large Language Models (LLM) in the healthcare sector has become popular, and already, the models are considered as effective diagnostic support, clinical documentation, triage support, patient communication and decision support devices. Such systems are marvellous in terms of language and inferences, but these applications present complex safety concerns that lie beyond the apparent accuracy. Medical decision-making should be a process that entails proper reasoning and alignment to clinical guidelines, hierarchies of evidence, and situational patient restrictions problems that may not be internalized by LLMs. This means that unsafe reasoning patterns may also be constituted turn out even where the outputs are both factually sound and linguistically coherent (Jiang et al., 2017). Such invisible mental traps may cause diagnoses that are incorrect, therapy recommendations that are not suitable, breached ethics, or guideline drift.

Traditional measures of evaluation like accuracy measure, hallucination, or ability to detect bias is inadequate to represent deep reasoning errors. Cognitive Hazard Mapping, in turn, suggests a systematic way of investigating how medical LLMs think unsafely and then making forecasts. The framework will determine interpretable, proactive and clinically aligned safety paradigm by detecting latent inference patterns that are clinically risky (Mehandru et al., 2024). This introduction explains why this new area is important and explains why reasoning-level safety is a fundamental demand to next-generation medical AI governance. As much as the introduction presents the emerging use of medical LLMs and the dangers of unsafe medicine, it is also necessary to place such issues in a wider context of the development of clinical AI safety research. The development of past safety frameworks can give the clue of how the drawbacks exist in present times and encourage the necessity of the reasoning-level analysis schemes like Cognitive Hazard Mapping. Thus, in the sections below, the historical evolution of AI safety in clinical setting will be reviewed and the major gaps in the area that support the proposed framework will be outlined.

1.1 Rise Of Medical LLMs

Due to the possibility to synthesize medical information, medical LLDs are becoming an increasing part of clinical ecosystems. Radiology reporting systems, Electronic Health Record (EHR) summarization tools, patient-facing chatbots, and telemedicine triage assistants, and solutions based on clinical decision support now include these models. With their high level of flexibility, they are able to derive symptoms, give different diagnoses, access clinical guidelines and generate structured documentation in seconds, which can be of significant benefit in terms of efficiency and accessibility (Moëll, Farestam, et al., 2025). Multimodal LLMs that have been advanced to the next level extend these features in that images, lab values, free-text notes, are processed concurrently. This has led to more hospitals, AI vendors and regulators to consider more widespread use of medical LLMs. However, this fast spread to practical application processes has surpassed the development of sound reasoning-level safety structures. Even though LLMs are pattern recognition experts in big data, their internal inference mechanisms are probabilistic and opaque, and prone to minor yet clinically relevant violations of medical standards (Abd-Alrazaq et al., 2023). The importance of critical evaluation of not only the output of the LLM but also the manner in which they build clinical reasoning becomes more critical with the increase in usage to provide patient safety.

1.2 Causes Of Unsafe Reasoning In Medical LLMs

Large-scale generative models have structural and data-related constraints that lead to unsafe reasoning in medical LLMs. Statistical pattern matching of LLMs as compared to mechanistic clinical reasoning makes them occasionally produce outputs that are credible, even when they are in general conflict with accepted guidelines or pathophysiological reasoning. The training datasets also have inconsistencies, outdated information, bias, and non-clinical language, which together predisposes internal representations of the model. Reasoning failures are further enhanced by domain shift, in which models get to work with unfamiliar populations, rare conditions or atypical presentations. Also, LLM does not have the ability to access dynamic clinical scenarios including patient history changes, longitudinal symptoms, drug interactions, and multi-morbidity profiles in real-time. The failure to establish causality, temporal evolution, or the strength of evidence cause their errors to include premature completion of diagnostic diagnoses, wrongful risk classification, imagined test results, or fabricated evidence courses (Ai/ML Enthusiast et al., 2025). Unsafe inferences can give an answer that appears to be right hence it is difficult to demonstrate. The stochastic quality of output generation is used to make small immediate adjustments to produce clinically divergent advice which proves reasoning paths to be unstable. All these structural vices make it important to emphasize the urgency to perform specific consideration of cognitive risks rather than using superficial performance indicators.

1.3 Need For Cognitive Hazard Mapping

Expansive evaluation measures (fact accuracy test, benchmark testing, and hallucination detection) are more output-focused since they do not question the reason processes on which a clinical recommendation is formed. These methods do not fit in high stakes environments as unsafe reasoning can be hidden even in cases where the outcomes of its use appear satisfactory. Cognitive Hazard Mapping brings about a systematic system of establishing, labeling, and predicting thinking-based risks within LLM outputs. The pattern of the systematic identification, such as diagnostic hallucination, guideline divergence, incomplete differentiation of reasoning or ethically inappropriate suggestions are identified in a systematic way with the use of the methodology where reasoning failures are considered cognitive hazards. This framework assists in the pro-active risk assessment by examining an inference process rather than individual responses so that clinicians and safety auditors can observe the latent failure modes. Furthermore, regulators are increasingly requiring transparent and auditable reasoning methods as AI governance within such programs as the FDA Good Machine Learning Practices (GMLP), the EU AI Act, and the WHO standards of trustworthy AI (Macmillan-Scott & Musolesi, 2024). Cognitive Hazard Mapping complies with these expectations through providing traceability, interpretability, and continuous monitoring. Finally, it offers a fundamental basis to warrant that the medical LLM should improve clinical decision-making and not create new safety weaknesses.

2. BACKGROUND TO THE STUDY

Cognitive hazards study in medical LLMs is based on the larger history of clinical AI safety studies, which conventionally have focused on quantifiable performance metrics, including accuracy, sensitivity, specificity, and bias measures. Although these indicators are useful, they are not the complete measure of clinical decision-making, in which the quality of reasoning and adherence to the evidence-based guidelines are essential. The growing complexity and independence of LLMs require a change in approach by moving past the analysis of model outputs to analyzing the way models make clinical inferences (Chow & Li, 2025). Previous studies on the science of diagnostic errors, human factors engineering and medical cognition prove that clinical errors are often caused by defective reasoning, and not knowledge deficiency.

Medical LLMs are not immune to such weaknesses, since they are based on reasoning patterns using large and imperfect datasets. With the integration of AI into healthcare infrastructure, regulators, healthcare practitioners, and patient safety all need to characterize and avoid failures on reasoning levels to maintain regulatory control, clinician acceptance, and patient safety (Han et al., 2024). This contextualizes Cognitive Hazard Mapping as a well-timed and needed medical AI safety development further than the traditional performance analysis to a richer, mechanistic appreciation of the many ways in which clinical reasoning is formed in AI systems. Despite the achievements that have been made in assessing AI in healthcare, the existing methods of validation are not enough to determine the risks of medical LLM on the reasoning level. Thus, the following section introduces the research goals that the Cognitive Hazard Mapping framework would be developed based on.

2.1 Clinical AI Safety Evolution

Clinical AI safety has also experienced a shift in the last ten years, moving beyond algorithm-specific evaluation to a larger evaluation of workflow integration, ethical adherence, and reliability of the system broadly. The early computer-aided diagnostic systems were mostly concerned with the static statistical models with safety analysis being based on the representativeness of the dataset and model calibration. When deep learning emerged, some new issues of opacities, adversarial vulnerability, and bias in datasets were raised, which prompted the invention of fairness audit, robustness verification, and post-hoc explainability methods. Newer and more complicated problems arise with the emergence of the use of generative AI and LLMs because they have an open-ended output space and can produce in-depth clinical narratives. Reasoning quality is a key safety issue, unlike traditional predictive models which can only generate recommendations, interpret symptoms, and suggest management plans (Diao et al., 2025). The regulatory agencies have countered it by stressing on transparency, interpretability, and human sensitivity in AI systems. However, current models do not consider the internal inferential processes that are specific to LLMs comprehensively. This development shows that it is necessary to consider methods that explicitly analyze the risk pathways of cognition, which makes Cognitive Hazard Mapping the next step in terms of clinical AI safety assessment. The figure 1 represents the gradual change in the clinical AI safety, starting with the initial model calibration and bias issues to the sophisticated sets of AI-guaranteed reasoning-level controls provided by Cognitive Hazard Mapping.

Figure 1. Evolution of Clinical AI Safety Frameworks

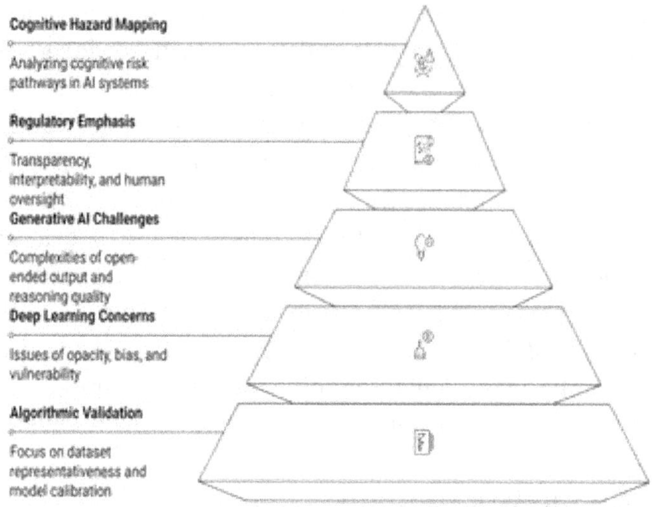

2.2 Gaps In Current Validation Approaches

The existing techniques of medical AI systems validation mainly test the correctness, reliability, and fairness of such systems, but does not explore the logic structures, which produce clinical advice. The benchmark tests, clinical vignettes and Hallucination measurements only reflect superficial performance, not how the reasoning of a model is consistent with clinical reasoning, evidence hierarchies, and patient safety principles. This loophole is especially dangerous to LLMs since they are capable of generating authoritative, consistent explanations that hide fallacious and unsafe reasoning. In addition, most validation processes rely on predetermined datasets that do not suit the dynamism and contextual nature of clinical interactions (Belkhouribchia and Pen, 2025). They do not make use of adversarial cases, variations in symptoms development over time, multi- morbidity interactions or counterfactual reasoning conditions all of which are needed to determine the caliber of the reasoning. Another weakness, which is also the lack of Instruments to separate small factual mistakes with more core risks of premature conclusion or misperception of risk factors, is also present. Unless auditors of safety check the internal inference paths, they have no way of determining whether model output results are founded on sound reasoning or an educated guess. These gaps demonstrate the necessity of a method that would consider reasoning structure and not result only, which justifies the significance of Cognitive Hazard Mapping.

2.3 Importance Of Reasoning-Level Safety

Evidence-based, consistent, and transparent reasoning is essential to the whole process of clinical decision-making. Unsafe reasoning even when using final recommendations that seem right can result in contraindications being ignored, improper sequence of treatment, or risk stratification. To avoid unsafe clinical judgment and ensure adherence to clinical logic, it is necessary to ensure reasoning-level safety. One should not monitor accuracy to guard against latent risks, particularly at boundary cases or uncommon situations, or ambiguous cases (Abikenari et al., 2025). With LLMs, thinking patterns are stimulated based on statistical associations and not on mechanistic medical knowledge, which exposes one to hazardous conclusions that sound plausible. Safety on the reasoning level, in turn, is necessary in a way that is not only aimed at avoiding harm but also will promote trust between clinicians, regulatory authorities, and healthcare providers. It facilitates risk identification in advance of deployment and other post-integration real workflows. Moreover, as the AI regulations continue to focus more on explainability, accountability, and auditability, models should be able to prove the consistency of their processes of inference with the accepted medical standards. It turns out to be a basic part of responsible development, implementation, and regulation of medical AI (Ravikumar, Aarthi, Olimbaevich, et al., 2025).

3. RESEARCH OBJECTIVES

This chapter hopes to develop a strict structure of the interpretation and control of unsafe thinking by medical LLMs. Traditional assessment is more concerned with the accuracy of output, whereas emerging clinical risks are associated with other pathways of inference that are more hidden and need to be systematically studied. The research objectives hence stress the identification, mapping, and control of cognitive hazards, which will see medical LLMs run transparently, reliably and clinically aligned in various healthcare functions.

- To identify and characterize cognitive hazards that arise from unsafe or clinically inconsistent reasoning patterns in medical LLMs.
- To develop a structured Cognitive Hazard Mapping framework capable of detecting, predicting, and categorizing reasoning-level risks.

- To analyze the inferential pathways of medical LLMs using multi-layer evaluation techniques such as counterfactual testing, uncertainty analysis, and logic consistency checks.
- To integrate clinician and auditor expertise into a human-in-the-loop assessment model, enhancing interpretability and real-world clinical applicability.
- To support clinical governance, auditing, and regulatory compliance by providing a traceable, explainable system for continuous monitoring of LLM reasoning safety.

4. CONCEPTUAL MODEL

Cognitive Hazard Mapping introduces a theoretical framework in which the root cause of unsafe medical reasoning in medical LLMs and the methodical identification, categorization and removal of such cases is possible. It is composed of multiple layers of analysis, which trace the inference paths of the model, reconcile them with clinical reasoning and graphical possibilities of breaking, which may lead to patient harm. The model notes that non-factual cognitive hazard are not limited to the errors in factual nature but encompass some of the subtle reasoning errors such as incomplete differential diagnosis, causal misalignment, time errors, guideline deviation and inappropriate order of therapeutic interventions. By using the visual representation of these hazards in the form of interconnected nodes of a clinical risk flow, the model illustrates how a small mistake during inference can cause severe clinical outcomes (Reddy et al., 2024). This structure also implicates medical LLM reasoning within a broader framework of decision-making within which the human clinicians, auditors, and safety engineers interact with the system.

Cognitive Hazard Mapping therefore plays a mediatory role between computation inference pattern as well as clinical anticipation of the prediction so as to detect reasoning weaknesses before they take place within the patient care setting. This theory is used in the medical applications to explain, control, and ensure constant safety during its application. Figure 2 presents the fundamental elements of the Cognitive Hazard Mapping model, where detection, categorization, explainability, mitigation, compliance and the ongoing monitoring collaborate with one another to establish a safe LLM reasoning in clinical practice. Although the development of the conceptual model describes the conceptual framework of Cognitive Hazard Mapping, its practical application needs a strict methodological framework that will be able to assess the processes of LLM reasoning in a variety of clinical situations. The following section thus outlines the research methodology with which the conceptual model is operationalized and the reasoning level risks are assessed systematically.

Figure 2. Cognitive Hazard Mapping Conceptual Model

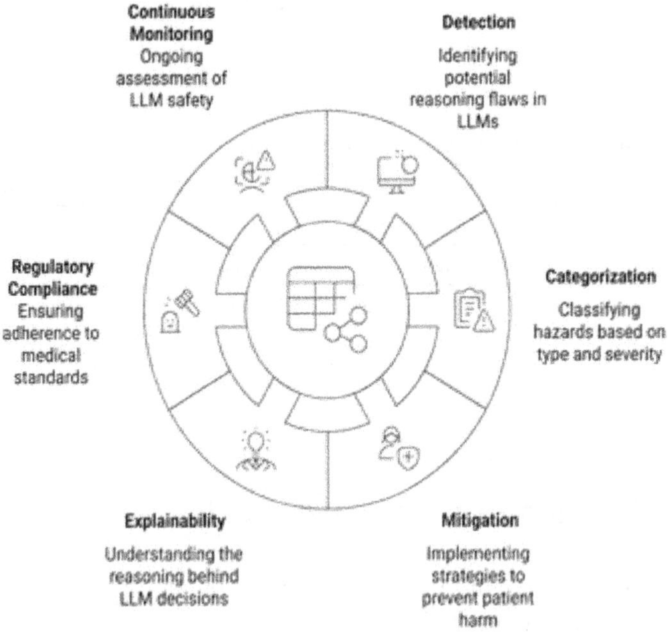

4.1 Components Of Cognitive Hazard Mapping

Cognitive Hazard Mapping model is developed on the basis of three major components namely inference pathway analysis, hazard detection mechanism, and risk mapping structure. Inference pathway analysis is a method that studies the derivation of the medical conclusion by the LLM, by tracking the sequence of reasoning in between, and determining whether the internal transitions of the model is based on logical, evidence-based clinical norms. The mechanism of hazard detection is performed at various levels such as factual verification, structural reasoning evaluation and guideline conformity checks (Wu et al., 2019). The patterns that are detected by these mechanisms include diagnostic overconfidence, premature closure, overlook of crucial red flags, or unsuitable escalation of therapy. Risk mapping formats transform the identified hazards into visual or table formats that demonstrate where failure can occur and how the failure can affect the clinical result. The relationships between reasoning errors and downstream risks are identified in this mapping to help clinicians and auditors to recognize how minor interpretations lapses can result in unsafe recommendations. However, when combined together, these elements form a powerful analytical mechanism that can be used to discover the latent cognitive structure underlying the outputs of the LLM and convert opaque logic into clinical governance-relevant, actionable information. Table 1 indicates the elementary components of the CHM framework.

Table 1. Components Of Cognitive Hazard Mapping

Component	Function	Outcome
Inference Pathway Analysis	Traces how LLM forms reasoning	Reveals hidden logic steps
Hazard Detection Layer	Identifies unsafe reasoning patterns	Flags risk points
Risk Mapping Structure	Visualizes hazard flow	Supports clear interpretation
Human Expert Review	Clinicians audit reasoning steps	Ensures clinical validity
Guideline Consistency Check	Compares output with standards	Detects divergence

4.2 Hazard Categories & Clinical Risk Flow

Medical LLM cognitive hazards (can be structured into categories that represent various types of unsafe reasoning). They are diagnostic hallucination, incomplete differential construction, rule divergence, therapeutic divergence, fabricated chains of evidence, temporal inconsistency, loss of context when providing longitudinal care. The categories themselves are indicative of a failure regarding a particular aspect of clinical reasoning so that it can be granularly classified and mitigated accordingly. Clinical risk flow is a description of the spread of these hazards through a series of decisions. As an illustration, a misunderstood symptom can cause a wrong diagnosis route, which in turn will translate into the wrong suggestion of tests, wrong treatment schedule or missing contraindications (Chen et al., 2024). Through the modeling of this flow, hazard mapping shows how clinical risks are increased in the downstream due to early reasoning errors. Also highlighted in the clinical risk flow are dependency among reasoning steps: an error in assessment of causality can lead to the misjudging of risk stratification, and misunderstanding of time can nullify follow-up recommendations. This systematic categorization and flow modeling allows evaluators to not only spot individual reasoning problems but also patterns which are systemic and which pose a risk to patient safety. Basic overview of significant medical cognitive pitfalls in medical LLMs. The following table 2 is an overview of the significant types of cognitive hazards that can arise during medical LLM reasoning and describes their definitions and the clinical risks of each type of error in reasoning.

Table 2. Cognitive Hazards Overview

Hazard Type	Meaning	Possible Clinical Risk
Diagnostic Hallucination	Model invents findings not in input	Wrong diagnosis or unnecessary tests
Guideline Divergence	Not following clinical protocols	Unsafe or incorrect treatment
Premature Closure	Stops reasoning too early	Missed critical differentials
Temporal Error	Misreads timing of symptoms	Incorrect risk assessment
Causal Misalignment	Wrong cause–effect logic	Faulty medical explanation
Context Loss	Forgets key patient details	Inconsistent recommendations

4.3 LLM Reasoning Process Vs. Clinical Pathways

The difference between the process of LLP and clinical pathways lies within the core of the reasoning, thus, harmonization between the two to ensure safety is critical. Clinical pathways are designed patterns that are based on evidence-based guidelines, risk levels, causal factors, and patient-related variables. Conversely, the thinking of LLM is speculative and motivated by statistical trends in training data as opposed to mechanical knowledge. The difference between this gives a chance of reasoning drift, in which the model can make plausible but clinically invalid suggestions. The gap between cognitive hazards and the pathways proposed by the LLM is filled by Cognitive Hazard Mapping which compares the inferred pathway to the expected clinical pathway of the recommendation made by the LLM. This comparison will demonstrate whether the model takes into account the key risk factors, has rational decision sequences, and complies with conventional care protocols (Cabral et al., 2024). Misalignment can be observed through the lack of diagnostic steps, incorrect prioritization of therapeutic steps, or sequencing of interventions. The awareness of these divergences allows the auditors to be aware of the safety of the internal logic of the model. This process creates a break between computational inference and clinical reasoning to justify that the results of the LLM are accurate but founded on rational and clinically consistent reasoning.

5. RESEARCH METHODOLOGY

The Cognitive Hazard Mapping is a methodology of research computational analysis of unsafe reasoning patterns in medical LLMs, which is clinically validated and reviewed by humans. It involves a multi-layered approach which begins with the systematic elucidation of the inference pathways through systematic discussion by use of structured prompts, clinical vignettes and variants of synthetic cases. To determine these outputs, the evaluation of their outputs is conducted in accordance with the analytical mechanisms such as uncertainty quantification, counterfactual testing, adversarial prompting and guideline consistency checking in order to identify the latent reasoning defects. The domain experts the clinicians, safety auditors and AI governance specialists are also integrated in the methodology as they check the clinical consistency and potential risks of each pattern of reasoning. They summarize what they observe into a hazard mapping framework that is illustrative of the risk flow and logic deviation (Berry et al., 2025). The methodological framework helps in the pre-deployment model audits and the ongoing real-world application whereby the model behavior and safety limits can undergo the refinement on an iterative basis. This ambivalent governance approach ensures that the identification of risks is grounded on computational knowledge besides clinical knowledge and a reasonable foundation of the level of safety of medical LLM. The methodology framework offers means to assess medical LLM reasoning safety. The subsequent section summarizes the literature available on the errors in reasoning, safety measures, and shortcomings in the current LLM assessment methods.

5.1 Multi-Layer Reasoning Evaluation

Multi-layer reasoning evaluation is the correlation of the evaluation mechanism of Cognitive Hazard Mapping. It evaluates the reasoning of the LLM on a variety of levels: surface output accuracy, structural coherence and alignment to guidelines, causal logic integrity and sequencing of clinical decisions. This is initiated by the production of responses in a variety of clinical situations, such as typical cases, unusual situations, high-risk presentation, and uncertain symptoms. The responses undergo a breakdown into steps of reasoning to find out whether the model is pursuing the right diagnostic and therapeutic directions. Coherence checks Structural A structural coherence checks determine the logical soundness of reasoning transitions, whereas guideline coherence checks determine compliance with evidence-based standards of medicine (Beidas et al., 2019). The evaluation of causal logic identifies whether the model has a correct comprehension of relationships among the symptoms, diseases, and the interventions or not. Lastly, sequencing analysis is done to determine whether prescribed measures go according to clinically anticipated orders. The multi-layered test reveals both blatant and hidden reasoning errors, which allow a systematic build of the types of cognitive hazard. The methodology offers more information on the reliability of LLDs in a wide range of clinical conditions through the assessment of reasoning, not only the results. Table 3 Displays layers involved in analysis of LLM reasoning.

Table 3. Multi-Layer Reasoning Evaluation Criteria

Evaluation Layer	What It Checks	Why It Is Important
Surface Accuracy	Basic correctness	Ensures factual validity
Structural Logic	Coherence of reasoning	Detects reasoning gaps
Clinical Guideline Match	Alignment with protocols	Ensures safe care
Causal Reasoning	Cause–effect logic	Prevents unsafe assumptions
Differential Completeness	Coverage of possibilities	Avoids missed diagnoses

5.2 Tools: Uncertainty, Counterfactuals, Adversarial Inputs

A collection of computing software complements hazard identification through stress-testing the reasoning of the LLM stability and soundness. Uncertainty quantification measures the level of confidence in the recommendations made by the model, to detect cases of high-confidence but erroneous thinking, which would carry a high clinical risk. Counterfactual testing looks at the responses to changes in the reasoning of a model when minor, clinically significant alterations are made to the input, e.g. symptom onset, severity, or patient demographics. This shows whether the model is updating its inferential pathway in a correct way using new evidence or not. Adversarial prompting: This method actively resistantly prompts on purpose; its aim is to uncover boundary failures, e.g. misguided symptom descriptions, incomplete histories, or conflicting clinical hints (Kim et al., 2023). All these assist in showing the reasoning drift, instability, and inconsistency and signal the situations under which the model may be hallucinating, ignoring the guidelines, or misinterpreting the clinical scenario. The combination of that will offer full evaluation of their reasoning power in real and stressful circumstances.

5.3 Human Expert Review Process

The human expert review is an important component of the hazard mapping method which provides the clinical expertise which is not captured in computer tools. The expert reviewers assess the reasoning steps in the LLM to establish whether the reasoning steps are consistent with medical guidelines, diagnostic heuristics that are identified and safe therapeutic practices. Clinicians consider logical consistency, red flags existence, correctness of risk stratification, and the fact that risk stratification considers the specifics of a patient. The compliance with the regulatory requirements and documentation principles and ethical demands are examined by safety auditors. In their checks, their observation is of minor such risks, such as an inappropriate tone of voice when reaching out to the patients, morally doubtful recommendations, or a violation of the clinical standards that are difficult to uncover using algorithms (Sorich et al., 2024). The review process also includes consensus scoring where there is a decision of two or three experts on the same pattern of reasoning so that bias is reduced, and reliability is improved. The clinical judgment is actually a component of the framework as the knowledge is entered into the hazard map by the human reviewers. It can be enhanced by such combination of human expertise to provide a better level of interpretability, which can be enhanced by a better degree of regulatory compliance and a tool that can be credibly used with medical LLMs.

6. LITERATURE REVIEW

The rapid implementation of Large Language Models (LLMs) in clinical practice has also resulted in a wealth of research in the area of the accuracy, robustness, fairness, and explainability of models. However, the new literature also identifies the fact that the majority of the performance appraisals fail to give the sufficient attention to the deeper meaning of the model results. Medical decision-making is a multifaceted phenomenon, which entails rational sequence, adherence to guidelines, cause-and-effect logic, and an interpretation of the patient (Banyi et al., 2025). With the rise of the use of LLMs in diagnosis, triage, and therapeutic advice, it is important to comprehend how they make their reasoning decisions. The current literature demonstrates that such models often produce clinically plausible yet slightly flawed reasoning schemes, which indicate some weaknesses in current safety paradigms. This review summarizes the existing data on reasoning errors in LLMs, assesses safety methods that have been developed to address those errors, and pinpoints some of the limitations that have remained in the process of detecting latent cognitive risks.

6.1 Reasoning Errors In LLMs

According to the recent studies, it is easy to find that the LLM may make errors not only due to the fact that they are unable to find the information but also due to the failures of reasoning. These fallacies are of diverse types. Diagnostic hallucination is an occurrence in which the model releases the signs, symptoms, or test results that are not present in the input. The human diagnosis error of premature closure is also replicated in the LLMs that cease at a diagnosis but without differentials. Experts who published their studies as late as 20232024 show that the generated differential diagnoses by LLM could overlook significant and uncommon conditions or high-risk possibilities, especially in obscure presentations. The other notable failure is causal misalignment in which the model confounds correlation with causation hence risk is estimated in an unrealistic manner (Rahav Koren et al., 2017). Also, there exist temporal reasoning errors, such as the fallacious repetitive reading of symptom onset sequences, the failure to update reasoning under longitudinal context. Moreover, LLMs are prone to domain shift: they give their outputs, which relies on statistical biases in the training data, which is not representative of the clinical reasoning. Studies on emergency medicine and cancer research, and studies on critical care, note that models sometimes generate pedagogical yet artificial links of evidence, and give an impression of correct reasoning and hides unreasonable thinking. These findings imply that the errors arising as a result of reasoning is systemic and could not be addressed adequately by the conventional measures of performance.

6.2 Existing Safety Techniques

A number of initiatives to enhance safety and reliability in LLM-based clinical uses have been designed. One of the earliest approaches is guardrail prompting and instruction tuning, which is aimed at containing the medical responses that are considered appropriate. Although such means minimise open hallucinations, they do not adequately inhibit inner reasoning mechanisms. The fact-checking systems such as the Retrieval-Augmented Generation (RAG) can assist with grounding the output on the known trusted clinical sources but fail in cases where inference or interpretation of the input requires multiple steps or is outside the scope of the retrieved information (Woo et al., 2025). Explainability algorithms, including chain-of-thought prompting or attribution heatmap, give partial explanations of the logic of models, yet recent studies caution that even chain-of-thought-generated explanations by LLMs may be hallucinatory. Other safety levels such as uncertainty estimation methods such as confidence scoring and probability calibration can be used to indicate high-risk outputs. In the meantime, other alignment methods, such as Human-Feedback-Reinforcement Learning (RLHF) can mitigate harmful behavior but cannot ensure transparency in reasoning. Regulation programs including the FDA Good Machine Learning Practices, as well as EU AI act, promote continued monitoring, documentation and risk management, but do not yet specify how reasoning-level verification should be done. Even though such approaches are useful as guardrails, they are generally focused on the rightness of output or surface behavior, and not on deep inferential structure.

6.3 Limitations In Detecting Hidden Hazards

Although some progress has been made, the state of the art of contemporary safety mechanisms are not able to detect and avert hidden cognitive risks hidden sources of reasoning error that can lead to dangerous clinical inferences even in cases where surface-level products are coherent and true to fact. Some of the shortcomings include the overuse of benchmark-style-testing which is analysis of performance in a relatively nonclinical dataset, and does not reflect the real clinical complexity. This kind of tests fails to detect the reasoning drift where the models fail to follow the logic, with which they are expected to act in uncertain or adversarial circumstances. The existing tools are not analyzed much to identify the presence of the intermediate reasoning steps that correspond to the clinical pathway that leads to the incompleteness of the error detection, such as omission of diagnostic steps or misleading associations of the symptoms. Although useful, explainability methods tend to generate narratives that are biased by the model as opposed to underlying internal reasoning (Kleebayoon & Wiwanitkit, 2024). Also, most safety frameworks do not include longitudinal assessment mechanisms, which makes it challenging to identify hazards, which arise during multi-step interactions or patient follow-up sequences. The fact that reasoning errors are not taxonomized has also a counter of systematic hazard detection. Finally, the use of the human expert review is seldom used systematically to the existing assessment pipelines, and it introduces clinical interpretability gaps. These limitations explain the need of Cognitive Hazard Mapping a paradigm where the reasoning strategies are evaluated, the latent risks identified and resolved to match the model predictions and clinical reasoning.

7. CASE STUDY SECTION

Experiments in the real world with medical LLM show that errors at the reasoning level can still be concealed by well-sounding clinical language and pose a threat when it is not explicitly measured through conventional accuracy-based evaluation. Case studies give a practical understanding of the appearance of cognitive hazards in the daily operations of a medical facility and how unsafe reasoning turned out to be detrimental in a real-life context. The cases below consider the 2024-2025 cases and discuss examples of LLM behavior in the high-stakes clinical settings of oncology and emergency medicine and their critical aspects of diagnostic accuracy and guideline compliance (Dinc et al., 2025). All of the cases reveal a unique type of hazard, such as diagnostic hallucination, unfinished differentials, and a guideline divergence. These cases illustrate the extent to which simple reasoning can be derailed by revealing the extent to which any form of reasoning may lead to a recommendation that is clinically unsafe. The combination of the two gives empirical support to the Cognitive Hazard Mapping model and accentuates the importance of active-level safety measures concerning the reasoning on a case-by-case basis in a variety of medical settings. The case studies are the real-life examples of how the unsafe reasoning patterns may affect clinical decision-making. Based on these observations, the next section of this paper discusses the findings made by Cognitive

Hazard Mapping, and how they can be used to enhance safety, transparency and trust in medical LLM systems.

7.1 Case Study A: Oncology Report Misinterpretation (2024–2025)

In 2024, a major hospital system tested a system that used LLM to assist clinicians in the oncology department by giving an initial version of the radiology report about the potential presence of lung cancer. In one of the cases, a patient with a 2.3 cm pulmonary nodule, CT was performed and a summary created by the LLM that revealed that the lesion has irregular borders that point to early metastasis. The radiology report given at the beginning only said that there was mild lobulation at the margins and none of the invasion. The reference to metastasis in the hallucinated LLM was a result of reasoning drift in the training of the model associated with statistical correlation between phrases containing nodules and phrases containing the metastasis (Benary et al., 2023). The model wrongly made its conclusions, which were allegedly based on anatomical considerations of metastatic behavior.

Closer analysis of its reasoning chain revealed several cognitive hazards:

- Diagnostic Hallucination – inventing clinical features absent from the source report.
- Premature Closure – failing to consider alternative benign explanations such as granuloma or post-inflammatory scarring.
- Guideline Divergence – skipping the recommended Fleischner Society risk stratification steps.

The incorrect conclusion had an effect on downstream recommendations: the LLM has recommended some urgency in PET-CT and oncology referral, but in reality, there was no such urgency. A reviewing clinician was able to identify the mistake before escalation was prevented unnecessarily. The Cognitive Hazard Mapping indicated that the LLM was grossly dependent on linguistic trends more than organised radiologic guidelines, and that it was important to adhere to the directives of guided inference and cross-validation mechanisms when processing high-risk oncology data. The Figure 3 shows how an LLM generated hallucination in an oncology report is uncovered and fixed during a clinician review and Cognitive Hazard Mapping.

Figure 3. Oncology Case Study Workflow

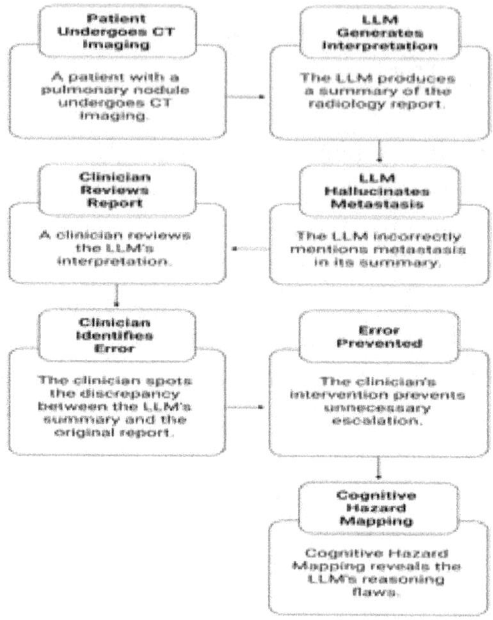

7.2 Case Study B: Emergency Medicine – Wrong Differential Diagnosis (2024–2025)

An LLM was applied in a trial, in which the triage notes were pre-generated with preliminary differential diagnoses in an emergency department in 2025. The patient introduced himself with acute chest pains, dizziness, and sweat, which may be signs of potentially fatal heart diseases. The LLM produced a different list with panic attack, dehydration, and musculoskeletal strain having the highest priority, with Acute Coronary Syndrome (ACS) being the fourth option. This prioritization contradicted emergency medicine practice in which it is assumed to have ACS unless it is clearly excluded. An audit on the reasoning showed a number of cognitive hazards. To start with, it was observed that the model contributed to the loss of context, i.e. the symptoms were considered in isolation, as opposed to the identification of the high-risk cluster that is characteristic of cardiac emergencies (Wang et al., 2024). Second, failure at temporal reasoning happened when it disregarded the fact that the patient described the onset of pain when he exercised, in a great deal, a red flag of ischemic pathology. Third, there was the causal misalignment whereby the model focused more on stress related etiologies because of the over representative of the same cases in the data.

The discrepancy was reported by the triage nurse, and the further examination revealed ST-Elevation Myocardial Infarction (STEMI). Without the review of the differential provided by the LLM, the patient would have experienced a lot of delay before getting life-saving intervention. Cognitive Hazard Mapping found that the inference process of the LLM did not account for key decision rules, such as, heuristics of HEART score and risk pathways of chest-pain (Savage et al., 2024). The case shows that there is a risk of relying on LLMs in high stakes situations without reasoning level precautions in place and that more systematic hazard analysis can be valuable when deploying emergency medicine systems. The figure 4 demonstrates that erroneous LLM-generated differential diagnosis of a case of chest-pain is detected, fixed, and processed by Cognitive Hazard Mapping to avoid clinical risks in the future.

Figure 4. Emergency Medicine Differential Diagnosis Error Workflow

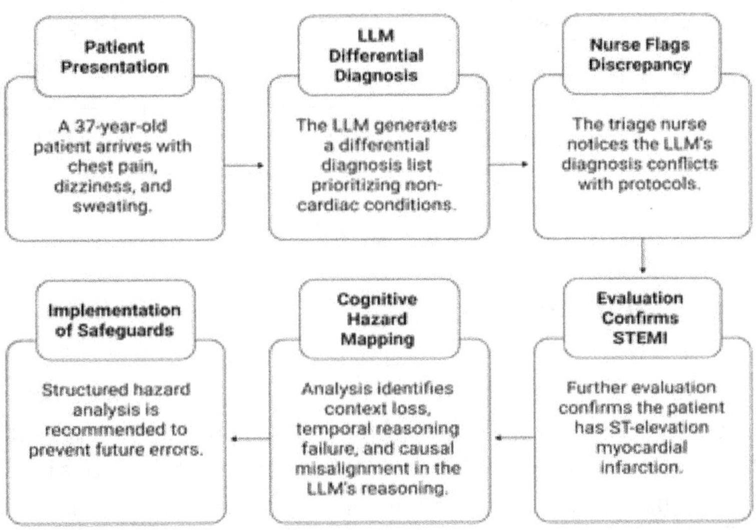

7.3 Key Lessons And Hazard Patterns

The two case studies have identified common recurring hazard patterns that cannot be detected by the traditional accuracy metrics. Although the two cases show that LLMs can generate logic that is coherent yet clinically unsafe in instances where probabilistic associations have overridden logic guided by guidelines. Hazards that were observed were diagnostic hallucination, premature closure, omission of high-risk differentials, loss of time, and loss of context. They also demonstrate that minor mistakes in reasoning can be spread into damaging suggestions, and that organised inference pathway audits are required, as opposed to evaluation of results as an end (Gao et al., 2025). Notably, human supervision was very important in intervening with dangerous reasoning. Combined, these examples prove that Cognitive Hazard Mapping is necessary to detect latent risks, enhance system transparency, and make safe the application of LLMs in different clinical processes. Table 4 Hazards in Case Study A and B Summarised.

Table 4. Hazards Identified in Case Studies (A & B)

Case Study	Main Hazard	Simple Explanation	Clinical Impact
Oncology Misinterpretation	Diagnostic Hallucination	Added metastasis not in report	Unnecessary tests/ referral
Oncology Misinterpretation	Guideline Divergence	Skipped Fleischner steps	Incorrect risk stratification
Emergency Medicine	Context Loss	Ignored symptom cluster	Missed high-risk ACS
Emergency Medicine	Temporal Error	Ignored exertion onset	Incorrect severity judgment
Emergency Medicine	Causal Misalignment	Prioritized stress factors	Delayed lifesaving treatment

8. RESULTS / DISCUSSION

The application of the Cognitive Hazard Mapping framework demonstrated reasonable results in regards to the procedure undertaken in the behavior of medical LLMs as far as their reasoning in relation to different clinical situations is concerned. As the findings indicate, inferential pathway analysis establishes latent mode of thinking that would have otherwise been identified by the more classical metrics of accuracy or rates of hallucinations. The recurrent patterns on hazard maps were seen as over-simplification of diagnosis, misplaced emphasis on risk and use of statistically significant but irrelevant association clinically. Instead of the original understanding and the recommendations to be done in future, the visualization of these risks gave one a better comprehension of how mistakes spread. Moreover, human expert inspection helped to make the distributions of hazards more accessible, which underpinned the role of clinicians in AI validation (van Nuland et al., 2024).

The discussion reveals that systematic mapping may also be employed to enhance model auditing, help to discover unsafe reasoning patterns at an earlier stage and contribute to more transparent AI governance. Finally, one may also integrate hazard knowledge with regulative systems and this fact proves that Cognitive Hazard Mapping can also serve as the foundation allowing implementing medical LLM in a more secure and consistent manner. Although the findings support the usefulness of Cognitive Hazard Mapping as a tool to detect risks at the reasoning level, the current technological and business regulatory trends imply that there are a number of areas, where future research can be conducted. The following section discusses possible research directions in the future to increase predictive safety measures and continuous monitoring capacities.

8.1 Cognitive Hazard Maps And Risk Visualization

Cognitive hazard maps encode the patterns of complicated reasoning into a visual format comprehensible to people that highlights where and how unsafe reasoning occurs. The maps illustrate the inference pathways, decision nodes, and hazard cluster using graphical illustrations that are easy to interpret by the clinicians and auditors. Hazard maps can be used to trace the flow of reasoning of a model to identify abnormalities in a set of clinical pathways the model should follow, like omitted diagnostic processes, misplaced causal hypotheses, or unsuitable order of therapy. Interactions among hazards are also visualized, that is, how premature closure can interact with incomplete construction of the difference to arrive at unsafe recommendations (Cantini et al., 2025). This kind of clarity enables the stakeholders to identify areas of failure in a short time, and put in place specific mitigation strategies. Moreover, the hazard maps allow making comparative analyses between various models, versions or clinical domains, and benchmarking this systematic comparisons. Such a visual solution would not only make the interpretation process more intuitive but also more trustworthy as the black box reasoning process would be more transparent to the health care professionals, safety auditors, and regulators.

8.2 Improvement In Safety, Accuracy, And Trust

Cognitive Hazard Mapping has a quantifiable beneficial safety, accuracy, and trust in medical LLM systems. Refining model behaviour, retraining on particular failure modes, and incorporating corrective guardrails can be used by organizations to identify latent reasoning errors before deployment and thus improve them. This will decrease the prevalence of high-risk hallucinations, increase the completeness of diagnostics, and increase compliance with clinical guidelines. Also, hazard mapping improves accuracy, not by emphasizing on the accuracy of the output, but the accuracy of the reasoning process. The more logical and clinically based the reasoning becomes, the more confident the users are in the system. A potential obstacle to AI implementation, clinician trust, is more likely to grow as models provide evidence of a traceable logic and predictable behavior when subjected to different clinical circumstances (Frutuoso, 2025). In addition, the hazard-intelligence can be used to create automated risk-scoring devices that indicate potentially unsafe outputs in real time. In general, Cognitive Hazard Mapping leads to a better, more credible, and clinically agreeable AI ecosystem. Table 5 illustrates that Cognitive Hazard Mapping enhances the means of detecting hazards of reasoning by examining inference pathways other than output correctness.

Table 5. Hazard Detection Improvement with CHM

Evaluation Method	Hazards Detected	Detection Rate (%)	Reasoning-Level Errors Identified	Safety Interpretation
Traditional Output-Based Evaluation (Accuracy / Hallucination Checks)	11	48%	Limited detection of reasoning errors	Many hidden reasoning hazards remain undetected
Explainability-Based Evaluation (Chain-of-Thought / Attribution)	14	61%	Partial identification of reasoning inconsistencies	Some reasoning errors detected but not systematically classified
Cognitive Hazard Mapping (CHM Framework)	19	83%	Comprehensive detection of reasoning hazards including hallucination, guideline divergence, and temporal errors	Significantly improved reasoning-level safety analysis

8.3 Alignment With FDA, EU AI ACT, WHO

Medical AI systems transparency, auditability, and safety are receiving increasing attention by the regulation agencies. One theory that is conforming to the international regulatory standards is Cognitive Hazard Mapping whose capacity to offer the formalized account of the thinking process and well-known risk areas. The FDA Good Machine Learning Practices (GMLP) require continuous monitoring, human factor, and rigorous pre-deployment analysis, which is caused by hazard mapping processes. The EU AI act holds that high-risk AI systems ought to be evaluated concerning risk, the documentation of decisions logic as well as explainability; in absence of hazard visualization and reasoning analysis, all these considerations are enabled (Clusmann et al., 2023). The WHO guidelines on credible AI state that the safety assurance, clinical relevance, and mitigation of bias must be provided, and they can be operationalized with the help of the framework, demonstrating unsafe forms of inferences. Cognitive Hazard Mapping has the benefit of increasing compliance, enabling audit trails and enabling transparent reporting between developers and hospitals and regulators, through demonstrating reasoning-level safety (Ravikumar, Aarthi, Atamuratova, et al., 2025). It is due to this fit that the framework is a powerful tool to pursue the new world guidelines in medical AI governance. Table 6 Shows the backing of CHM to regulatory compliance.

Table 6. Regulatory Alignment Overview

Regulatory Body	Key Requirement	How CHM Helps
FDA (GMLP)	Transparency & continuous monitoring	Provides mapped reasoning pathways
EU AI Act	High-risk AI documentation	Hazard maps serve as audit evidence
WHO	Trustworthy & safe AI	Identifies unsafe reasoning early
National Health Agencies	Clinical validation	Enables structured clinician review

9. FUTURE RESEARCH

The prospects in future research reposition Cognitive Hazard Mapping to forecasting as well as automated surveillance and open-source logic frameworks. Although the existing implementations are centered around the idea of post-hoc analysis of reasoning errors, future approaches can potentially be used to identify the risks and avert them prior to affecting the results in the outputs. Further modeling methods may also include machine learning methods that forecast dangerous lines of thought in response to initial indicators of inference. Also, embracing the framework to the continuous monitoring systems would aid in real-time evaluation of implemented LLMs in dynamic clinical conditions. This especially matters towards the domain shift, workload variability, and medical evidence development. Future reasoning safety might further need stronger interconnection with interpretable modeling systems, such as hybrid symbolic-neural systems, which encode clinical logic in model reasoning (Pashangpour & Nejat, 2024). The research should also focus on scalability to make sure that hazard analysis can be used with large-scale deployments of hospitals. Finally, the future developments will aid in designing the LLM systems that not only will be safe but also inherently based on the clinical cognition and ethical medical practice. The developments in predictive hazard systems and monitoring will determine the use and regulation of AI in healthcare organizations.

As a result, one should convert these findings of research to pragmatic recommendations to the stakeholders tasked with the deployment of the medical AI systems.

9.1 Cognitive Hazard Prediction Models

Cognitive hazard prediction models are a logical development of the existing hazard mapping methodology since they allow proactive instead of reactive safety assurance. Rather than detecting hazards when reasoning has already been performed, predictive models examine signals of early-stage inference, e.g. token-level uncertainty behaviors or anomalous reasoning behaviors or deviations of clinical logic, to predict whether the end-result will contain a hazard. Annotated Hazard Corpora and training Machine learning algorithms used to train machine learning encompass sequence modeling, anomaly detectors and meta-reasoning classifiers can be trained on annotated hazard corpora obtained by previous audits (Tan et al., 2025). Such predictive systems could in turn produce real time warnings or impose safe-guarded intervention routes in case dangerous patterns of reasoning are found. The combination of prediction models and clinical decision support systems would provide timely clinician supervision, decrease the latency of identifying risks, and avoid high-impact errors prior to their entry into clinical processes (Ravikumar & Aarthi, 2025). This orientation is a great boost to the preventability of medical AI safety frameworks.

9.2 Live Monitoring And Safety Pipelines

Cognitive Hazard Mapping is operational on Live monitoring systems. The performance of the models is monitored through such systems and in case of abnormal output trends, the systems apply measures of safety when they are applied in real time. The pipelines monitors may also contain automatic scoring of risk, checks of compliance and drift capabilities that detects the change of reasoning behavior over time. Such systems are particularly sensitive to clinical settings, where the demographics of incoming patients, strange manifestation of rare diseases and new evidence may alter the behavior of the model without any prior warning. Live monitoring ensures that risks that are introduced by domain shift, model aging or system updates are monitored in good time (Botross et al., 2024). In addition, automated audit logs can also log logic records, flagged hazards and clinician overrides to enable regulatory compliance, and post incident review. With the inclusion of real-time monitoring and hospital IT infrastructure, one has the chance of having a more resilient and adaptable AI ecosystem that could assist in saving lives of the patients throughout the life cycle of the model. The Figure 5 shows the monitoring workflow diagram that is constantly being used to monitor the behavior of the model, identify drift, enforce safety checks, and ensure that the performance of the deployed medical LLM systems is guided by guidelines.

Figure 5. Continuous Monitoring Pipeline for Medical LLM Safety

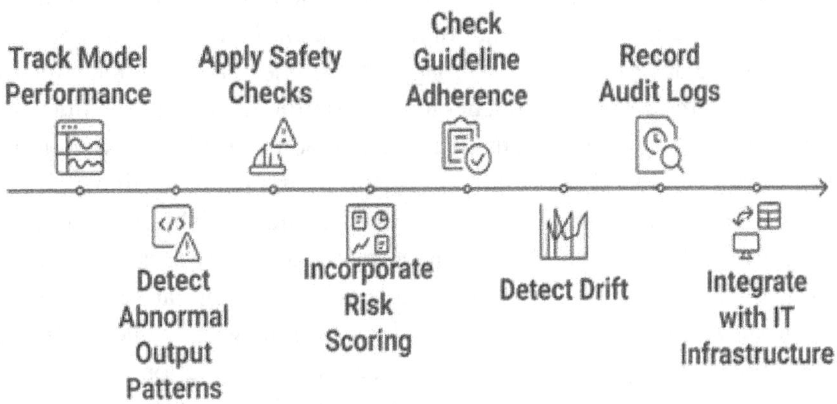

9.3 FULLY TRANSPARENT REASONING SYSTEMS

One of the long-term research objectives is creation of AI systems which are able to produce fully transparent reasoning, that is, internal inference paths can be explained, clinically explained and consistent with medical logic. The neural LLM architectures can be used to implement the transparent reasoning systems that can be integrated with the symbolic reasoning modules, clinical guideline engines or structured knowledge graphs that provide logical consistency. This combination method decreases the use of probabilistic association and encourages the use of proven medical pathways (Moëll, Sand Aronsson, et al., 2025). Also, transparent systems can have self-verification techniques, like automatic consistency checking, causal reasoning modules or explicit differential diagnosis generators, which enable the models to test the quality of their own reasoning. Full transparency can also help in achieving the results of clinician trust, compliance, and ethical governance (Ravikumar, et al., 2025). These developments would technically be difficult, but they would turn LLMs into scorecards rather than probabilistic text generators, making them useful clinical decision makers.

10. MANAGERIAL IMPLICATIONS

The managerial implications of Cognitive Hazard Mapping of the implementation of medical LLM by hospitals, developers, and regulatory bodies are grave and should be implemented in a responsible way. In the example of hospitals, the framework would help to introduce AI tools in the clinical workflow safer, not only in terms of visibility of the quality of reasoning but also through the passage of targeted oversight controls. To developers, hazard mapping provides practical understanding of the weaknesses of the models and encourages continuous periods of improvement in line with regulatory requirements. Regulatory bodies find it convenient to have systematic evidence to aid in compliance testing, post-market testing, and incident testing (Leypold et al., 2024). The managers of any industry should understand that reasoning-level safety cannot be guaranteed by the accuracy measures only, as the constant audits, training of employees, and government-regulating procedures are crucial. Organizations can create trusted AI ecosystems with the help of Cognitive Hazard Mapping through the embedded procurement, validation, and deployment processes, which improve patient care without creating systemic risk. The managerial lessons offered in the above sections indicate the practical significance of reasoning-level safety to hospitals, developers and regulators. The final part of the chapter is a summary of the main findings of the chapter and a reflection on the general implications of Cognitive Hazard Mapping of integrating large language models into the healthcare sector safely. Table 7 Provides useful recommendations to hospitals, developers and regulators.

Table 7. Managerial Implications Across Stakeholders

Stakeholder	Responsibility	Benefit of CHM
Hospitals	Ensure safe AI adoption	Detect unsafe outputs early
Developers	Improve model reasoning	Identify failure patterns
Regulators	Enforce safety standards	Use hazard maps for audits
Clinicians	Review AI decisions	Gain transparent insights
IT Governance Teams	Monitor AI tools	Maintain ongoing compliance

10.1 Implications For Hospitals

Hospitals are strained to use AI tools and ensure safety of patients, efficiency of employees, as well as regulation. The Cognitive Hazard Mapping is beneficial to the hospital administrators in the sense that the logic of action of the deployed

LLMs can be clearly seen. This eases the process of undertaking informed decisions during procurement and evaluation, which implies that hospitals can decide the models that can align with the hospital policies of internal safety. During deployment, hazard mapping can be utilized to inform triage plans, escalation plans and clinician management plans (Krishna & Gupta, 2025). It is also good in reducing the risks where the high-risk output is present in real-time and the frontline staff is not overworked. In addition, the knowledge of the hazards can be applied to develop certain training programs in which clinicians are trained to have a critical approach towards the reactions created by AI. The concept of hazard analysis as an inbuilt element into the structures of managing hospitals is effective in enhancing accountability, building trust in clinicians, and tackling the safety of patients in different departments.

10.2 Implications For Developers

To AI developers, Cognitive Hazard Mapping provides a systematic way of enhancing the robustness of a model, its interpretability and regulatory preparedness. It allows developers to detect patterns of recurrent failures and focus their attention on model retraining of clinically significant hazards. Through reasoning deviations, developers are able to optimize model architecture, selection of training data and alignment strategies to achieve safer outputs. The communication with clinical partners is also made easier through the use of hazard mapping that gives interpretation evidence of model behavior (van Tongeren et al., 2020). Hazard insights can be applied by developers to develop automated safety layers, chain-of-thought verification modules and enhance uncertainty calibration. Also, the framework enhances adherence to new rules whereby risk mitigation, decision-making, and constant monitoring must be documented. In general, Cognitive Hazard Mapping can be used to help build clinically viable and governance-ready AI systems.

10.3 Implications For Regulators

Regulators are progressively putting pressure on stringent evidence of safety, transparency, and accountability of medical AI. Cognitive Hazard Mapping offers a framework through which it is possible to assess risks of reasoning level, which enables a regulator to determine whether an LLM acts in a manner that reflects clinical practice and ethics. Hazard maps can be used to provide auditable records of inference pathways, used to support compliance reviews to approve, to support post-marketing surveillance and adverse event investigation. They also enable compliance with the world regulatory standards, such as FDA, EU AI act, and WHO guidelines (Warraich et al., 2025). By asking developers to submit hazard analyses, the regulators can make them implement proactive safety measures as opposed to the use of output-based measures. Hazard mapping, therefore, allows oversight to be more sophisticated facilitating responsible innovation and protecting the health of the population.

11. CONCLUSION

The conceptual framework is Cognitive Hazard Mapping (CHM), which aims to detect, examine, and remove the unsafe reasoning behaviors of medical Large Language Models (LLMs). Current AI assessment methods in the medical field mostly concentrate on the accuracy of outputs and identifying hallucinations, but they are not very effective to evaluate reasoning-level weaknesses that might result in unsafe clinical guidelines. The discussion identifies that reasoning errors, including diagnostic hallucination, guideline divergence, temporal misinterpretation, and causal misalignment may be a serious clinical risk despite their seeming sense of coherence and plausibility in their model outputs. CHM fills this gap with a systematic approach to identifying the presence of hidden reasoning errors with the help of hazard identification, analysis of inference pathways, and visual risk mapping. The framework assists in making medical AI systems more transparent and systematically evaluated by examining the way in which recommendations are produced as opposed to the final result alone.

The methodology combines several methods of analysis such as multi-layer reasoning evaluation, adversarial testing, uncertainty quantification, and human expert review, establishing an overall auditing process as a distribution between the analysis of computation and clinical expertise. This makes it easier to interpret, increases clinician confidence and promotes regulatory compliance because opaque model reasoning is converted into interpretable clinical knowledge. Moreover, CHM can help to create safer AI governance processes, as it allows to perform continuous monitoring and organized hazard analysis in healthcare settings. Further studies are necessary in the area of large-scale empirical validation, the creation of computer-based algorithms of hazard-detection systems, and the incorporation of real-time monitoring pipelines into hospital systems. Since LLMs are still being incorporated into diagnostic support, triage, medical documentation, and communication with the patient, the integrity and transparency of their reasoning processes will become more and more important. Therefore, Cognitive Hazard Mapping is an important step towards the realization of credible, interpretable, and clinically compatible AI systems in contemporary healthcare.

REFERENCES

Abd-Alrazaq, A., AlSaad, R., Alhuwail, D., Ahmed, A., Healy, P. M., Latifi, S., Aziz, S., Damseh, R., Alabed Alrazak, S., & Sheikh, J. (2023). Large language models in medical education: Opportunities, challenges, and future directions. *JMIR Medical Education, 9*, e48291. DOI: 10.2196/48291 PMID: 37261894

Abikenari, M., Awad, M. H., Korouri, S., Mohseni, K., Abikenari, D., Freichel, R., Mukadam, Y., Tanzim, U., Habib, A., & Kerwan, A. (2025). *Reframing clinical AI evaluation in the era of generative models: Toward multidimensional, stakeholder-informed, and safety-centric frameworks for real-world health care deployment.* Premier Journal of Science., DOI: 10.70389/PJS.100089

Ai/ML Enthusiast, U. S. A., Sivalingam, E., & Chinnachamy, T. (2025a). Explainable GENAI techniques to interpret and visualize LLM reasoning. INTERNATIONAL JOURNAL OF SCIENTIFIC RESEARCH IN ENGINEERING AND MANAGEMENT, 09(10), 1–9. https://doi.org/DOI: 10.55041/IJSREM53123

Banyi, N., Ma, B., Amanian, A., Bur, A., & Abdalkhani, A. (2025). Applications of natural language processing in otolaryngology: A scoping review. *The Laryngoscope, 135*(9), 3049–3063. DOI: 10.1002/lary.32198 PMID: 40309961

Beidas, R. S., Volpp, K. G., Buttenheim, A. N., Marcus, S. C., Olfson, M., Pellecchia, M., Stewart, R. E., Williams, N. J., Becker-Haimes, E. M., Candon, M., Cidav, Z., Fishman, J., Lieberman, A., Zentgraf, K., & Mandell, D. (2019). Transforming mental health delivery through behavioral economics and implementation science: Protocol for three exploratory projects. *JMIR Research Protocols, 8*(2), e12121. DOI: 10.2196/12121 PMID: 30747719

Belkhouribchia, J., & Pen, J. J. (2025). Large language models in clinical nutrition: An overview of its applications, capabilities, limitations, and potential future prospects. *Frontiers in Nutrition, 12*(1635682), 1635682. DOI: 10.3389/fnut.2025.1635682 PMID: 40851903

Benary, M., Wang, X. D., Schmidt, M., Soll, D., Hilfenhaus, G., Nassir, M., Sigler, C., Knödler, M., Keller, U., Beule, D., Keilholz, U., Leser, U., & Rieke, D. T. (2023). Leveraging large language models for decision support in personalized oncology. *JAMA Network Open, 6*(11), e2343689. DOI: 10.1001/jamanetworkopen.2023.43689 PMID: 37976064

Berry, P., Dhanakshirur, R. R., & Khanna, S. (2025). Utilizing large language models for gastroenterology research: A conceptual framework. *Therapeutic Advances in Gastroenterology, 18*, 17562848251328576. DOI: 10.1177/17562848251328577 PMID: 40171241

Botross, M., Mohammadi, S. O., Montgomery, K., & Crawford, C. (2024). Performance of Google's artificial intelligence chatbot "Bard" (now "Gemini") on ophthalmology board exam practice questions. *Cureus, 16*(3), e57348. DOI: 10.7759/cureus.57348 PMID: 38690460

Cabral, S., Restrepo, D., Kanjee, Z., Wilson, P., Crowe, B., Abdulnour, R.-E., & Rodman, A. (2024). Clinical reasoning of a generative artificial intelligence model compared with physicians. *JAMA Internal Medicine, 184*(5), 581–583. DOI: 10.1001/jamainternmed.2024.0295 PMID: 38557971

Chen, D., Huang, R. S., Jomy, J., Wong, P., Yan, M., Croke, J., Tong, D., Hope, A., Eng, L., & Raman, S. (2024). Performance of multimodal artificial intelligence chatbots evaluated on clinical oncology cases. *JAMA Network Open, 7*(10), e2437711. DOI: 10.1001/jamanetworkopen.2024.37711 PMID: 39441598

Chow, J. C. L., & Li, K. (2025). Large language models in medical chatbots: Opportunities, challenges, and the need to address AI risks. *Information (Basel), 16*(7), 549. DOI: 10.3390/info16070549

Clusmann, J., Kolbinger, F. R., Muti, H. S., Carrero, Z. I., Eckardt, J.-N., Laleh, N. G., Löffler, C. M. L., Schwarzkopf, S.-C., Unger, M., Veldhuizen, G. P., Wagner, S. J., & Kather, J. N. (2023). The future landscape of large language models in medicine. *Communications Medicine, 3*(1), 141. DOI: 10.1038/s43856-023-00370-1 PMID: 37816837

Diao, M., Li, R., Liu, S., Liao, G., Wang, J., Cai, X., & Xu, W. (2025). SEAS: Self-Evolving Adversarial Safety optimization for Large Language Models. Proceedings of the ... AAAI Conference on Artificial Intelligence. AAAI Conference on Artificial Intelligence, 39(22), 23778–23786. DOI: 10.1609/aaai.v39i22.34549

Dinc, M. T., Bardak, A. E., Bahar, F., & Noronha, C. (2025). Comparative analysis of large language models in clinical diagnosis: Performance evaluation across common and complex medical cases. *JAMIA Open, 8*(3), ooaf055. Advance online publication. DOI: 10.1093/jamiaopen/ooaf055 PMID: 40510808

Frutuoso, J. (2025). Building a safe and transparent workflow for large language model (LLM)-assisted clinical trials and prediction models: A technical report. *Cureus, 17*(9), e92571. DOI: 10.7759/cureus.92571 PMID: 41111869

Gao, Y., Li, R., Croxford, E., Caskey, J., Patterson, B. W., Churpek, M., Miller, T., Dligach, D., & Afshar, M. (2025). Leveraging medical knowledge graphs into large language models for diagnosis prediction: Design and application study. *JMIR AI*, *4*, e58670. DOI: 10.2196/58670 PMID: 39993309

Han, T., Adams, L. C., Bressem, K. K., Busch, F., Nebelung, S., & Truhn, D. (2024). Comparative analysis of multimodal large language model performance on clinical vignette questions. *Journal of the American Medical Association*, *331*(15), 1320–1321. DOI: 10.1001/jama.2023.27861 PMID: 38497956

Jiang, F., Jiang, Y., Zhi, H., Dong, Y., Li, H., Ma, S., Wang, Y., Dong, Q., Shen, H., & Wang, Y. (2017). Artificial intelligence in healthcare: Past, present and future. *Stroke and Vascular Neurology*, *2*(4), 230–243. DOI: 10.1136/svn-2017-000101 PMID: 29507784

Kim, M., Sohn, H., Choi, S., & Kim, S. (2023). Requirements for trustworthy artificial intelligence and its application in healthcare. *Healthcare Informatics Research*, *29*(4), 315–322. DOI: 10.4258/hir.2023.29.4.315 PMID: 37964453

Kleebayoon, A., & Wiwanitkit, V. (2024). Re: Investigating the impact of innovative AI chatbot on post-pandemic medical education and clinical assistance: a comprehensive analysis. *ANZ Journal of Surgery*, *94*(3), 492. DOI: 10.1111/ans.18717 PMID: 37749857

Krishna, A., & Gupta, M. (2025). Next-gen 3rd party cybersecurity risk management practices. In Advancing IT Audits Through Integrative Approaches and Emerging Technologies (pp. 1–30). IGI Global Scientific Publishing. DOI: 10.4018/979-8-3373-3078-5.ch001

Leypold, T., Lingens, L. F., Beier, J. P., & Boos, A. M. (2024). Integrating AI in lipedema management: Assessing the efficacy of GPT-4 as a consultation assistant. *Life (Basel, Switzerland)*, *14*(5), 646. DOI: 10.3390/life14050646 PMID: 38792666

Macmillan-Scott, O., & Musolesi, M. (2024). (Ir)rationality and cognitive biases in large language models. *Royal Society Open Science*, *11*(6), 240255. DOI: 10.1098/rsos.240255 PMID: 39100158

Mehandru, N., Miao, B. Y., Almaraz, E. R., Sushil, M., Butte, A. J., & Alaa, A. (2024). Evaluating large language models as agents in the clinic. *NPJ Digital Medicine*, *7*(1), 84. DOI: 10.1038/s41746-024-01083-y PMID: 38570554

Moëll, B., Farestam, F., & Beskow, J. (2025). Swedish Medical LLM Benchmark: Development and evaluation of a framework for assessing large language models in the Swedish medical domain. *Frontiers in Artificial Intelligence*, *8*(1557920), 1557920. DOI: 10.3389/frai.2025.1557920 PMID: 40718621

Moëll, B., Sand Aronsson, F., & Akbar, S. (2025). Medical reasoning in LLMs: An in-depth analysis of DeepSeek R1. *Frontiers in Artificial Intelligence*, *8*, 1616145. DOI: 10.3389/frai.2025.1616145 PMID: 40607450

Pashangpour, S., & Nejat, G. (2024). The future of intelligent healthcare: A systematic analysis and discussion on the integration and impact of robots using large language models for healthcare. *Robotics (Basel, Switzerland)*, *13*(8), 112. DOI: 10.3390/robotics13080112

Rahav Koren, R., Suriu, C., Yakir, O., Akria, L., Barhoum, M., & Braester, A. (2017). Physicians' lack of knowledge - a possible reason for red blood cell transfusion overuse? *Israel Journal of Health Policy Research*, *6*(1), 49. Advance online publication. DOI: 10.1186/s13584-017-0173-0 PMID: 29228989

Ravikumar, A. Olimbaevich, I. R., Mashkhura, S., & Musayeva, S. (2025). Transforming Healthcare with Large Language Models and AI agents. In Advances in Computational Intelligence and Robotics (pp. 51–82). IGI Global Scientific Publishing. DOI: 10.4018/979-8-3373-2008-3.ch003

Ravikumar, A. S., Atamuratova, Z., Ashirova, A., Jurayev, K., & Hayitova, M. (2025). Comprehensive evaluation of AI-driven systems in modern hospital environments. In Advances in Computational Intelligence and Robotics (pp. 61–88). IGI Global Scientific Publishing. DOI: 10.4018/979-8-3373-2787-7.ch003

Ravikumar, R. S., Manujakshi, Aarthi, S., Urazbaeva, Y., & Tamilselvi, S. (2025). Navigating data privacy, security, and regulatory challenges in healthcare AI ensuring fairness, bias mitigation, interpretability, and trust. In Transformative Role of Transformer Models in Healthcare (pp. 25–54). IGI Global Scientific Publishing. DOI: 10.4018/979-8-3373-2038-0.ch002

Ravikumar, R. N., & Aarthi, S. (2025). AI-powered synergistic robotics and IoT ecosystems for predictive and preventive healthcare. In *Robotics and IoT Synergy in Next-Generation Healthcare* (pp. 1–32). IGI Global Scientific Publishing., DOI: 10.4018/979-8-3373-5447-7.ch001

Reddy, S., Lebrun, A., Chee, A., & Kalogeropoulos, D. (2024). Discussing the role of explainable AI and evaluation frameworks for safe and effective integration of large language models in healthcare. *Telehealth and Medicine Today*, *9*(2). Advance online publication. DOI: 10.30953/thmt.v9.485

Savage, T., Nayak, A., Gallo, R., Rangan, E., & Chen, J. H. (2024). Diagnostic reasoning prompts reveal the potential for large language model interpretability in medicine. *NPJ Digital Medicine*, *7*(1), 20. DOI: 10.1038/s41746-024-01010-1 PMID: 38267608

Sorich, M. J., Menz, B. D., & Hopkins, A. M. (2024). Quality and safety of artificial intelligence generated health information. *BMJ (Clinical Research Ed.)*, *384*, q596. DOI: 10.1136/bmj.q596 PMID: 38508683

Tan, T. F., Thirunavukarasu, A. J., Quek, C., & Ting, D. S. W. (2025). Evaluation of ophthalmic large language models: Quantitative vs. qualitative methods. *Current Opinion in Ophthalmology*, *36*(6), 466–471. DOI: 10.1097/ICU.0000000000001171 PMID: 40910897

van Nuland, M., Lobbezoo, A.-F. H., van de Garde, E. M. W., Herbrink, M., van Heijl, I., Bognàr, T., Houwen, J. P. A., Dekens, M., Wannet, D., Egberts, T., & van der Linden, P. D. (2024). Assessing accuracy of ChatGPT in response to questions from day to day pharmaceutical care in hospitals. *Exploratory Research in Clinical and Social Pharmacy*, *15*(100464), 100464. DOI: 10.1016/j.rcsop.2024.100464 PMID: 39050145

van Tongeren, J. M. Z., Harkes-Idzinga, S. F., van der Sijs, H., Atiqi, R., van den Bemt, B. J. F., Draijer, L. W., Hiel, D., Kerremans, A., Kremers, B., de Leeuw, M., Olthoff, M. V., Pham, T. K.-L., Valentijn-Robertz, R., Tsoi, K., Wichers, I., de Wit, M., & Borgsteede, S. D. (2020). The development of practice recommendations for drug-disease interactions by literature review and expert opinion. *Frontiers in Pharmacology*, *11*, 707. DOI: 10.3389/fphar.2020.00707 PMID: 32499701

Wang, H., Gao, C., Dantona, C., Hull, B., & Sun, J. (2024). DRG-LLaMA : Tuning LLaMA model to predict diagnosis-related group for hospitalized patients. *NPJ Digital Medicine*, *7*(1), 16. DOI: 10.1038/s41746-023-00989-3 PMID: 38253711

Warraich, H. J., Tazbaz, T., & Califf, R. M. (2025). FDA perspective on the regulation of artificial intelligence in health care and biomedicine. *Journal of the American Medical Association*, *333*(3), 241–247. DOI: 10.1001/jama.2024.21451 PMID: 39405330

Woo, B. F. Y., Song, J., Middleton, E., Fijačko, N., & Cato, K. (2025). Teaching critical thinking in the age of AI: Safeguarding clinical reasoning in healthcare documentation. *International Nursing Review*, *72*(3), e70102. DOI: 10.1111/inr.70102 PMID: 40845221

Wu, X., Huang, Y., Liu, Z., Lai, W., Long, E., Zhang, K., Jiang, J., Lin, D., Chen, K., Yu, T., Wu, D., Li, C., Chen, Y., Zou, M., Chen, C., Zhu, Y., Guo, C., Zhang, X., Wang, R., & Lin, H. (2019). Universal artificial intelligence platform for collaborative management of cataracts. *The British Journal of Ophthalmology*, *103*(11), 1553–1560. DOI: 10.1136/bjophthalmol-2019-314729 PMID: 31481392

KEY TERMS AND DEFINITIONS

Adversarial Prompting: Inputs designed to intentionally test LLM robustness and expose hidden weaknesses.

Causal Misalignment: Incorrect interpretation of cause-and-effect relationships in clinical reasoning.

Cognitive Hazard: A hidden reasoning error in an LLM that appears logical but can lead to unsafe clinical decisions.

Context Loss: Failure of the model to maintain or use key patient information across multi-step interactions.

Counterfactual Testing: Evaluating model reasoning by slightly changing input details to observe response shifts.

Diagnostic Hallucination: The model invents symptoms, findings, or diagnoses that were not provided in the input.

Guideline Divergence: When the LLM's recommendations deviate from established clinical guidelines or protocols.

Hazard Map: A visual representation of reasoning errors and their potential clinical impacts.

Human-in-the-Loop Review: Clinicians and experts reviewing model reasoning to ensure safety and correctness.

Premature Closure: The model settles on one diagnosis too early without evaluating full differentials.

Reasoning Drift: Gradual deviation of the model's reasoning from expected clinical logic under different conditions.

Regulatory Alignment: Ensuring AI behavior complies with standards such as FDA GMLP, EU AI Act, and WHO guidance.

Risk Flow: The path through which a small reasoning error grows into a clinically harmful recommendation.

Temporal Reasoning Error: Misunderstanding or ignoring the order, timing, or progression of symptoms or events.

Uncertainty Quantification: Methods to measure how confident the model is in its outputs.

Chapter 14
Safety Assurance Through Red-Teaming, MLOps, and Continuous Monitoring for Medical LLMs

Adarsh Kumar Pandey
http://orcid.org/0009-0002-1364-6903
Poornima University, India

Sakshi Sharma
http://orcid.org/0000-0002-7754-7974
Poornima University, India

Rocky Kumar
http://orcid.org/0009-0002-6995-2037
Poornima University, India

Gaurav Kumar
http://orcid.org/0009-0004-6126-8526
Poornima University, India

ABSTRACT

The rapid introduction of Large Language Models (LLMs) into clinical practice offers both opportunities and threats that require the use of stringent evaluation, governance, and management, and constant control. In this chapter, the relationships between red-teaming and MLOps practices and pervasive monitoring of models get researchers closer to all the key building blocks of the safety, reliability, and

DOI: 10.4018/979-8-3373-7862-6.ch014

compliance with regulations of medical LLM in practical healthcare facilities. Even before clinical implementation, red-teaming has probably been identified as a pre-emptive strategy that needs to be taken to draw attention to an asset of vulnerabilities, hallucinations, unsafe guidance and adversarial hazards in the behaviour of LLM. However, it is impossible to use red-teaming without formal operational systems.

1. INTRODUCTION

The fast development of Large Language Models (LLMs) in the medical field is one of the most significant changes in the history of medical informatics, clinical decision support, and the digital health industry. With artificial intelligence-based tools available in a variety of forms applicable to diagnosis, clinical documentation, triage, and patient engagement, the role of LLMs in healthcare systems changed as an experimental system became a functional element of a clinical process. In direct contrast to the past machine learning models that works with a fundamentally limited set of predictive tasks, LLMs are generative, interactive, and can produce complex unstructured outputs that have the potential to have a direct impact on clinical reasoning and decision-making (Bommasani et al., 2021; Krittanawong et al., 2023). The given paradigm shift has a significant potential of enhancing efficiency, care accessibility, and quality, but on the other hand, it brings new and critical risks. Such risks are hallucinated medical data, biases and misleading prescriptions, leaking privacy, and over-confident production that can reduce patient safety and ethics, when unaddressed (Nori et al., 2023; Shen et al., 2023).

The introduction of LLM as a component of medical context, thus, requires a radical reconsideration of the definition, regulation, and implementation of clinical AI safety. The conventional medical software has been traditionally governed within the established frameworks including the digital health guidelines made by the World Health Organization, the Software as a Medical Device (SaMD) framework done by the United States Food and Drug Administration, and the European Union AI Act. These are based on risk-classification, traceability, validation and post-market surveillance principles, to promote safety, accountability (WHO, 2021; FDA, 2022; European Commission, 2024). Nevertheless, the use of LLMs questions these regulatory paradigms because of their probabilistic nature, non-deterministic response and continuous learning abilities as well as dynamic user interactions. In experimental studies, medical LLMs have been shown to produce responses that seem to be authoritative, but which have factual inaccuracies or dangerous clinical advice. They can evolve as a result of hallucination phenomena, lack of full contextual penetration or biases within training data. Recent research comparing state-of-the-art models like GPT-4 and Med-PaLM have revealed that despite their ability to perform well to medical standard, their consistency in reasoning as well as safety is inconsistent in real-world clinical settings (Singhal et al., 2023; Shen et al., 2023). More recent studies have also pointed to the fact that AI systems created as generative agents used in clinical settings can have random reasoning patterns, which must be managed with well-organized safety governance frameworks, which unify evaluation, operational control, and continuous monitoring mechanisms (Zhang et al., 2024; Awasthi et al., 2025; Jindal et al., 2025).

More recent studies have added to the stress of the need of safety evaluation of medical LLMs. Research papers published post-2023 have shown that generative AI systems in clinical settings may have unpredictable reasoning behavior, and need systematic governance systems which integrate evaluation, operational control, and continuous monitoring systems (Zhang et al., 2024; Thawani et al., 2023; Singhal et al., 2023; Awasthi et al., 2025; Jindal Recent assessment systems and clinical research indicate that conventional benchmarking approaches may not be adequate to represent real-world risks in healthcare AI systems, or that in-depth evaluation plans are necessary to evaluate the quality of reasoning, safety, trustworthiness, and clinical reliability of AI systems before implementation in the patient-facing setting.

To address such difficulties, three pillars of managing the safety of LLM in clinical settings are becoming more unified in the literature: red-teaming, MLOps, and constant observer of the model. These elements combine to offer a lifecycle-based approach to the management of safety that is not limited to pre-deployment validation. Red-teaming is an offensive and preventive assessment technique used to understand potential weaknesses, resilience test model behaviour, and failure mode uncovering prior to clinical implementation (Ganguli et al., 2023). With medical LLM, red-teaming are no longer limited to common security practices, such as timely adversarial testing and clinically realistic simulated environment, but also proactive investigation of hallucinations, bias, and unsafe suggestions. It is indicated that this kind of specific assessment has the potential to reveal clinically relevant errors that would otherwise remain hidden by routine benchmark data and performance indicators (Wang et al., 2024).

Although red-teaming is critical to identify risks during pre-deployment, it will not adequately achieve continued safety in practice in the clinical environment. The dynamic and flexible process of the LLM requires the presence of robust operational infrastructures that can ensure the safety, transparency, and accountability of the entire model lifecycle. MLOps (Machine Learning Operations) is a way to satisfy this need by applying the DevOps concepts to the specifics of machine learning systems. MLOps has a focus on version control, auto testing, secure data pipelines, audit tracing, and workflow automation to be able to keep model development and deployment in a controlled and traceable state (Lwakatare et al., 2020; Nguyen et al., 2022). Medical facilities MLOps frameworks are essential in recording model updates, the provenance of training data, performance change validation, and regulatory requirements. The implementation of LLM may make the deployment of MLOps opaque, difficult to audit, and out of line with well-known clinical safety guidelines (Benjamens et al., 2022).

The third pillar, continuous model monitoring, is a final pillar in a safety lifecycle since it allows overseeing of the behaviour of LLM in real-time once it is deployed to real-life conditions. Goodness-of-fit monitors can be used to trace performance change, shift of the distribution, abnormality output and changes in interaction patterns which might only manifest themselves in practical large-scale clinical applications. It is expected based on the dynamism of healthcare, which is defined by a varying number of patients, an ever-changing medical knowledge base, and varying operational conditions (Wang and Sontak, 2023). The regulatory landscape is starting to impose such control: EU AI Act is obligatory to monitor high-risk AI systems post-market; FDA insists on ongoing monitoring of products of approved SaMD (FDA, 2022; European Commission, 2024). Monitoring provides sufficient time to identify the spikes in hallucinations, clinical reasoning degradation, or inappropriate recommendations, as well as gives feedback signals used to inform MLOps pipelines to run retrained, rollback, or remediation.

Together, red-teaming, MLOps, and continuous monitoring are interrelated with each other and create a unified system of safeguarding the safety throughout the lifecycle that guarantees that the technical aspects of the process are aligned with the clinical governance considerations. Although the individual components have been examined, recently, they have also placed a strong emphasis on bringing together these practices into a coherent framework, which encompasses design, development, deployment, and post-deployment (Long et al., 2023). This type of integration will result in timely detection of risk, ongoing operational control and never-ending learning due to clinical application in the real world.

This chapter will set out to give an in-depth analysis of the medical LLMs lifecycle safety management by reference to these three pillars. It starts with the description of the peculiar safety issues of generative AI in healthcare, and then proceeds to discuss the red-teaming techniques as applied to clinical situations in detail. This chapter then proceeds to discuss an MLOps frameworks that are used to facilitate regulatory adherence and operational governance and explores an approach to continuous monitoring strategies to ensure long-term model reliability. Lastly, an integrated safety framework is suggested, backed by the practical examples, supporting it by the case studies and policy implications. The analysis will enable the chapter to contribute to the existing debate on the use of LLMs in healthcare through ensuring their implementation is a safe, transparent, and trustworthy process.

The safety issues mentioned above indicate that the implementation of generative AI systems in healthcare involves more than traditional techniques of assurance.

Rather, an approach to safety that follows a lifecycle is required to make sure that the risks are detected, addressed, and monitored at all times during the process of model development and deployment. The sections below thus will analyze the principles of clinical safety of medical LLM, regulatory standards, the principles of human-AI interaction, and the new risk landscape of the presence of generative AI in healthcare settings.

2. FOUNDATIONS OF CLINICAL SAFETY FOR MEDICAL LLMS

To guarantee clinical safety with the application of Large Language Models (LLM), the effectiveness of the intersection of risk, reliability, accountability, and clinical governance must be thoroughly understood in medical facilities. In contrast to conventional medical software, LLMs are generative, probabilistic, and flexible and generate results that can appear similar to clinical reasoning but have no deterministic guarantees. Since their outputs may have a direct influence on the accuracy of the diagnosis, the direction of treatment, and communication with patients, before implementing LLMs in any healthcare process, it is critical to provide solid grounds of clinical safety. This part of the paper will describe the theoretical and regulatory foundation of the clinical safety, the risk environment that LLMs create, and the specific areas in which LLMs need to be evaluated in order to guarantee patient safety and adherence to clinical best practices.

All of the expanding literature on AI in healthcare highlights the importance of safety not relying on an accurate algorithm, but on systems-level designs that include regulation, human factor, technical controls, and constant assessment (Benjamens et al., 2022; Nori et al., 2023). Since the role of LLMs continues to expand in their interaction with clinicians and patients, their safety bases should be based on the principles related to the field of clinical governance, regulations of medical devices, and digital health ethics. These pillars direct subsequent stages of lifecycle (red-teaming, MLOps systems and ongoing monitoring).

2.1 The Unique Risk Landscape of Medical LLMs

Generative, to some extent, is the reason that LLLs are riskier than the previous generations of clinical AI. These risks may be in form of subtle occurrences and may not be detected by normal model evaluation guidelines. The three categories of risks prevail: informational risks, behavioural risks, and interactional risks.

Informational risks come in place as the model creates false, wrong, or old medical knowledge. LLM hallucinations may be in the forms of wrong medication dosage, perceived contraindications, misinterpreted clinical patterns, or fake clinical guidelines (Ayoub et al., 2023). Even small hallucinations may have disproportional effects during clinical practice.

The behavioural risks are related to the nature of the model that entails the creation of responses that are unwarrantedly confident, emotionally compelling, or anthropomorphic in nature. The most dangerous characteristic of medical LLM is over-confidence because clinicians can end up believing confident prose as evidence of something right (Nori et al., 2023).

Interactional risks happen to human-AI communication, where the model might not grasp the intention of the user, or cannot read ambiguous/incomplete entries or react to complex clinical situations subpar. The dynamics of interaction have potential to create compounding errors, particularly when the use of LLMs is incorporated in the high-paced clinical workflow.

All of these risk groups demonstrate the importance of safety foundations being holistic and ongoing over time and not fixed.

These categories of risks are conceptually different, but in the real-clinical setting, they tend to interact. As an example, a behavioural overconfidence might be used to increase the intensity of informational hallucinations, and the clinician will rely on incorrect answers. In the same way, interactional misunderstandings can initiate the wrong mode of thinking and result in erroneous clinical recommendations. These interdependencies imply that safety evaluation structures should cease to focus on individual measures of performance and instead they have to evaluate the overall sociotechnical framework within which medical LLMs are functional. The primary risk categories associated with medical LLMs are illustrated in Figure 1.

Figure 1. Risk Categories in Medical LLM Safety Foundations

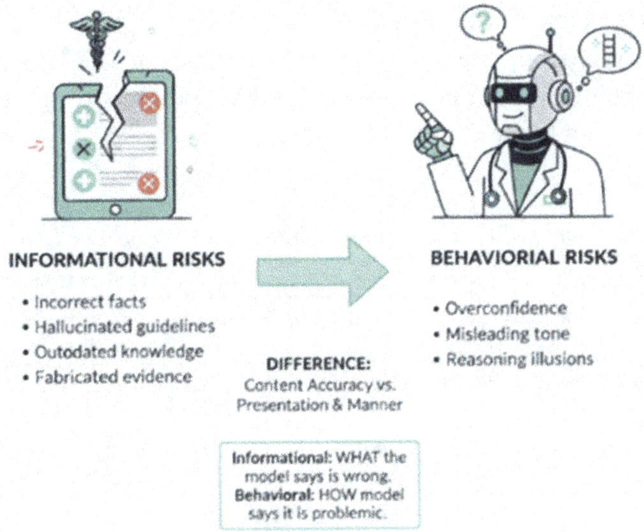

Figure 1 illustrates the three primary categories of risk that shape foundational safety requirements for medical LLMs (adapted from Nori et al., 2023; Ayoub et al., 2023).

2.2 Regulatory and Governance Frameworks for Medical LLM Safety

Generative, to some extent, is the reason that LLLs are riskier than the previous generations of clinical AI. These risks may be in form of subtle occurrences and may not be detected by normal model evaluation guidelines. The three categories of risks prevail: informational risks, behavioural risks, and interactional risks.

Informational risks come in place as the model creates false, wrong, or old medical knowledge. LLM hallucinations may be in the forms of wrong medication dosage, perceived contraindications, misinterpreted clinical patterns, or fake clinical guidelines (Ayoub et al., 2023). Even small hallucinations may have disproportional effects during clinical practice.

The behavioural risks are related to the nature of the model that entails the creation of responses that are unwarrantedly confident, emotionally compelling, or anthropomorphic in nature. The most dangerous characteristic of medical LLM is over-confidence because clinicians can end up believing confident prose as evidence of something right (Nori et al., 2023).

Interactional risks happen to human-AI communication, where the model might not grasp the intention of the user, or cannot read ambiguous/incomplete entries or react to complex clinical situations subpar. The dynamics of interaction have potential to create compounding errors, particularly when the use of LLMs is incorporated in the high-paced clinical workflow.

All of these risk groups demonstrate the importance of safety foundations being holistic and ongoing over time and not fixed. Table 1 presents key global governance frameworks relevant to medical LLM safety.

Table 1. Global Governance Frameworks Relevant to Medical LLM Safety

Framework / Body	Scope	LLM Safety Relevance
FDA (United States)	SaMD regulation; clinical AI approval	Requires validation, post-market surveillance, and risk classification
EU AI Act (Europe)	High-risk AI systems	Mandates continuous monitoring, transparency, audit logs, and lifecycle safety controls
WHO Guidance on AI in Health	Ethics and governance principles	Emphasizes accountability, fairness, inclusiveness, and human oversight
ISO/IEC 62304	Software lifecycle processes	Provides structure compatible with MLOps-based lifecycle governance for medical LLMs

2.3 Human–AI Interaction Principles and Clinical Workflow Integration

More complexities are also brought about by clinical workflow integration. Medical workers work in high-stake environments, where time constraints, mental and intellectual workload, and multidisciplinary duties are present. These workflows have to be empowered by LLLMs, not overwhelmed. The concept of safety has been closely associated with the ways of human perception and isolation on AI results which have been previously widely reported in the studies of human-factors engineering (Sarter and Woods, 1995).

A major challenge is possible due to the effect of the automation bias, which is the human desire to place trust in AI-generated recommendations despite the contradiction with intuition. Research has indicated that there is a possibility of clinicians overweighting AI outputs, particularly in terms of their presentation using confident language (Jacobs et al., 2021). Automation bias might diminish the situational awareness of clinicians with time.

A different obstacle is the fact that there must be suitable transparency. Excessive technicality may disorient the clinicians whereas insufficient transparency may not allow effective accountability. A balance between showing uncertainty, evidence sources and clinical rationale should be achieved through effective human-AI interaction.

It also involves the use of powerful fallback mechanisms in workflow integration. The clinicians should be in a position to override, challenge or ignore outputs in an un strained manner. The implementation of LLDAs into systems where direct human judgment is essential should therefore be introduced.

While regulatory governance and clinical workflow design provide essential safety foundations, proactive evaluation techniques are required to identify potential vulnerabilities in medical LLM behavior before deployment. One widely adopted approach in AI safety research is red-teaming, which involves systematically testing models under adversarial or high-risk scenarios to uncover hidden failure modes. The following section examines how red-teaming methodologies can be applied to healthcare-focused LLM systems.

3. RED-TEAMING FOR MEDICAL LLM SAFETY

One of the most essential mechanisms of assessing the safety, robustness, and reliability of large language models (LLMs) before their incorporation into clinical settings has become red-teaming. Although traditionally used in regards to cybersecurity penetration testing, red-teaming when applied to LLMs does mean organized adversarial testing that has tried to provoke harmful, biased, or factually incorrect or otherwise unsafe behaviour. Red-teaming in the medical context is not only aimed at testing accuracy but it is more of a stress-testing of the systems in the conditions that are comparable with the real-world conditions of the clinical problems, edge cases, hostile misuse, and human-AI interaction dynamics. Red-teaming during pre-deployment is necessary to identify the failures modes that still types of benchmarks fail to detect as LLMs retrieve more and more clinical summaries (or/and triage assistance) or offer patient-facing information (Ganguli et al., 2023; Wang et al., 2024).

3.1 Types of Red-Teaming in Medical LLM Contexts

Red-teaming is not a single-dimensional process. Instead, it is composed of a number of categories which address various elements of the LLM behaviour. Four prevailing types of red-teaming are used in a medical context and are important to evaluative processes, and they include: clinical adversarial testing, safety and toxicity probing, bias and fairness evaluation, and misuse/abuse scenario testing.

Clinical adversarial testing is aimed at testing the understanding of medical knowledge by the model. Such adversarial example tasks recapitulate complicated clinical situations that may be characterized by uncommon illnesses, uncertain signs and symptoms, comorbidities, or complicated drug interactions. This type of testing indicates the ability of the model to be coherent and accurate in instances outside of cases that are frequently seen in training data (Krittanawong et al., 2023).

Bias and fairness analysis determines differences in model behaviours that interact with demographic factors like race, gender, age, socioeconomic background or disability. The problem of medical bias has always been an issue contributing to health disparities, and LLMs being trained on biased datasets endanger supporting damaging stereotypes or unequal care guidelines (Chen et al., 2023).

The misuse and abuse scenario testing looks into the capability of the model to be influenced in a way that will make it give dangerous commands. As an example, it can happen that prompts are urging the LLM to provide an explanation of how they can abuse prescriptions or evade medical check-ups. To avoid unintentional or targeted malicious uses in patient-facing applications of LLM, the vulnerability of this instrument to manipulation must be evaluated (Ganguli et al., 2023).

All such red-teaming has developed a strong evaluation matrix that documents the extent of dangers that exists in the interaction of medical LLMs with medical stakeholders. The major categories of red-teaming approaches are shown in Figure 2.

Figure 2. Categories of Medical LLM Red-Teaming

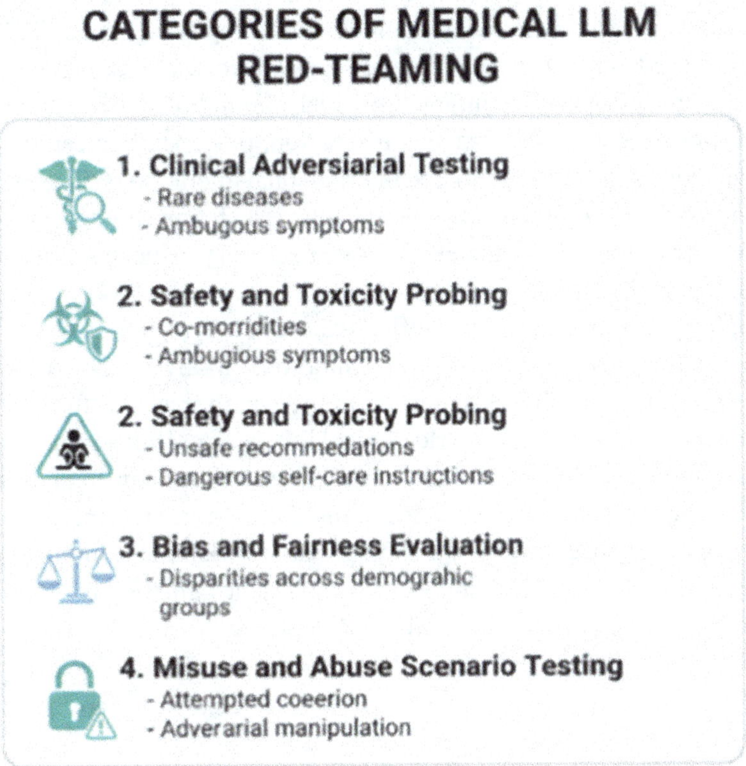
CATEGORIES OF MEDICAL LLM RED-TEAMING
1. Clinical Adversiarial Testing
- Rare diseases
- Ambugous symptoms
2. Safety and Toxicity Probing
- Co-morridities
- Ambugious symptoms
2. Safety and Toxicity Probing
- Unsafe recommedations
- Dangerous self-care instructions
3. Bias and Fairness Evaluation
- Disparities across demograhic groups
4. Misuse and Abuse Scenario Testing
- Attempted coeerion
- Adverarial manipulation

Figure 2 summarizes four critical dimensions of red-teaming tailored for medical LLM evaluation (adapted from Ganguli et al., 2023; Chen et al., 2023).

3.2 Methods and Frameworks for Conducting Red-Teaming in Healthcare

Red-teaming has to involve meticulous methodologies that would be integrated in evaluation. Clinical expertise, technical model analysis, and ethical considerations should be incorporated into red-teaming used in healthcare. There are usually three methodological pillars that can lead to effective medical red-teaming, which include prompt-based adversarial generation, scenario-based clinical simulation, and domain-expert adversarial review.

Prompt-based adversarial generation: This deals with creating huge amounts of prompts that can be used to cause hallucinations, incorrect reasoning, or unsafe clinical advice. Human-generated prompts can be provided with automated adversarial prompt generators, although experts need to play a crucial role in making sure that scenarios are presented as real clinical risk. Timely engineering methods like perturbations, conflicting instructions, or advanced medical histories have the ability to uncover the inconsistency in model reasoning (Zeng et al., 2023).

Scenario-based clinical simulation augments adversarial assessment by modelling simulated patient-provider interaction. Such simulations reflect actual hospital experiences: emergency calls, triage conversation, postoperative care and chronic disease management advice. Simulated interpersonal interaction red-teaming evaluates the conversational dynamics, emotional tone, escalation strategy, and uncertain recognition capabilities of the model which are necessary to make safe use in clinical practice (Long et al., 2023).

Although red-teaming has proven effective in uncovering model vulnerabilities, current methodologies still face several limitations. Many adversarial evaluation techniques rely on manually designed prompts, which may not fully capture the diversity and complexity of real-world clinical interactions. Furthermore, standardized evaluation benchmarks for healthcare LLM safety remain limited, making it difficult to compare results across institutions. Future research therefore needs to develop domain-specific adversarial testing frameworks that combine automated prompt generation with clinician-guided scenario design. Figure 3 presents the lifecycle safety framework for medical LLM deployment.

Figure 3. Lifecycle Safety Framework for Medical LLM Deployment

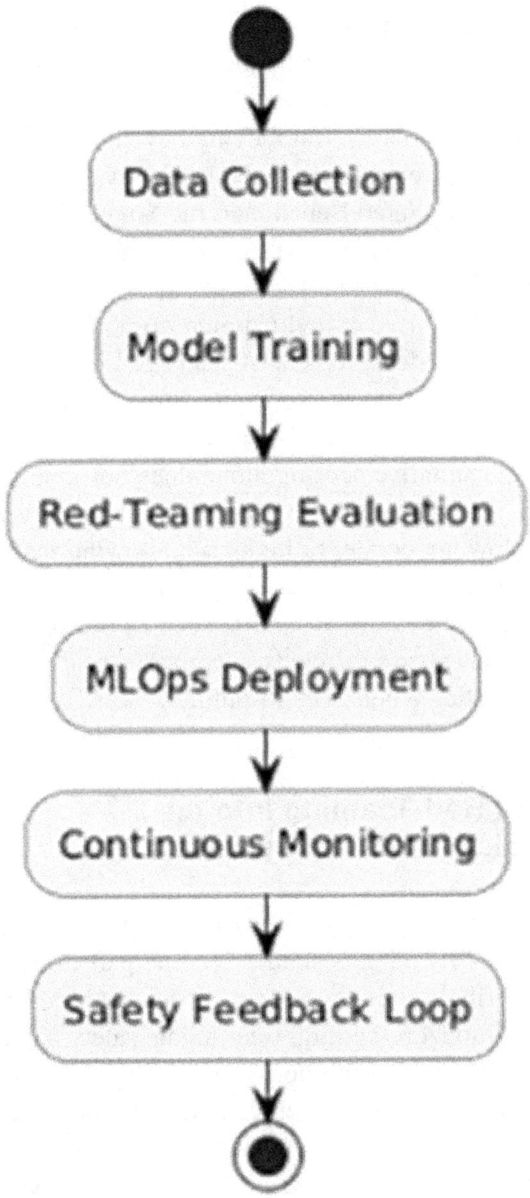

3.3 Tools and Evaluation Metrics Used in Red-Teaming

A number of tools and metrics are created to facilitate systematic red-teaming of LLMs. Such tools typically combine model probing user interfaces, logging, and analytics dashboards. MedQA, PubMedQA, and MedMCQA are useful starting points because safety benchmarks, but moving beyond these fixed benchmarks is necessary to conduct the adversarial evaluation of safety evaluation (Jin et al., 2021). New tools like RedQueen, SafetyBench, and the Stanford HELM framework are offering platforms to produce adversarial expertise and detect trends of breakdown in a variety of regions (Li et al., 2023).

Measures of evaluation used in red-teaming do not necessarily coincide with accuracy-based measures. Measurement of safety can be hallucination rate, score of clinical rightness, classification of severity of error, percentage of generation of harmful contents and vulnerability to manipulation. Even in most situations within the clinical setting, quantitative scoring alone does not give sufficient insight as compared to qualitative assessment by experts. Error-based scales determine the categories of errors low, moderate, or high-risk, allowing institutions to focus on mitigation plans (Chen et al., 2023).

Beyond this, measures of time-to-failure, such as the speed at which a model makes an unstable output when subjected to adversarial prompting, are now a metric of interest as a diagnostic. When time-to-failure is less, it is more susceptible to misuse in reality.

3.3 Integration of Red-Teaming into the Lifecycle of Medical LLM Deployment

Red-teaming is not an independent exercise; but it is the initial step in a lifecycle continuity safety model. Its outputs should become part of MLOps pipelines and direct ongoing monitoring activities. An exegetic when red-teaming detects vulnerabilities, this requires model retraining, fine-tuning, safety patching, or immediate template adjustments. Then the continuous monitoring can be used to verify that the model behaves consistently after its deployment, particularly after version change.

Red-teaming therefore is a cycle that should be repeated to identify weaknesses, put in place mitigation measures, re-test, monitor and improve. On that note, red-teaming is, in this regard, not just a defensive mechanism but an active kind of safety governance which is focused on pre-empting failures prior to their reaching patients.

4. MLOps FOR MEDICAL LLM GOVERNANCE AND SAFETY

MLOps or the Machine Learning Operations became the foundation of safe, reproducible, and auditable machine learning in the business world, and its significance is multiplied in the medical sphere where medical LLMs play with personal patient information, alter diagnostics, and may cause health interventions. Medical MLOps pipelines, in contrast to the conventional software engineering pipelines, should combine strict regulatory control, lifecycle management, human verification, and model versioning, to guarantee reliability and clinical acceptability of the insights provided by LLM (Kreuzberger et al., 2023). Since medical LLMs are constantly improved, whether by fine-tuning or training on a new guideline, MLOps offers the framework that guarantees the consistency, reproducibility, and safety of each deployment cycle. Since these systems are becoming more automated on elements of clinical decision support or medication summative, or diagnostic support, opioid governance structures vested in MLOps pipelines are a critical ingredient of medical AI risk management (Amann et al., 2020).

The MLOps practices are getting more popular in medical institutions striving to match the demands of, say, FDA and EMA. Unlike general-purpose AI pipelines, clinical MLOps pipelines should have the provenance of every model and dataset lineage, dataset annotation specification, bias analyses, and audit trails explicitly documented (Sendak et al., 2020). This subsection investigates MLOps pipeline architecture, components and safety capabilities of MLOps pipelines in medical LLM deployments. It also gives you a conceptual figure, which can be transferred to the complete chapter.

4.1 MLOps Architecture Tailored for Medical LLMs

The basic medical MLOps pipeline is usually constituted of interlinked layers such as data source, data governance, model building, validation, deployment, monitoring and integration of feedback. Every step is automatized with the help of the workflows and the established human control points. The role of these checkpoints is that clinical data and clinical interpretations cannot be assessed entirely based purely on the automated validators (Castiglioni et al., 2021).

An EHRS feeds LLMs with structured fields of data, free-text clinical notes, imaging reports, lab summaries, and ICD-coded medical data. All these sources must be strictly pre-processed and do not expose personal information to attacks due to the ability of LLMs to be unintentionally memorized or intentionally poured out (Carlini et al., 2023). In turn, MLOps pipelines built to operate on the LLMs include automated PHI-detecting tools, de-identification engines, and synthetic-data augmentation units which, in combination, decrease the probability of patient-specific memorizing or re-identification attempts.

Medical LLM designs are also designed to change regularly with new biomedical literature, new clinical directions and disease trends demanding timely changes to the models. MLOps supports such updates by version-controlling pipeline where every model version passes through regression frameworks and bias-detection tools, and only approved to pass through them, is deployed. The incorporation of those automated testing routines enables hospitals and research organisations to make sure that the updates of models comply with clinical evidence and inadvertently introduce adverse behaviour (Levine et al., 2023). Figure 4 illustrates different types of drift affecting medical LLM performance.

Figure 4. Conceptual Architecture of a Medical LLM MLOps Pipeline

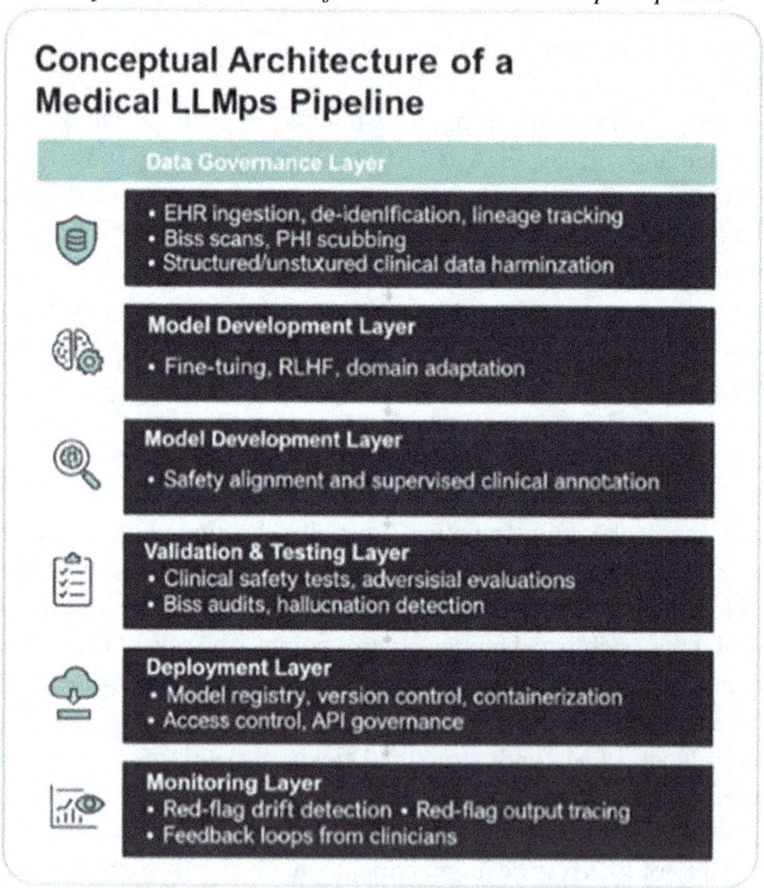

4.2 Data Governance and Clinical-Grade Dataset Management

One of the main pillars of clinical MLOps pipelines is data governance since medical LLMs rely on a high-quality, integrity, and ethical collection of clinical data extensively. The data governance lifecycle works in a medical setting with strict guidelines to control consent and any other necessary measures such as privacy assurance and traces of data use. Clinical narratives, e.g., discharge summaries, diagnostic impressions, and physician correspondence, are sensitive, which is why the risks of re-identification or improper use are particularly relevant (Price and Cohen, 2019).

A successful medical MLOps pipeline uses dataset lineage to record the exact origin, annotation procedure, transformation history, and storage place of the current version of the dataset. This lineage is central in retroactive audits especially when the regulators inspect the safety profiles of installed clinical AI systems (FDA, 2023). Due to the fact that most of the LLM fine-tuning datasets are gathered across various institutions, MLOps governance models will have to implement harmonization processes to align the terminologies of variables, coding guidelines and documentation formats. Harmonization helps in not only enhancing the performance of models but also minimizing the spread of systematic biases that are related to particular populations or different practices of the clinical process (Gianfrancesco et al., 2018).

Within an IT medical setting, data governance can similarly aid in ongoing updates to LLM by guaranteeing that newly obtained data including imaging reports, pathology summaries, and others is validated, anonymized, and integrated in manners that do not compromise fairness. The lack of such processes can result in the unconscious aggravation of the differences in diagnosis quality among population groups (Obermeyer et al., 2019). Consequently, data governance level of MLOps pipeline is turned into a core mechanism of fairness and bias.

4.3 Model Training, Fine-Tuning, and Alignment Workflows

Training medical LLMs In MLOps, a number of steps are followed: initial pre-training on biomedical corpora, supervised fine-tuning on clinical datasets, reinforcement learning from human feedback (RLHF) and alignment tuning to ensure clinical safety. Such stages are organized by using automated workflow managers, which orchestrate training jobs, do hyperparameter optimization and validate training results with the established safety metrics (Xu et al., 2024).

This is one of the areas of fine-tuning that are especially sensitive in healthcare since clinical datasets usually include language specialized to the domain where even minor nuances significantly vary in interpretation. Lack of alignment at this stage could result in high-confidence hallucination or unhealthy medical advice.

Therefore, medical MLOps workflows impose the gated approval models where clinical domain experts assess the initial output of the LLM and subsequently fine-tune the iterations (Li et al., 2023).

MLOps systems that train LLMs should also be able to comply with regulatory requirements on explain ability since black-box elements may negate trust on clinical systems (Doshi-Velez and Kim, 2017). In this way, workflow training processes include feature-importance estimation tools, or example-based explanation tools, and alignment metrics that emphasise risky behaviour. These systems are vital to address transparency needs on health AI oversight.

Despite the advantages of MLOps frameworks, implementing these pipelines in healthcare environments presents significant challenges. Clinical data governance requirements, strict regulatory oversight, and the need for human-in-the-loop validation often slow down deployment cycles compared to other industries. Additionally, integrating MLOps pipelines with existing hospital infrastructure such as electronic health record systems require careful architectural design and institutional coordination.

4.4 Deployment Governance and Model Registry Systems

Implementing a medical LLM would entail enforcing controlled pipelines to guarantee the interests of accessibility and stringent regulation mechanisms that would enhance the clinical reliability. The deployment of an MLOps workflow is associated with containerization approaches that help encapsulate the model environment, which minimise differences in behaviour across different hospital systems and guarantee consistent behaviour across deployments.

Model registries serve as the core as they maintain a list of all versions of the LLM, its training data sources, configuration, evaluation measures, and compliance reports. This registry serves as an audit log and traceability space, which meets regulatory requirements, equal to post-market surveillance measures in medical device regulation (European Medicines Agency, 2021).

Access control systems to restrict access to LLM outputs by what clinical personnel to request are also part of deployment governance. More crucially, the policies of output governance define the guidelines in accordance with which classes of suggestions should be examined by clinicians prior to the implementation. These regulations are specific to jurisdiction but usually echo human-in-the-loop needs advanced by prominent health AI regulatory programs (World Health Organization, 2021).

Besides regulatory compliance, deployment governance system encompasses user-facing safety controls, e.g., disclaimers, uncertainty warnings, and pre-structured response templates to reduce the risk of misleading content. A combination of these mechanisms constitutes a necessary level of protection in corresponding clinical AI implementations.

4.5 Continuous Monitoring, Drift Detection, and Safety Feedback Loops

Monitoring continuously is among the most significant MOLOps duties of the medical LLM lifecycle safety management. Monitoring can be defined as the process of identifying the changes in the input population structure, novel disease trends, a variation in clinical workflow, or a variation in clinical guidelines, all of which impact model reliability. Specifically, distribution shift or concept drift is quite perilous to medical LLMs since their outputs may seem authoritative even in cases when the model face new information (Widmer and Kubat, 1996).

MLOps pipelines combine various tools in monitoring that include real time sampling of model outputs, hallucination detection systems, and semantic drift analysis modules. These tools identify anomalies or unsafe reaction that are not in accordance with the historical trend. MLOps platforms can also automatically issue alerts to clinical governance teams when a deviation is identified or rollback procedures, restoring the system to a safer version, can be initiated (Zhang et al., 2024).

Continuous LLM also requires the existence of feedback loops. Such loops will enable clinicians to report unsafe responses, wrong interpretation or even cases of hallucination. MLOps pipelines design such reports into structured error categories that guide the following training and red-teaming procedures. In contrast to traditional monitoring systems, clinical AI feedback loops need to be properly developed to prevent the overcrowding of clinicians with overwhelming reporting in the future (Benjamens et al., 2022).

Bias detection is also involved in monitoring. The performance of the models of a specific institution should be regularly assessed in the subgroups of demographics to identify emerging heterogeneity early, before it causes any damage (Rajkomar et al., 2018). This is a proactive method in securing long-term clinical equity. Table 2 summarizes core MLOps functions supporting medical LLM governance.

Table 2. Core MLOps Functions Supporting Medical LLM Governance

MLOps Function	Clinical Significance	Safety Contribution
Data Governance	Controls data lineage, consent, and PHI protection	Prevents leakage, bias propagation
Model Registry	Tracks LLM versions and audit documentation	Ensures traceability and regulatory compliance
Automated Testing	Evaluates clinical safety, hallucinations, and bias	Detects unsafe updates before deployment
Drift Monitoring	Observes real-time model performance	Identifies emerging risks and shifts
Feedback Integration	Collects clinician reports	Guides retraining and alignment tuning

4.6 Regulatory Alignment and Compliance Considerations

MLOps is critical towards making medical LLMs adhere to procedures of regulation of machine learning in the healthcare sector. New AI-specific regulatory frameworks, e.g. the proposed Clinical Decision Support Systems rule by FDA and the AI Act of EU, focus on risk classification, documentation, monitoring, and transparency over performance These features are very compatible with MLOps features like increased monitoring, automated logging, and repeatable deployment of workflows.

Regulators are becoming more and more demanding that AI systems keep transparent records of the nature of the training data, the metrics of evaluation and analysis of risks and known limitations. MLOps structures facilitate these expectations in that documents are currently centralized in model registries and related metadata. More to the point, MLOps will enable post-market oversight of medical AI- a field where a continuous observation and safety feedback will be of paramount importance (FDA, 2023).

Some other areas of intersection between regulation and ethical requirements in clinical settings include patient safety, explain ability, autonomy, and fairness. MLOps structures that are focused on governance formally address these issues by supporting alignment workstations, red-teaming patterns, and routines of fairness, which jointly contribute to addressing downstream risks. Finally, MLOps can help the institutions comply with regulatory requirements, as well as providing the institutions a greater sense of confidence in medical LLM implementations by guaranteeing a steady safety monitoring throughout the model lifecycle.

5. CONTINUOUS MODEL MONITORING AND RISK MANAGEMENT FOR MEDICAL LLMS

One of the most important lifecycle governance aspects of medical LLMs is constant supervision of models. In contrast to fixed clinical software systems, LLMs are probabilistic and dynamic and continuously evolve in their behaviours with changing clinical conditions, changes in data distributions, and emerging medical vocabularies in addition to encountering new patterns of disease (Lu et al., 2022). As an illustration, the SARS-CoV-2 pandemic not only created vast drift unbroken by old model assumptions but also introduced new pathogens, which, in turn, necessitated changes in clinical terms, diagnostic and treatment guidelines, and so on (Liang et al., 2021). This is because tracking can identify such changes at the earliest, avoiding the spread of unsafe outputs to clinical workflows.

There are also the risks linked with medical LLP which includes hallucinations, amplification of bias, vague reasoning patterns and recommendations are not at par. Such models can also create domain-specific defects, including suggesting a drug drug interaction that is incorrect, giving incorrect triage guidance, or misunderstanding lab values (Singhal et al., 2023). Constant monitoring thus becomes necessary not only to determine the accuracy of the model but also to help detect any safety hazard that might arise before it can result in clinical damage in the real world(European Parliament, 2023).

Observation is also important in determining regulatory adherence to medical AI. Upon the adaptive AI/ML systems, agencies like FDA, EMA, MHRA, and WHO have also been urging on the need to have so-called post-market surveillance (FDA, 2023; WHO, 2021). Since medical LLMs are susceptible to degradation with age, which has been effectively demonstrated in other clinical ML systems, regulators expect institutions to use continuous monitoring pipelines that may detect, record and correct performance failures (Benjamens et al., 2022). Therefore, monitoring is not a technical process but a governance requirement to make sure that the deployed clinical AI tools are reliable, fair, and safe.

5.1 Dimensions of Drift in Medical LLMs

Model drift happens when the data distribution, clinical conditions, or interaction patterns of the user alter to reduce the model reliability. The use of LLMs in the healthcare environment presents several types of drifts that are unique to it.

A drift in data distribution takes place where the clinical inputs that the LLM is exposed to at the time of fine-tuning are not the same. This may arise due to the changing patient demographics, modifications in hospital documentation, new diagnoses, or variations among clinical specialists (Winkler et al., 2023). As an illustration, when an LLM is related on cardiology notes in particular but applied to various departments, the language and conceptual noise difference may result in more hallucinations or wrong medical interpretations.

Concept drift occurs when there is the change in the underlying meaning or clinical importance of medical concepts. This is more so in fields like oncology, infectious diseases and endocrinology where the lines of treatment vary very much. An LLM engaged with out-of-date causes of oncology principles might recommend the use of the out-of-date instance of chemotherapy unless updated or observed on schedule (Kocbek et al., 2020). Such drifts are identified through continuous monitoring by comparing the current model recommendations to modern clinical recommendations in order to overcome the drifts by early correction.

Semantic drift has an impact on the meaning of medical terminologies. With the development of clinical lingo, words can develop certain diagnostic or prognostic value. An example of this is that the term long COVID became part of medical terminology quickly and would not be represented using pre-2020 models. Semantically embeddable monitoring system can flag the moment that an LLM start to deal with unfamiliar words and fuze warnings to manage teams (Basu et al., 2022).

User behaviour drift is a change in the interaction with the system by clinicians or patients. The risk profile of the system changes when the usage patterns change, e.g., when there is greater dependence on LLMs to summarize medication or provide an interpretation of the diagnosis. The log of the kind and difficulty of user queries will assist in predicting new threats to safety and adjust the alignment mechanisms (Nori et al., 2023). Figure 5 shows the continuous monitoring and risk management cycle.

Figure 5. Types of Drift Affecting Medical LLM Performance

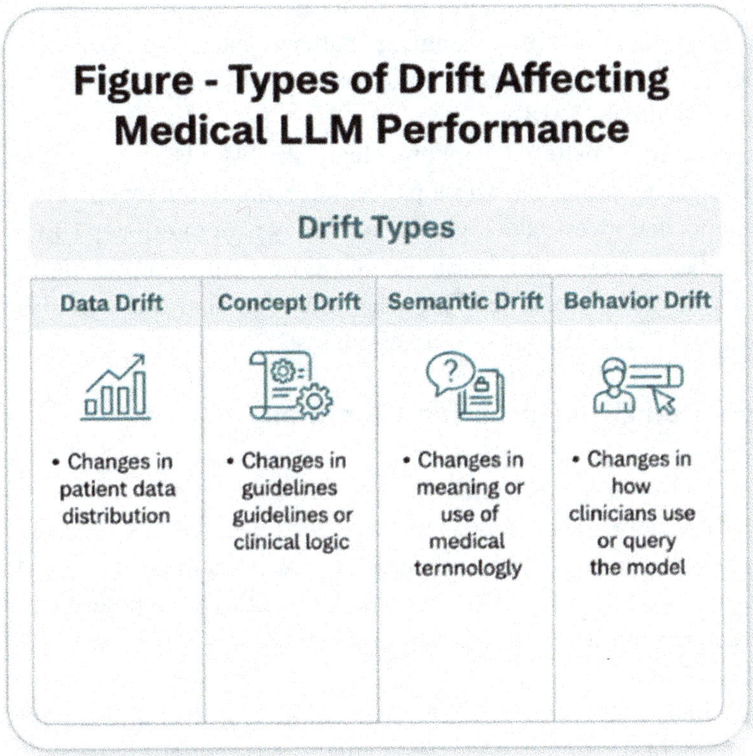

5.2 Monitoring Hallucinations, Bias, and Unsafe Reasoning Patterns

One of the key factors of the safety-based practices of LLM is hallucination monitoring. Medical hallucinations are particularly dangerous since they can provide fictitious clinical truths, not existing treatment advice, or false references that seem authoritative (Ji et al., 2023). Continuous monitoring uses algorithms (hallucination scoring) to compare responses generated to confirmed clinical knowledge bases including UpToDate, PubMed, SNOMED-CT or ICD-10. Any sources, which cannot be validated, are marked as under review.

Monitoring bias is also extremely important as medical LLMs can replicate or enhance inequality within their training samples. As an example (Levine et al., 2023), risk prediction tools have traditionally yielded biased results on minority groups, and the same phenomenon could be reflected in advice suggested by LLM (Obermeyer et al., 2019). Monitoring is done repeatedly over the demographic characteristics of prompts or determined by context, to identify harmful differentials in model responses. Although language patterns cannot reach protected attributes directly, subtle indications in the language patterns can result in biased generation despite the fact that the protection does not imply hiding the patterns altogether (Bender and Friedman, 2018).

Unsafe reasoning patterns happen when LLLMs justify their decisions by baseless medical assumptions. These patterns are monitored by coercive reasoning chain validators that investigate logical consistency over multi-step LLC reasoning, particularly, during a task of different diagnosis or medication titration (Wei et al., 2022). The validator raises a red flag when the argument line contains irrational links, forged statements, or missing assessments.

5.3 Automated Drift Detection Pipelines

Constant monitoring is executed via automated drift detection wherein the current model behaviour is compared with reference benchmarks. The pipelines use quantitative measures such as KL divergence, cosine similarity drift (Poursabzi-Sangdeh et al., 2021), changing the number of tokens through perplexity, and the semantic vectors should shift to detect premature failures in the model performance (Kumar et al., 2023).

Such pipelines are applied in an MLOps monitoring layer in the clinical setting, and they can run in streaming mode. When the LLMs generate the encodings of the incoming notes of a physician or clinical query, the input is encoded into embeddings, which are contrasted with the past distributions of outputs. Even slight drift in the semantic space indicates the beginning of drift (Chen et al., 2023). Since medical drift tends to creep in over time, the automated analysers prove higher in comparison to human reviewers only, as they can provide the additional data to identify easy changes in the very initial stages (Lu et al., 2022).

Automated drift detection also involves real-world clinical outcome data, such as comparing the prescription of medications as recommended by the model to what the physician actually prescribes as a dosage (Zhang et al., 2024). In case the discrepancies grow with time, drift detector amplifies the signal as a high-priority alarm. The integration of pipes with EHR systems enables them to record trends in vast groups of patients (Sendak et al., 2020). Table 3 highlights key drift indicators and their clinical impact.

Table 3. Core MLOps Functions Supporting Medical LLM Governance

Drift Indicator	Description	Example Clinical Impact
Perplexity Increase	Rising difficulty predicting token sequences	Incorrect medication summarization
Embedding Shift	Semantic drift in generated terminology	Misclassification of disease categories
Guideline Divergence	Deviation from clinical protocols	Outdated cancer treatment recommendations
Hallucination Spike	Sudden increase in fabricated content	Unsafe drug–drug interaction claims

Although automated drift detection techniques provide valuable early warning signals, interpreting these alerts in clinical contexts remains challenging. Not all detected drift necessarily leads to clinically significant errors, and excessive alerting may overwhelm governance teams. Therefore, monitoring systems must incorporate risk prioritization mechanisms that distinguish between minor performance fluctuations and safety-critical deviations. Table 4 presents monitoring tools used for ensuring medical LLM safety.

Table 4. Monitoring Tools for Medical LLM Safety

Monitoring Tool	Purpose	Example
Hallucination Detection	Detect fabricated clinical information	Knowledge verification
Bias Monitoring	Identify demographic bias	Fairness evaluation
Drift Detection	Detect distribution changes	KL divergence
Risk Scoring	Classify safety severity	Clinical risk analysis

5.4 Safety Feedback Loops and Human-in-the-Loop Governance

Medical LLM reliability is improved through safety feedback mechanisms that ensure an improvement in the reliability over time. These loops enable clinicians to record unsafe outputs, conflicting statements or logical fallacy. MLOps systems automatically group feedback reports in clusters of errors that include hallucinations, outdated guidelines, medication misinformation, and bias-related behaviour (Benjamens et al., 2022).

Human-in-the-loop governance paves the way to make sure clinicians have control over AI-assisted decision-making. The outputs of medical LLM should not be considered autonomous but advisory, and the feedback connections serve to remind clinicians to preserve this hierarchy by providing the ability to override or provide corrections to model recommendations. These corrections are in turn fed-back to the alignment tuning and red-teaming loops and enhance the safety profile of the system (Amann et al., 2020).

Additionally, feedback mechanisms facilitate the so-called continuous learning governance, which is a regulatory idea, according to which any model developments need to be publicly available, traceable, and defensible and then implementable (FDA, 2023). Once the clinicians complain of continuous mistakes in a specific area, referred to as misinterpreted radiology terminology (Thawani et al., 2023), the MLOps team performs model retraining or red-teaming that uses the LLM in particular.

5.5 Risk Scoring, Prioritization, and Escalation Mechanisms

Risk scoring systems assess the outputs of every LLM with an assessment of its likelihood to result in clinical harm. Depending on such dimensions as the severity of hallucinations, mismatches of guidelines, misalignment of confidence, sensitivity to demographic factors, and complexity of reasoning, these systems can be overlaid (Nori et al., 2023). Those that have a high-risk score in the output are blocked or sent back to human review, or identified as critical warning.

Pathways of escalation make sure that the risky outputs are responded to swiftly. Indicatively, risky outputs such as those associated with medication dosing error or wrong emergency triage directions are automatically activated and alerts sent to clinical safety officers. These routes resemble incident management systems involved in patient safety models (Kellogg et al., 2017).

Risk prioritization is also useful in the allocation of the organization resources. Low risk outputs might be reviewed during a batch, and the high-risk ones must be taken into account and analysed in-depth.

5.7 Post-Market Surveillance and Regulatory Compliance Monitoring

Regulators need to conduct continuous monitoring to make sure that adaptive medical AI systems do not pose a threat after implementation. Medical LLM post-market surveillance combines error logs, drift measures, clinician feedback, usage measures and re-training histories to develop an overall understanding of the system stability (European Medicines Agency, 2021).

Conduct pipelines produce timely safety reports that record their trends in hallucinations, drifts, and upgrades as well as mitigation measures. These reports are constitutive audit and compliance certification documents. Regulators are increasingly demanding clear records of how models change with time, particularly in the event of reinforcement learning or ongoing fine-tuning (European Parliament, 2023).

Monitoring should also be implemented as a part of regulatory systems to increase accountability and allow identification of the so-called silences failures, harmful behaviour that goes unattended by clinical supervision. Systematic oversight would assure the availability of consistent monitoring as a basis of AI safety governance.

Figure 6. Continuous Monitoring and Risk Management Cycle

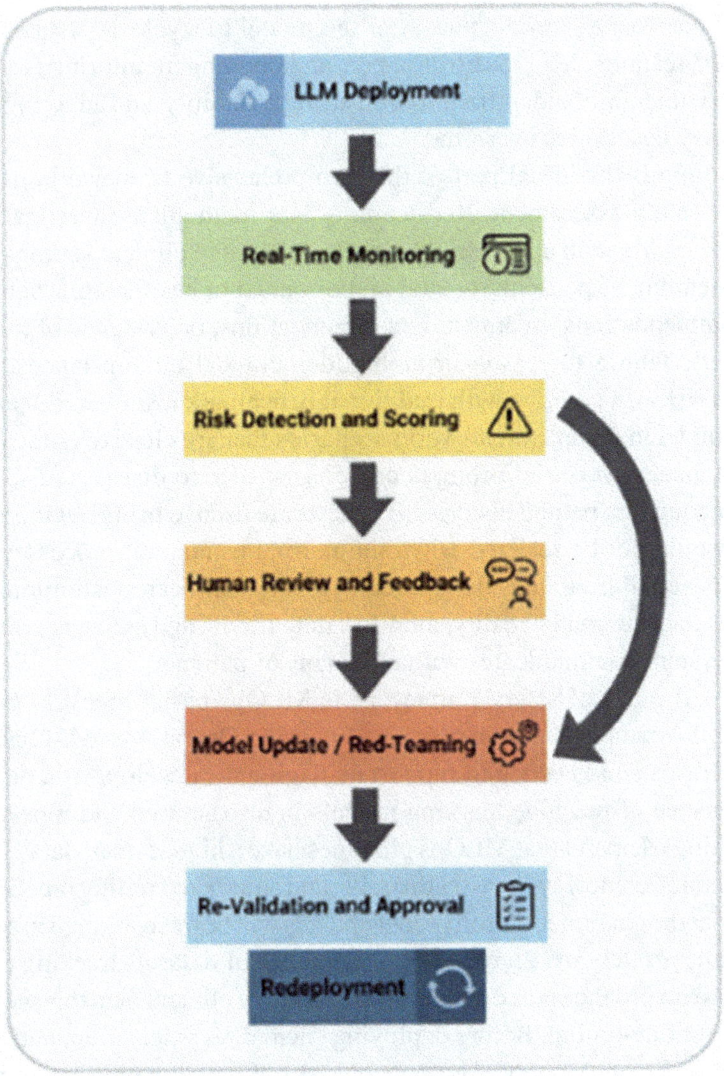

6. INTEGRATED SAFETY FRAMEWORK FOR MEDICAL LLM DEPLOYMENT

The recent adoption of large language models (LLMs) into healthcare facilities has led to a sense of urgency in terms of developing organized safety measures that would oversee the full lifecycle. In contrast to conventional medical software systems, generative AI models can generate probabilistic outputs that can change with context, user prompts, and changing data distributions. Consequently, to ensure the safety implementation of medical LLMs, coordinated safety controls need to be in place, which can act at various phases of the model lifecycle. A safety framework involving red-teaming, MLOps governance, and ongoing monitoring is an effective approach to vulnerability identification, ensuring reliability, and adhering to clinical and regulatory necessities over time.

Red-teaming is the initial part of this comprehensive framework, namely pre-deployment safety assessment. Red-teaming is a methodical investigation of the behaviour of LLMs with adversarial prompts, simulated clinical settings, and edge cases. Red-teaming is particularly vital in the context of healthcare, where the diagnostic recommendations, treatment recommendations, or evidence of hallucinated medical facts, failure to reason in ambiguous clinical circumstances, or biased diagnosis is risky. In contrast with traditional benchmark testing, red-teaming tries to test the model in complex real-world scenarios that are close to clinical practice. As one instance, adversarial prompts can consist of rare diseases, discrepant lab values, or incomplete patient histories. The tests are used to bring out the vulnerable areas that would not be realized when the normal evaluation processes are used. Detecting these failure modes before deployment, healthcare institutions can tune their models to better match reality, modify safety filters, and enhance training plans before the system communicates with clinicians or patients.

The second pillar of safety framework is MLOps-based lifecycle governance after pre-deployment evaluation. Machine Learning Operations (MLOps) is an operational infrastructure needed to support managing the development, deployment, and maintenance of machine learning models in a structured and repeatable way. Medical settings demand that MLOps pipelines have a high level of data governance practices, version control systems, audit trails, and automated testing pipelines. These elements offer the guarantee that all model updates will be traceable and in accordance with the clinical safety. As an example, the lineage of datasets tracking can enable institutions to record the source and pre-processing of clinical data that were applied in training and fine-tuning. Before deploying each new cycle, automated validation tests can be used to assess model outputs on risks of hallucination, patterns of bias, and adherence to guidelines. Model registries also facilitate transparency by keeping records of model configurations, training parameters and performance measures.

Collectively, these processes empower healthcare organizations to implement LLM systems in a responsible way and be accountable to regulations.

The other important feature of MLOps governance implementation is the integration of human-in-the-loop controls. Clinical decision-making is complex in nature, and AI systems are not supposed to replace professional judgment but assist in it. Consequently, safety frameworks integrated should have check points where domain analysts examine model products, assess safety reports, and endorse significant changes prior to execution. This team-building process assists in ensuring confidence in AI systems and at the same time ensures that automated procedures do not stray off course. The human control is also a significant factor when there is ambiguity in model output and in cases of subtle errors in reasoning that automatic evaluation tools might not be able to detect.

The third pillar in the integrated framework is ongoing checking of deployed models. After medical LLM becomes part of healthcare systems, the behaviour of these systems needs to be closely monitored to identify risks and performance decay. There are continuous monitoring mechanisms that monitor many indicators including frequency of hallucinations, adherence to guidelines, demographic equity and semantic drift in model outputs. There are dynamic aspects of healthcare settings, and the clinical guidelines, demographics of the patients, and medical knowledge are subject to continuous changes. These changes may result in changes in distribution that diminish the model reliability over time. To detect irregularities in model behaviour, pipelines therefore are monitored with statistical drift detectors, semantic analysis, and real-time logging systems.

Safety feedback loops are closely associated with continuous monitoring to enable clinicians and system administrators to report problematic model outputs. The incidents are classified and processed in the MLOps pipeline when unsafe responses or reasoning errors are detected. This feedback, in turn, feeds further updates to the model, retaining or re-training, or modification to safety policies. This cycle of improvement allows healthcare institutions to retain long-term model safety and meet the changes in clinics.

Notably, red-teaming, MLOps governance, and monitoring processes are integrated to make the safety management not a one-time assessment exercise but a process in the lifecycle. The integrated framework encourages continuous learning and risk reduction throughout the first-order operations of the AI system instead of applying only pre-deployment validation. This lifecycle methodology is parallel to new regulatory guidelines being released by government agencies like the U.S. Food and Drug Administration and the European Union AI Act, which also highlight the need to have post-deployment surveillance and openness in AI governance.

Overall, safe implementation of LLMs in healthcare needs a coordinated safety infrastructure that extends across the model life cycle. Red-teaming aids in identifying the weak points prior to its deployment, MLOps governance ensures the transparent and controlled system administration, and continuous monitoring allows identifying the new vulnerabilities early. These elements combine to create a holistic safety model that can facilitate a credible and accountable generative AI technology uptake in clinical application.

7. FUTURE RESEARCH DIRECTIONS IN MEDICAL LLM SAFETY

The recent accelerated development of big language models (LLMs) in medical institutions creates great possibilities to enhance clinical decision support and medical records, as well as communication with patients. Nevertheless, the safe and reliable utilization of these systems is still a challenge of a standalone task. The future studies should thus aim to come up with more resilient models of assessing and managing medical LLMs in their lifecycle.

A key area of research is in the development of standardized safety standards specifically in the field of healthcare. Although existing evaluation datasets (MedQA and PubMedQA) do offer valuable performance metrics, they tend to lack the capacity to reproduce real-life clinical complexity. Many different patient cases, uncommon conditions, vague symptoms, and ethical issues should be used in the future as benchmarks to improve the way models think and behave safely.

Advanced monitoring and risk detection systems development is another important sphere of study. In real-time clinical settings, continuous monitoring pipelines need to be developed to identify insidious manifestations of model drift, hallucinations, and biased output. The combination of monitoring tools with electronic health record systems and hospital governance platforms may enable healthcare organizations to better address possible safety concerns at earlier stages and react more efficiently.

There is also a need to conduct research that can enhance human-AI interaction in clinical procedures. Medical LLMs are not to be used as substitutes to professional judgment; they should be used as aids that can complement the decision-making process of clinicians. To preserve clinician trust and ensure responsible AI use, it will be necessary to design clear interfaces that convey model uncertainty, reasoning paths, and sources of evidence.

Lastly, the regulatory and ethical frameworks that could be used to balance between innovation and patient safety should be examined in the future. Since the health care AI systems are becoming more and more adjustable and data-driven, the regulators and the developers will have to cooperate in order to develop a set of guidelines that will help promote transparency, accountability, and ongoing safety assessment. The reinforcement of such governance arrangements will be critical in facilitating safe and sustainable uptake of LLM technologies into contemporary healthcare systems.

8. CONCLUSION

Implementing large language models in healthcare is a big breakthrough in medical AI. Nevertheless, to make them a safe part of clinical workflows, it is necessary to implement a perfect governance framework to respond to the special risks of generative AI. This chapter has discussed three of the three complementary medical LLM safety pillars, namely red-teaming, MLOps-based lifecycle governance, and continuous monitoring frameworks. Collectively, these methods furnish a methodical plan of locating vulnerabilities, preserving the reliability of operations, and identifying the emergent risks in the actual deployment. As the healthcare systems keep embracing the use of generative AI technologies, upcoming studies have to concentrate on the development of consistent safety standards, enhancement of transparency measures, and the creation of coordination between clinicians, AI developers, and regulatory bodies.

REFERENCES

Amann, J., Blasimme, A., Vayena, E., Frey, D., & Madai, V. I. (2020). Explainability for artificial intelligence in healthcare: A multidisciplinary perspective. *BMC Medical Informatics and Decision Making*, *20*(1), 310. DOI: 10.1186/s12911-020-01332-6 PMID: 33256715

Awasthi, R., Bhattad, A., Ramachandran, S. P., Mishra, S., Khanna, A. K., Cywinski, J. B., Maheshwari, K., Mahapatra, D., DiRosa, I., Cohen, A., Arshad, H., Atreja, A., Alshukaili, A., Vohra, A., Singh, N., Papay, F. A., Atreja, A., Kashyap, R., & Mathur, P. (2025). Human evaluation of large language models in healthcare. *Npj Health Systems*, *2*(1), 40. Advance online publication. DOI: 10.1038/s44401-025-00043-2

Ayoub, A.. (2023). Evaluating large language models for clinical decision support under adversarial conditions. *NPJ Digital Medicine*, *6*, 210. DOI: 10.1038/s41746-023-00928-3

Basu, S.. (2022). Monitoring semantic drift in clinical language models. *Journal of Biomedical Informatics*, *128*, 104039. DOI: 10.1016/j.jbi.2022.104039

Bender, E. M., & Friedman, B. (2018). Data statements for natural language processing: Toward mitigating system bias and enabling better science. *Transactions of the ACL*, *6*, 587–604. DOI: 10.1162/tacl_a_00041

Benjamens, S., Dhunnoo, P., & Meskó, B. (2022). The state of artificial intelligence–based FDA-approved medical devices and algorithms. *NPJ Digital Medicine*, *3*(1), 118. DOI: 10.1038/s41746-020-00324-0 PMID: 32984550

Bommasani, R., ... (2021). On the opportunities and risks of foundation models. *arXiv preprint arXiv:2108.07258*. https://doi.org//arXiv.2108.07258DOI: 10.48550

Carlini, N.. (2023). Extracting training data from large language models. *USENIX Security Symposium*. DOI: 10.48550/arXiv.2012.07805

Castiglioni, I.. (2021). Machine learning applied to medical imaging: A systematic review. *European Radiology*, *31*, 554–566. DOI: 10.1007/s00330-020-07214-4

Chang, Q.. (2025). Expert consensus on retrospective evaluation of large language model applications in clinical scenarios. *Chinese Medical Journal*.

Chen, I. Y., Johansson, F. D., & Sontag, D. (2023). Why is my classifier discriminatory? *ACM Conference on Fairness, Accountability, and Transparency*. DOI: 10.1145/3531146.3533233

Doshi-Velez, F., & Kim, B. (2017). Towards a rigorous science of interpretable machine learning. *arXiv preprint arXiv:1702.08608*. https://doi.org//arXiv.1702.08608DOI: 10.48550

European Commission. (2024). *Artificial Intelligence Act*. Official Journal of the European Union.

. European Parliament. (2023). AI Act: Regulatory framework for high-risk AI systems.

. FDA. (2022). Software as a Medical Device (SaMD): Clinical evaluation.

. FDA. (2023). Good Machine Learning Practice for Medical Device Development.

Ganguli, D., ... (2023). Red teaming language models to reduce harms. *arXiv preprint arXiv:2209.07858*. https://doi.org//arXiv.2209.07858DOI: 10.48550

Gianfrancesco, M. A., Tamang, S., Yazdany, J., & Schmajuk, G. (2018). Potential biases in machine learning algorithms using electronic health record data. *JAMA Internal Medicine*, *178*(11), 1544–1547. DOI: 10.1001/jamainternmed.2018.3763 PMID: 30128552

Jacobs, M.. (2021). The value of interpretability in machine learning for medicine. *Communications of the ACM*, *64*(1), 57–65. DOI: 10.1145/3348485

Ji, Z., Lee, N., Frieske, R., Yu, T., Su, D., Xu, Y., Ishii, E., Bang, Y. J., Madotto, A., & Fung, P. (2023). Survey of hallucination in natural language generation. *ACM Computing Surveys*, *55*(12), 1–38. Advance online publication. DOI: 10.1145/3571730

Jin, Q.. (2021). *PubMedQA: A dataset for biomedical research question answering*. EMNLP., DOI: 10.18653/v1/2021.emnlp-main.784

Jindal, M., ... (2025). SAGE: A generic framework for large language model safety evaluation. *Proceedings of the EMNLP Industry Track*. https://aclanthology.org/2025.emnlp-industry.2/

Kellogg, K. C.. (2017). Patient safety incident reporting systems. *BMJ Quality & Safety*, *26*(2), 96–105. DOI: 10.1136/bmjqs-2015-004386 PMID: 29217696

Kocbek, S.. (2020). Text mining electronic hospital records to automate clinical coding. *Journal of Biomedical Informatics*, *102*, 103374. DOI: 10.1016/j.jbi.2019.103374

Kreuzberger, D., Kühl, N., & Hirschl, S. (2023). Machine learning operations (MLOps): Overview and challenges. *IEEE Access : Practical Innovations, Open Solutions*, *11*, 30920–30938. DOI: 10.1109/ACCESS.2023.3262138

Krittanawong, C.. (2023). ChatGPT in cardiovascular medicine. *Nature Reviews. Cardiology*, *20*, 593–594. DOI: 10.1038/s41569-023-00819-8

Levine, D. M.. (2023). Monitoring deployed clinical AI systems. *NPJ Digital Medicine*, *6*, 55. DOI: 10.1038/s41746-023-00760-9

Li, Y., ... (2023). SafetyBench: Evaluating the safety of large language models. *arXiv preprint arXiv:2309.07045*. https://doi.org//arXiv.2309.07045DOI: 10.48550

Long, J.. (2023). Evaluating AI systems under real-world clinical conditions. *Nature Medicine*, *29*, 202–210. DOI: 10.1038/s41591-022-02043-7

Lu, J.. (2022). Learning under concept drift: A review. *IEEE Transactions on Knowledge and Data Engineering*, *34*(9), 4287–4312. DOI: 10.1109/TKDE.2020.3042330

Lwakatare, L. E.. (2020). DevOps in practice: A multiple case study. *Information and Software Technology*, *114*, 106–118. DOI: 10.1016/j.infsof.2019.06.009

Nguyen, G.. (2022). Machine learning lifecycle management. *IEEE Software*, *39*(2), 42–49. DOI: 10.1109/MS.2021.3135619

Nori, H.. (2023). Capabilities of GPT-4 in medicine. *NPJ Digital Medicine*, *6*, 98. DOI: 10.1038/s41746-023-00788-x

Obermeyer, Z.. (2019). Dissecting racial bias in health algorithms. *Science*, *366*(6464), 447–453. DOI: 10.1126/science.aax2342 PMID: 31649194

Poursabzi-Sangdeh, F.. (2021). Manipulating and measuring model interpretability. *CHI Conference*. DOI: 10.1145/3411764.3445315

Rajkomar, A., Hardt, M., Howell, M. D., Corrado, G., & Chin, M. H. (2018). Ensuring fairness in machine learning to advance health equity. *Annals of Internal Medicine*, *169*(12), 866–872. DOI: 10.7326/M18-1990 PMID: 30508424

Sendak, M. P.. (2020). A path for translation of machine learning products into healthcare delivery. *NPJ Digital Medicine*, *3*, 109. DOI: 10.1038/s41746-020-00349-5

Shen, Y.. (2023). Large language models in medicine: Evaluation and deployment. *Nature Medicine*, *29*, 26–36. DOI: 10.1038/s41591-022-02116-7

Singhal, K., Azizi, S., Tu, T., Mahdavi, S. S., Wei, J., Chung, H. W., Scales, N., Tanwani, A., Cole-Lewis, H., Pfohl, S., Payne, P., Seneviratne, M., Gamble, P., Kelly, C., Babiker, A., Schärli, N., Chowdhery, A., Mansfield, P., Demner-Fushman, D., & Natarajan, V. (2023). Large language models encode clinical knowledge. *Nature*, *620*(7972), 172–180. DOI: 10.1038/s41586-023-06291-2 PMID: 37438534

Wei, J., ... (2022). Chain-of-thought prompting elicits reasoning in LLMs. *NeurIPS*. https://doi.org//arXiv.2201.11903DOI: 10.48550

. WHO? (2021). Ethics and governance of artificial intelligence for health.

Widmer, G., & Kubat, M. (1996). Learning in the presence of concept drift. *Machine Learning*, *30*(1), 69–101. DOI: 10.1023/A:1018046501280

Zhang, Y.. (2024). Real-time monitoring of large language models in healthcare. *IEEE Journal of Biomedical and Health Informatics*. Advance online publication. DOI: 10.1109/JBHI.2024.3341125

Compilation of References

Abbas, S. R., Abbas, Z., Zahir, A., & Lee, S. W. (2024). Federated learning in smart healthcare: A comprehensive review on privacy, security, and predictive analytics with IoT integration. *Healthcare (Basel)*, *12*(24), 2587. DOI: 10.3390/healthcare12242587

Abd-Alrazaq, A., AlSaad, R., Alhuwail, D., Ahmed, A., Healy, P. M., Latifi, S., Aziz, S., Damseh, R., Alrazak, S. A., & Sheikh, J. (2023). Large language models in medical education: Opportunities, challenges, and future directions. *JMIR Medical Education*, *9*(1), e48291. DOI: 10.2196/48291 PMID: 37261894

Abd-Alrazaq, A., Safi, Z., Alajlani, M., Warren, J., Househ, M., & Denecke, K. (2020). Technical metrics used to evaluate health care chatbots: Scoping review. *Journal of Medical Internet Research*, *22*(6), e18301. DOI: 10.2196/18301 PMID: 32442157

Abdelwanis, M., Alarafati, H. K., Tammam, M. M. S., & Simsekler, M. C. E. (2024). Exploring the risks of automation bias in healthcare AI applications: A Bowtie analysis. *Journal of Safety Science and Resilience = An Quan Ke Xue Yu Ren Xing (Ying Wen)*, *5*(4), 460–469.

Abikenari, M., Awad, M. H., Korouri, S., Mohseni, K., Abikenari, D., Freichel, R., Mukadam, Y., Tanzim, U., Habib, A., & Kerwan, A. (2025). *Reframing clinical AI evaluation in the era of generative models: Toward multidimensional, stakeholder-informed, and safety-centric frameworks for real-world health care deployment.* Premier Journal of Science., DOI: 10.70389/PJS.100089

Adams, S. J., Mikhael, P., Wohlwend, J., Barzilay, R., Sequist, L. V., & Fintelmann, F. J. (2023). Artificial Intelligence and Machine Learning in Lung Cancer Screening. *Thoracic Surgery Clinics*, *33*(4), 401–409. DOI: 10.1016/j.thorsurg.2023.03.001 PMID: 37806742

Agarwal, R.. (2024). Evaluating the reliability of large language models in clinical settings. *Nature Medicine*, *30*(2), 245–252.

Agency for Healthcare Research and Quality. (2024). Patient safety indicators technical specifications (AHRQ Publication No. 24-0001). U.S. Department of Health and Human Services. https://qualityindicators.ahrq.gov/Archive/psi_techspec/icd10_v2024

Ai/ML Enthusiast, U. S. A., Sivalingam, E., & Chinnachamy, T. (2025a). Explainable GENAI techniques to interpret and visualize LLM reasoning. INTERNATIONAL JOURNAL OF SCIENTIFIC RESEARCH IN ENGINEERING AND MANAGEMENT, 09(10), 1–9. https://doi.org/DOI: 10.55041/IJSREM53123

Ajmera, P., Dillard, R., Kline, T., Missert, A., Korfiatis, P., & Khandelwal, A. (2025). FDA-approved artificial intelligence products in abdominal imaging: A comprehensive review. *Current Problems in Diagnostic Radiology, S0363018825000829*. Advance online publication. DOI: 10.1067/j.cpradiol.2025.04.011 PMID: 40287285

Akinci D'Antonoli, T., Tejani, A. S., Khosravi, B., Bluethgen, C., Busch, F., Bressem, K. K., Adams, L. C., Moassefi, M., Faghani, S., & Gichoya, J. W. (2025). Cybersecurity Threats and Mitigation Strategies for Large Language Models in Health Care. *Radiology. Artificial Intelligence*, *7*(4), e240739. Advance online publication. DOI: 10.1148/ryai.240739 PMID: 40366259

Al Nazi, Z., & Peng, W. (2024). Large Language Models in Healthcare and Medical Domain: A Review. *Informatics (MDPI)*, *11*(3), 57. DOI: 10.3390/informatics11030057

Alaa, A., Hartvigsen, T., Golchini, N., Dutta, S., Dean, F., Raji, I. D., & Zack, T. (2025). Position: Medical large language model benchmarks should prioritize construct validity. In *Proceedings of the 42nd International Conference on Machine Learning (ICML)*.

Alami, H., Lehoux, P., Papoutsi, C., Shaw, S. E., Fleet, R., & Fortin, J. P. (2024). Understanding the integration of artificial intelligence in healthcare organisations and systems through the NASSS framework: A qualitative study in a leading Canadian academic centre. *BMC Health Services Research*, *24*(1), 701. DOI: 10.1186/s12913-024-11112-x PMID: 38831298

Alber, F.. (2023). Challenges of implementing LLMs in clinical practice: Perspectives. *Journal of Clinical Medicine*, *14*(17), 6169. DOI: 10.3390/jcm14176169

Alboksmaty, A., Aldakhil, R., Hayhoe, B. W. J., Ashrafian, H., Darzi, A., & Neves, A.-L. (2025). The impact of using AI-powered voice-to-text technology for clinical documentation on quality of care in primary care and outpatient settings: A systematic review. *EBioMedicine*, *118*, 105861. DOI: 10.1016/j.ebiom.2025.105861 PMID: 40694861

Alcalá Minagorre, P. J., Salmerón Fernández, M. J., Domingo Garau, A., Díaz Pernas, P., Nebot Marzal, C. M., Pino Ramírez, R. M., & Madrid Rodríguez, A. (2025). Strategies for improving diagnostic safety and clinical reasoning. *Anales de Pediatría (English Ed.), 102*(4), 503827. DOI: 10.1016/j.anpede.2025.503827 PMID: 40246601

Aljohani, M., Hou, J., Kommu, S., & Wang, X. (2025). A comprehensive survey on the trustworthiness of large language models in healthcare. 6720–6748. DOI: 10.18653/v1/2025.findings-emnlp.356

Alkalbani, A. M., Alrawahi, A. S., Salah, A., Haghighi, V., Zhang, Y., Alkindi, S., & Sheng, Q. Z. (2025). A systematic review of large language models in medical specialties: Applications, challenges and future directions. *Information (Basel), 16*(6), 489. DOI: 10.3390/info16060489

Allen, A. M., Younossi, Z. M., Diehl, A. M., Charlton, M. R., & Lazarus, J. V. (2024). Envisioning how to advance the MASH field. *Nature Reviews. Gastroenterology & Hepatology, 21*(10), 726–738. DOI: 10.1038/s41575-024-00938-9 PMID: 38834817

Alowais, S. A., Alghamdi, S. S., Alsuhebany, N., Alqahtani, T., Alshaya, A. I., Almohareb, S. N., Aldairem, A., Alrashed, M., Bin Saleh, K., Badreldin, H. A., Al Yami, M. S., Al Harbi, S., & Albekairy, A. M. (2023). Revolutionizing healthcare: The role of artificial intelligence in clinical practice. *BMC Medical Education, 23*(1), 689. DOI: 10.1186/s12909-023-04698-z PMID: 37740191

Al-Qerem, W., Eberhardt, J., Jarab, A., Al Bawab, A. Q., Hammad, A., Alasmari, F., Alazab, B., Husein, D. A., Alazab, J., & Al-Beool, S. (2023). Exploring knowledge, attitudes, and practices towards artificial intelligence among health professions' students in Jordan. *BMC Medical Informatics and Decision Making, 23*(1), 288. DOI: 10.1186/s12911-023-02403-0 PMID: 38098095

Amann, J., Blasimme, A., Vayena, E., Frey, D., & Madai, V. I. (2020). Explainability for artificial intelligence in healthcare: A multidisciplinary perspective. *BMC Medical Informatics and Decision Making, 20*(1), 1–9. DOI: 10.1186/s12911-020-01332-6 PMID: 33256715

Amodei, D., Olah, C., Steinhardt, J., Christiano, P., Schulman, J., & Mané, D. (2023). *Concrete problems in AI safety*. arXiv. https://arxiv.org/abs/1606.06565

Anyaso, K., & Okoye, V. (2024). The impact of big data and predictive analytics on U.S. healthcare delivery: Opportunities, challenges, and future directions. *World Journal of Advanced Research and Reviews, 24*(1), 2275–2287. DOI: 10.30574/wjarr.2024.24.1.3266

Aramaki, E., Wakamiya, S., Yada, S., Hisada, S., & Tamayo, L. P. V. (2025). NTCIR-18 MedNLP-CHAT: Determining medical, ethical, and legal risks in patient-doctor conversations. In *Proceedings of the NTCIR-18 Conference*.

Aravazhi, P. S., Gunasekaran, P., Benjamin, N. Z. Y., Thai, A., Chandrasekar, K. K., Kolanu, N. D., Prajjwal, P., Tekuru, Y., Brito, L. V., & Inban, P. (2025). The integration of artificial intelligence into clinical medicine: Trends, challenges, and future directions. *Disease-a-Month : DM*, *71*(6), 101882. DOI: 10.1016/j.disamonth.2025.101882 PMID: 40140300

Arora, A., Kaffee, L., & Augenstein, I. (2023). Probing Pre-Trained Language Models for Cross-Cultural Differences in Values. *Proceedings of the First Workshop on Cross-Cultural Considerations in NLP (C3NLP)*, 114–130. DOI: 10.18653/v1/2023.c3nlp-1.12

Arora, R. K.. (2025). HealthBench: Evaluating large language models towards improved human health. *arXiv*. https://arxiv.org/abs/2505.08775

Asgari, E.. (2025). Safety evaluation frameworks for AI in healthcare: A systematic review. *IEEE Journal of Biomedical and Health Informatics*, *29*(1), 112–125.

Asgari, E., Montaña-Brown, N., Dubois, M., Khalil, S., Balloch, J., Au Yeung, J., & Pimenta, D. (2025). A framework to assess clinical safety and hallucination rates of LLMs for medical text summarisation. npj. *Digital Medicine*, *8*(1), 274. DOI: 10.1038/s41746-025-01670-7 PMID: 40360677

Awasthi, R., Bhattad, A., Ramachandran, S. P., Mishra, S., Khanna, A. K., Cywinski, J. B., Maheshwari, K., Mahapatra, D., DiRosa, I., Cohen, A., Arshad, H., Atreja, A., Alshukaili, A., Vohra, A., Singh, N., Papay, F. A., Atreja, A., Kashyap, R., & Mathur, P. (2025). Human evaluation of large language models in healthcare. *Npj Health Systems*, *2*(1), 40. Advance online publication. DOI: 10.1038/s44401-025-00043-2

Ayaan, A., & Ng, K. W. (2025). Automated grading using natural language processing and semantic analysis. *MethodsX*, *103395*, 103395. Advance online publication. DOI: 10.1016/j.mex.2025.103395 PMID: 40529512

Ayoub, A.. (2023). Evaluating large language models for clinical decision support under adversarial conditions. *NPJ Digital Medicine*, *6*, 210. DOI: 10.1038/s41746-023-00928-3

Azamfirei, R., Kudchadkar, S. R., & Fackler, J. (2023). Large language models and the perils of their hallucinations. *Critical Care : The Official Journal of the Critical Care Forum*, *27*(1), 120. DOI: 10.1186/s13054-023-04393-x PMID: 36945051

Banyi, N., Ma, B., Amanian, A., Bur, A., & Abdalkhani, A. (2025). Applications of natural language processing in otolaryngology: A scoping review. *The Laryngoscope*, *135*(9), 3049–3063. DOI: 10.1002/lary.32198 PMID: 40309961

Basu, S.. (2022). Monitoring semantic drift in clinical language models. *Journal of Biomedical Informatics*, *128*, 104039. DOI: 10.1016/j.jbi.2022.104039

Beam, A. L., & Kohane, I. S. (2020). Big data and machine learning in health care. *Journal of the American Medical Association*, *319*(13), 1317–1318. DOI: 10.1001/jama.2017.18391 PMID: 29532063

Beauchamp, T., & Childress, J. (2021). Principles of biomedical ethics: Marking its fortieth anniversary. *The American Journal of Bioethics : AJOB*, *19*(11), 9–12. DOI: 10.1080/15265161.2019.1665402 PMID: 31647760

Bedi, S., Liu, Y., Orr-Ewing, L., Dash, D., Koyejo, S., Callahan, A., Fries, J. A., Wornow, M., Swaminathan, A., Lehmann, L. S., Hong, H. J., Kashyap, M., Chaurasia, A. R., Shah, N. R., Singh, K., Tazbaz, T., Milstein, A., Pfeffer, M. A., & Shah, N. H. (2025). Testing and evaluation of health care applications of large language models: A systematic review. *Journal of the American Medical Association*, *333*(4), 319–328. DOI: 10.1001/jama.2024.21700 PMID: 39405325

Bednarczyk, L., Reichenpfader, D., Gaudet-Blavignac, C., Ette, A. K., Zaghir, J., Zheng, Y., Bensahla, A., Bjelogrlic, M., & Lovis, C. (2025). Scientific evidence for clinical text summarization using large language models: Scoping review. *Journal of Medical Internet Research*, *27*, e68998. DOI: 10.2196/68998 PMID: 40371947

Beidas, R. S., Volpp, K. G., Buttenheim, A. N., Marcus, S. C., Olfson, M., Pellecchia, M., Stewart, R. E., Williams, N. J., Becker-Haimes, E. M., Candon, M., Cidav, Z., Fishman, J., Lieberman, A., Zentgraf, K., & Mandell, D. (2019). Transforming mental health delivery through behavioral economics and implementation science: Protocol for three exploratory projects. *JMIR Research Protocols*, *8*(2), e12121. DOI: 10.2196/12121 PMID: 30747719

Belkhouribchia, J., & Pen, J. J. (2025). Large language models in clinical nutrition: An overview of its applications, capabilities, limitations, and potential future prospects. *Frontiers in Nutrition*, *12*(1635682), 1635682. DOI: 10.3389/fnut.2025.1635682 PMID: 40851903

Benary, M., Wang, X. D., Schmidt, M., Soll, D., Hilfenhaus, G., Nassir, M., Sigler, C., Knödler, M., Keller, U., Beule, D., Keilholz, U., Leser, U., & Rieke, D. T. (2023). Leveraging large language models for decision support in personalized oncology. *JAMA Network Open*, *6*(11), e2343689. DOI: 10.1001/jamanetworkopen.2023.43689 PMID: 37976064

Bender, E. M., & Friedman, B. (2018). Data statements for natural language processing: Toward mitigating system bias and enabling better science. *Transactions of the ACL, 6*, 587–604. DOI: 10.1162/tacl_a_00041

Bender, E. M., Gebru, T., McMillan-Major, A., & Shmitchell, S. (2021). On the dangers of stochastic parrots: Can language models be too big? In *Proceedings of the 2021 ACM Conference on Fairness, Accountability, and Transparency* (pp. 610–623). DOI: 10.1145/3442188.3445922

Benjamens, S., Dhunnoo, P., & Meskó, B. (2022). The state of artificial intelligence–based FDA-approved medical devices and algorithms. *NPJ Digital Medicine, 3*(1), 118. DOI: 10.1038/s41746-020-00324-0 PMID: 32984550

Berry, P., Dhanakshirur, R. R., & Khanna, S. (2025). Utilizing large language models for gastroenterology research: A conceptual framework. *Therapeutic Advances in Gastroenterology, 18*, 17562848251328576. DOI: 10.1177/17562848251328577 PMID: 40171241

Bhimani, M., Miller, A., Agnew, J. D., Ausin, M. S., Raglow-Defranco, M., Mangat, H., Voisard, M., Taylor, M., Bierman-Lytle, S., Parikh, V., Ghukasyan, J., Lasko, R., Godil, S., Atreja, A., & Mukherjee, S. (2025). Real-world evaluation of large language models in healthcare (RWE-LLM): A new realm of AI safety & validation. DOI: 10.1101/2025.03.17.25324157

Botross, M., Mohammadi, S. O., Montgomery, K., & Crawford, C. (2024). Performance of Google's artificial intelligence chatbot "Bard" (now "Gemini") on ophthalmology board exam practice questions. *Cureus, 16*(3), e57348. DOI: 10.7759/cureus.57348 PMID: 38690460

Broch Porcar, M. J., & Castellanos-Ortega, Á. (2025). Patient safety, what does clinical simulation and teaching innovation contribute? *Medicina intensiva, 49*(3), 165–173. DOI: 10.1016/j.medin.2024.03.017 PMID: 38797620

Brown, T. B., Mann, B., & Ryder, N.. (2020). Language models are few-shot learners. *Advances in Neural Information Processing Systems, 33*, 1877–1901.

Bruner, L. P., White, A. M., & Proksell, S. (2023). Inflammatory bowel disease. *Primary Care, 50*(3), 411–427. DOI: 10.1016/j.pop.2023.03.009 PMID: 37516511

Busch, F., Hoffmann, L., dos Santos, D. P., Makowski, M. R., Saba, L., Prucker, P., Hadamitzky, M., Navab, N., Kather, J. N., Truhn, D., Cuocolo, R., Adams, L. C., & Bressem, K. K. (2024). Large language models for structured reporting in radiology: Past, present, and future. *European Radiology, 35*(5), 2589–2602. DOI: 10.1007/s00330-024-11107-6 PMID: 39438330

Cabral, S., Restrepo, D., Kanjee, Z., Wilson, P., Crowe, B., Abdulnour, R.-E., & Rodman, A. (2024). Clinical reasoning of a generative artificial intelligence model compared with physicians. *JAMA Internal Medicine, 184*(5), 581–583. DOI: 10.1001/jamainternmed.2024.0295 PMID: 38557971

Caliskan, A., Bryson, J. J., & Narayanan, A. (2020). Semantics derived automatically from language corpora contain human-like biases. *Science, 356*(6334), 183–186. DOI: 10.1126/science.aal4230 PMID: 28408601

Caner, V. (2025). Profiling safety behavior in clinical laboratory environments. *Frontiers in Public Health, 13*, 1681513. DOI: 10.3389/fpubh.2025.1681513 PMID: 41080846

Carlini, N., Tramer, F., Wallace, E., Jagielski, M., Herbert-Voss, A., Lee, K., Roberts, A., Brown, T., Song, D., Erlingsson, U., Oprea, A., & Raffel, C. (2021). Extracting training data from large language models. *arXiv preprint arXiv:2012.07805.*

Carlini, N.. (2023). Extracting training data from large language models. *USENIX Security Symposium.* DOI: 10.48550/arXiv.2012.07805

Castiglioni, I.. (2021). Machine learning applied to medical imaging: A systematic review. *European Radiology, 31*, 554–566. DOI: 10.1007/s00330-020-07214-4

Chang, K. W., Prabhakaran, V., & Ordonez, V. (2019). Bias and fairness in natural language processing. In *Proceedings of the 2019 Conference on Empirical Methods in Natural Language Processing.*

Chang, Q.. (2025). Expert consensus on retrospective evaluation of large language model applications in clinical scenarios. *Chinese Medical Journal.*

Chang, Y., Yin, J., Li, J., Liu, C., Cao, L., & Lin, S. (2024). Applications and Future Prospects of Medical LLMs: A Survey Based on the M-KAT Conceptual Framework. *Journal of Medical Systems, 48*(1), 112. DOI: 10.1007/s10916-024-02132-5 PMID: 39725770

Char, D. S., Shah, N. H., & Magnus, D. (2023). Implementing machine learning in health care—Addressing ethical challenges. *The New England Journal of Medicine, 378*(11), 981–983. DOI: 10.1056/NEJMp1714229 PMID: 29539284

Chau, M., Rahman, M. G., & Debnath, T. (2025). From black box to clarity: Strategies for effective AI informed consent in healthcare. *Artificial Intelligence in Medicine, 167*, 103169. DOI: 10.1016/j.artmed.2025.103169 PMID: 40446592

Chen, L., & Lee, S. (2023). Large language model empowered privacy-protected framework for PHI annotation in clinical notes. *IOS Press*. https://pubmed.ncbi.nlm.nih.gov/40775983/

Chen, D., Huang, R. S., Jomy, J., Wong, P., Yan, M., Croke, J., Tong, D., Hope, A., Eng, L., & Raman, S. (2024). Performance of multimodal artificial intelligence chatbots evaluated on clinical oncology cases. *JAMA Network Open*, *7*(10), e2437711. DOI: 10.1001/jamanetworkopen.2024.37711 PMID: 39441598

Chen, I. Y., Johansson, F. D., & Sontag, D. (2023). Why is my classifier discriminatory? *ACM Conference on Fairness, Accountability, and Transparency*. DOI: 10.1145/3531146.3533233

Chen, L. (2024). Building trust and interpretability in medical AI through explainable models. *Journal of AI in Healthcare and Medicine*, *4*(1).

Chen, S., Gao, M., Sasse, K., Hartvigsen, T., Anthony, B., Fan, L., Aerts, H., Gallifant, J., & Bitterman, D. S. (2025). When helpfulness backfires: LLMs and the risk of false medical information due to sycophantic behavior. npj. *Digital Medicine*, *8*(1), 605. DOI: 10.1038/s41746-025-02008-z PMID: 41107408

Chen, Z., Liang, N., Zhang, H., Li, H., Yang, Y., Zong, X., Chen, Y., Wang, Y., & Shi, N. (2023). Harnessing the power of clinical decision support systems: Challenges and opportunities. *Open Heart*, *10*(2), e002432. DOI: 10.1136/openhrt-2023-002432 PMID: 38016787

Chow, J. C. L., & Li, K. (2025). Large language models in medical chatbots: Opportunities, challenges, and the need to address AI risks. *Information (Basel)*, *16*(7), 549. DOI: 10.3390/info16070549

Chuang, Y.-S., Sarkar, A. R., Hsu, Y.-C., Mohammed, N., & Jiang, X. (2025). Robust privacy amidst innovation with large language models through a critical assessment of the risks. *Journal of the American Medical Informatics Association : JAMIA*, *32*(5), 885–892. DOI: 10.1093/jamia/ocaf037 PMID: 40112189

Clusmann, J., Kolbinger, F. R., Muti, H. S., Carrero, Z. I., Eckardt, J.-N., Laleh, N. G., Löffler, C. M. L., Schwarzkopf, S.-C., Unger, M., Veldhuizen, G. P., Wagner, S. J., & Kather, J. N. (2023). The future landscape of large language models in medicine. *Communications Medicine*, *3*(1), 141. DOI: 10.1038/s43856-023-00370-1 PMID: 37816837

Collins, F. S., & Varmus, H. (2020). A new initiative on precision medicine. *The New England Journal of Medicine*, *372*(9), 793–795. DOI: 10.1056/NEJMp1500523 PMID: 25635347

Colombel, J.-F., Narula, N., & Peyrin-Biroulet, L. (2017). Management strategies to improve outcomes of patients with inflammatory bowel diseases. *Gastroenterology*, *152*(2), 351–361. DOI: 10.1053/j.gastro.2016.09.046 PMID: 27720840

Coye, L., Jones, M. A., Gaza-Bulseco, G., Chitikila, C., Clavier, S., Fougeron, D., Grimaldi, C., Hurkmans, K., Hutchinson, R., Kellogg, B., Liu, X., Palackal, N., Tank, M., Valax, P., Waerner, T., Wang, F., Zhang, Y., Zhao, Y., Sloan, S., & de Zafra, C. Z. (2025). Host Cell Protein Clinical Safety Risk Assessment-An Updated Industry Review. *Biotechnology and Bioengineering*, *122*(11), 3229–3248. DOI: 10.1002/bit.70029 PMID: 40757641

Czarnowska, P., Vyas, Y., & Shah, K. (2021). Quantifying social biases in NLP: A generalization and empirical comparison of extrinsic fairness metrics. *Transactions of the Association for Computational Linguistics*, *9*, 1249–1267. DOI: 10.1162/tacl_a_00425

Daneshjou, R., Vodrahalli, K., Novoa, R. A., Jenkins, M., Liang, W., Rotemberg, V., Ko, J., Swetter, S. M., Bailey, E. E., Gevaert, O., Mukherjee, P., Phung, M., Yekrang, K., Fong, B., Sahasrabudhe, R., Allerup, J. A. C., Okata-Karigane, U., Zou, J., & Chiou, A. (2022). Disparities in dermatology AI performance on a diverse, curated clinical image set. *Science Advances*, *8*(32), eabq6147. Advance online publication. DOI: 10.1126/sciadv.abq6147 PMID: 35960806

Dang, A. (2023). Real-world evidence: A primer. *Pharmaceutical Medicine*, *37*(1), 25–36. DOI: 10.1007/s40290-022-00456-6 PMID: 36604368

Davahli MR, Karwowski W, Fiok K, Wan T, Parsaei HR. Controlling Safety of Artificial Intelligence Based Systems in Healthcare. Symmetry (Basel). 2021

Davenport, T., & Kalakota, R. (2020). The potential for artificial intelligence in healthcare. *Future Healthcare Journal*, *6*(2), 94–98. DOI: 10.7861/futurehosp.6-2-94 PMID: 31363513

De Vito, G., Ferrucci, F., & Angelakis, A. (2025). LLMs for drug-drug interaction prediction: A comprehensive comparison. *arXiv preprint arXiv:2502.06890.*

Dhade, P., & Shirke, P. (2023). Federated learning for healthcare: A comprehensive review. *Engineering Proceedings*, *59*(1), 230. DOI: 10.3390/engproc2023059230

Di Vita, A., Fusco, G., Lorenzon, L., Tognoni, P., & Maggi, A. (2025). The Model–Context–Relation framework for clinical AI evaluation. *JMIR Formative Research*, *9*, e62845. DOI: 10.2196/62845

Diao, M., Li, R., Liu, S., Liao, G., Wang, J., Cai, X., & Xu, W. (2025). SEAS: Self-Evolving Adversarial Safety optimization for Large Language Models. Proceedings of the ... AAAI Conference on Artificial Intelligence. AAAI Conference on Artificial Intelligence, 39(22), 23778–23786. DOI: 10.1609/aaai.v39i22.34549

Dinc, M. T., Bardak, A. E., Bahar, F., & Noronha, C. (2025). Comparative analysis of large language models in clinical diagnosis. *JAMIA Open*, *8*(3), ooaf055. DOI: 10.1093/jamiaopen/ooaf055 PMID: 40510808

Doherty, C., Baldwin, M., Keogh, A., Caulfield, B., & Argent, R. (2024). Keeping pace with wearables: A living umbrella review of systematic reviews evaluating the accuracy of consumer wearable technologies in health measurement. *Sports Medicine*, *54*(11), 2907–2926. DOI: 10.1007/s40279-024-02077-2 PMID: 39080098

Donnelly, H. K., Brown, G. K., Green, K. L., Vurgun, U., Hwang, S., Schriver, E., Steinberg, M., Reilly, M. E., Mehta, H., Labouliere, C., Oquendo, M. A., Mandell, D., & Mowery, D. L. (2026). Automated Safety Plan Scoring in Outpatient Mental Health Settings Using Large Language Models: Exploratory Study. *JMIR Mental Health*, *13*(1), e79010. DOI: 10.2196/79010 PMID: 41505705

Drăgoi, A.-L., & Neme , R.-M. (2023). The "Electronic Pediatrician (EPed®)" – A clinically tested prototype software for computer-assisted pathophysiologic diagnosis and treatment of ill children. *International Journal of Medical Informatics*, *178*, 105169. DOI: 10.1016/j.ijmedinf.2023.105169 PMID: 37562316

El Hassani, I., Masrour, T., Kourouma, N., Motte, D. C., & Tavčar, J. (2024). Integrating large language models for improved failure mode and effects analysis (FMEA): A framework and case study. *Proceedings of the Design Society*, *4*, 2019–2028. DOI: 10.1017/pds.2024.204

Emanuel, E. J., Wachter, R. M., & Grady, C. (2020). Artificial intelligence in health care: Ethical considerations. *Journal of the American Medical Association*, *323*(6), 509–510. PMID: 31845963

European Commission. (2021). Proposal for a regulation laying down harmonized rules on artificial intelligence (Artificial Intelligence Act). *European Union.*

European Commission. (2021). *Proposal for a regulation laying down harmonized rules on artificial intelligence*. Artificial Intelligence Act.

European Commission. (2024). *Artificial Intelligence Act*. Official Journal of the European Union.

European Parliament. (2024). Regulation (EU) 2024/1689 of the European Parliament and of the Council of 13 June 2024 laying down harmonised rules on artificial intelligence (Artificial Intelligence Act). Official Journal of the European Union, L 2024/1689. https://eur-lex.europa.eu/legal-content/EN/TXT/?uri=OJ:L_202401689

Farquhar, S., Kossen, J., Kuhn, L., & Gal, Y. (2024). Detecting hallucinations in large language models using semantic entropy. *Nature*, *630*(8017), 625–630. DOI: 10.1038/s41586-024-07421-0 PMID: 38898292

Feldman, M. J., Hoffer, E. P., Conley, J. J., Chang, J., Chung, J. A., Jernigan, M. C., Lester, W. T., Strasser, Z. H., & Chueh, H. C. (2025). Dedicated AI expert system vs generative AI with large language model for clinical diagnoses. *JAMA Network Open*, *8*(5), e2512994. DOI: 10.1001/jamanetworkopen.2025.12994 PMID: 40440012

Feretzakis, G., & Verykios, V. S. (2024). Trustworthy AI: Securing Sensitive Data in Large Language Models. *AI*, *5*(4), 2773–2800. DOI: 10.3390/ai5040134

Ferrer, X., Van Nuenen, T., Such, J. M., & Criado, N. (2021). Discovering and Categorising Language Biases in Reddit. *Proceedings of the International AAAI Conference on Web and Social Media, 15*, 140–151. DOI: 10.1609/icwsm.v15i1.18048

Festor, P., Nagendran, M., Gordon, A. C., Faisal, A. A., & Komorowski, M. (2025). Safety of human-AI cooperative decision-making within intensive care: A physical simulation study. *PLOS Digital Health*, *4*(2), e0000726. DOI: 10.1371/journal.pdig.0000726 PMID: 39992918

Finlayson, S. G., Subbaswamy, A., Singh, K., Bowers, J., Kupke, A., Zittrain, J., Kohane, I. S., & Saria, S. (2021). The clinician and dataset shift in artificial intelligence. *The New England Journal of Medicine*, *385*(3), 283–286. DOI: 10.1056/NEJMc2104626 PMID: 34260843

Food and Drug Administration (FDA). (2023). *Artificial intelligence and machine learning in software as a medical device*. U.S. FDA.

Frutuoso, J. (2025). Building a safe and transparent workflow for large language model (LLM)-assisted clinical trials and prediction models: A technical report. *Cureus*, *17*(9), e92571. DOI: 10.7759/cureus.92571 PMID: 41111869

Gaber, D. A., Mayer, M. A., Lau, A. Y. S., & Neves, A. L. (2025). Governance of retrieval-augmented generation in clinical chatbots: Framework and evaluation criteria. npj. *Digital Medicine*, *8*(1), 112. DOI: 10.1038/s41746-025-01234-9 PMID: 39966675

Gaber, F.. (2025). Evaluating large language model workflows in clinical decision support for triage and referral. *npj. Digital Medicine*, *8*, 263. PMID: 40346344

Gaber, F., Shaik, M., Allega, F., Bilecz, A. J., Busch, F., Goon, K., Franke, V., & Akalin, A. (2025). Evaluating large language model workflows in clinical decision support for triage, referral, and diagnosis. *NPJ Digital Medicine*, *8*(1), 263. DOI: 10.1038/s41746-025-01684-1 PMID: 40346344

Gallegos, I. O., Rossi, R. A., Barrow, J., Research, A., Kim, S., Dernoncourt, F., Yu, T., Zhang, R., & Ahmed, N. K. (2024). Bias and Fairness in Large Language Models: A Survey Md Mehrab Tanjim under a Creative Commons Attribution-NonCommercial-NoDerivatives 4.0 International (CC BY-NC-ND 4.0) license. *Computational Linguistics*, *50*(3).

Gallifant, J., Chen, S., Moreira, P., Munch, N., Gao, M., Pond, J., Aerts, H., Celi, L. A., Hartvigsen, T., & Bitterman, D. S. (2024). Language models are surprisingly fragile to drug names in biomedical benchmarks. In *Findings of the 2024 Conference on Empirical Methods in Natural Language Processing* (pp. 12448–12465). DOI: 10.18653/v1/2024.findings-emnlp.726

Gama, F., Tyskbo, D., Nygren, J., Barlow, J., Reed, J., & Svedberg, P. (2022). Implementation frameworks for artificial intelligence translation into health care practice: Scoping review. *Journal of Medical Internet Research*, *24*(1), e32215. DOI: 10.2196/32215 PMID: 35084349

Gao, Y., Li, R., Croxford, E., Caskey, J., Patterson, B. W., Churpek, M., Miller, T., Dligach, D., & Afshar, M. (2025). Leveraging medical knowledge graphs into large language models for diagnosis prediction: Design and application study. *JMIR AI*, *4*, e58670. DOI: 10.2196/58670 PMID: 39993309

Garrido-Muñoz, I., Montejo-Ráez, A., Martínez-Santiago, F., & Ureña López, L. A. (2021). A survey on bias in deep NLP. *Applied Sciences (Basel, Switzerland)*, *11*(7), 3184. DOI: 10.3390/app11073184

Gehman, S., Gururangan, S., Sap, M., Choi, Y., & Smith, N. A. (2020). RealToxicityPrompts: Evaluating neural toxic degeneration in language models. *arXiv preprint arXiv:2009.11462*. DOI: 10.18653/v1/2020.findings-emnlp.301

Gehrmann, S., Clark, E., & Sellam, T. (2023). Repairing the cracked foundation: A survey of obstacles in evaluation practices for generated text. *Journal of Artificial Intelligence Research*, *77*, 103–166. DOI: 10.1613/jair.1.13715

Gerke, S., Minssen, T., & Cohen, G. (2020). Ethical and legal challenges of artificial intelligence-driven healthcare. In Bohr, A., & Memarzadeh, K. (Eds.), *Artificial intelligence in healthcare* (pp. 295–336). Academic Press., DOI: 10.1016/B978-0-12-818438-7.00012-5

Gero, Z., Singh, C., Xie, Y., Zhang, S., Subramanian, P., Vozila, P., Naumann, T., Gao, J., & Poon, H. (2024). Attribute structuring improves LLM-based evaluation of clinical text summaries. *arXiv preprint arXiv:2407.17778*.

Ghassemi, M., Oakden-Rayner, L., & Beam, A. L. (2021). The false hope of current approaches to explainable artificial intelligence in health care. *The Lancet. Digital Health, 3*(11), e745–e750. DOI: 10.1016/S2589-7500(21)00208-9 PMID: 34711379

Ghnemat, R.. (2026). Governance and compliance strategies for AI in healthcare systems. *Journal of Medical Systems, 50*(3), 45–60.

Ghosh, A., Sridhar, S., Ravi, R. K., Muhsin, M., Saha, S., & Agarwal, C. (2025). CLINIC: Evaluating Multilingual Trustworthiness in Language Models for Healthcare. *ArXiv*. https://arxiv.org/abs/2512.11437

Gianfrancesco, M. A., Tamang, S., Yazdany, J., & Schmajuk, G. (2018). Potential biases in machine learning algorithms using electronic health record data. *JAMA Internal Medicine, 178*(11), 1544–1547. DOI: 10.1001/jamainternmed.2018.3763 PMID: 30128552

Goel, R., Jaiswal, U. K., Singh, P., Yadav, S. P., & Upadhyay, P. (2025). Deep learning for early brain tumor detection: A Keras-Based approach using MRI and CT imaging. In *Demystifying the role of natural Language processing (NLP) in mental health* (pp. 145-180). IGI Global Scientific Publishing. DOI: 10.4018/979-8-3693-4203-9.ch009

Goh, E., Gallo, R., Strong, E., Weng, Y., Kerman, H., Freed, J., Cool, J. A., Kanjee, Z., Lane, K. P., Parsons, A. S., Ahuja, N., Horvitz, E., Yang, D., Milstein, A., Olson, A. P. J., Hom, J., Chen, J. H., & Rodman, A. (2024). *Large Language Model Influence on Management Reasoning: A Randomized Controlled Trial*. https://doi.org/DOI: 10.1101/2024.08.05.24311485

Gong, E. J., Bang, C. S., Lee, J. J., & Baik, G. H. (2025). Knowledge-practice performance gap in clinical large language models: Systematic review of 39 benchmarks. *Journal of Medical Internet Research, 27*, e84120. DOI: 10.2196/84120 PMID: 41325597

Gong, L., Fang, W., & Yang, T.. (2026). MedDialogRubrics: Benchmark and evaluation framework for multi-turn medical consultations in large language models. *arXiv*. https://arxiv.org/abs/2601.03023

Goodman, B., & Flaxman, S. (2017). European Union regulations on algorithmic decision-making and a "right to explanation.". *AI Magazine, 38*(3), 50–57. DOI: 10.1609/aimag.v38i3.2741

Goodrum, H., Roberts, K., & Bernstam, E. V. (2020). Automatic classification of scanned electronic health record documents. *International Journal of Medical Informatics*, *144*, 104302. DOI: 10.1016/j.ijmedinf.2020.104302 PMID: 33091829

Gosak, L., Štiglic, G., San, W. T. W., & Vrbnjak, D. (2025). Human-led and artificial intelligence-automated critical appraisal of systematic reviews: Comparative evaluation. *Nurse Education in Practice*, *89*, 104614. DOI: 10.1016/j.nepr.2025.104614 PMID: 41202494

Granstedt, L.. (2025). Hallucination in large language models: Risks and mitigation strategies. *Artificial Intelligence in Medicine*, *134*, 102345.

Gururangan, S., Marasović, A., Swayamdipta, S., Lo, K., Beltagy, I., Downey, D., & Smith, N. A. (2020). Don't stop pretraining: Adapt language models to domains and tasks. In *Proceedings of the 58th Annual Meeting of the Association for Computational Linguistics* (pp. 8342–8360). DOI: 10.18653/v1/2020.acl-main.740

Hager, P., Jungmann, F., Holland, R., Bhoelan, S., Ruber, T., Scherer, J., Baader, S., Braren, R., Kaissis, G., & Rueckert, D. (2024). Evaluation and mitigation of the limitations of large language models in clinical decision-making. *Nature Medicine*, *30*(9), 2613–2622. DOI: 10.1038/s41591-024-03097-1 PMID: 38965432

Han, T., Adams, L. C., Bressem, K. K., Busch, F., Nebelung, S., & Truhn, D. (2024). Comparative analysis of multimodal large language model performance on clinical vignette questions. *Journal of the American Medical Association*, *331*(15), 1320–1321. DOI: 10.1001/jama.2023.27861 PMID: 38497956

Han, T., Kumar, A., Agarwal, C., & Lakkaraju, H. (2024). MedSafetyBench: Evaluating and improving the medical safety of large language models. *arXiv*. https://arxiv.org/abs/2403.03744

Han, X., Shen, A., Cohn, T., Baldwin, T., & Frermann, L. (2022). Systematic evaluation of predictive fairness. In *Proceedings of the Association for Computational Linguistics*.

Higgins, D., & Madai, V. I. (2020). From Bit to Bedside: A Practical Framework for Artificial Intelligence Product Development in Healthcare. *Advanced Intelligent Systems*, *2*(10), 2000052. DOI: 10.1002/aisy.202000052

Holm, J. E. J., Ruppert, J. G., & Ramsden, S. D. (2022). Impact of Changing Regulations and the Dynamic Nature of European Risk Management Plans for Human Medicines on the Lifecycle of Safety Concerns. *Pharmaceutical Medicine*, *36*(1), 33–46. DOI: 10.1007/s40290-021-00414-8 PMID: 35099785

Holzinger, A., Carrington, A., & Müller, H. (2022). Measuring the quality of explanations: The system causability scale (SCS). *Wiley Interdisciplinary Reviews. Data Mining and Knowledge Discovery*, *12*(2), e1436.

Holzinger, A., Langs, G., Denk, H., Zatloukal, K., & Müller, H. (2020). Causability and explainability of artificial intelligence in medicine. *Wiley Interdisciplinary Reviews. Data Mining and Knowledge Discovery*, *9*(4), e1312. DOI: 10.1002/widm.1312 PMID: 32089788

Holzinger, A., Saranti, A., Molnar, C., Biecek, P., & Samek, W. (2022). Explainable AI methods for safe and trustworthy healthcare AI. *IEEE Computer*, *55*(4), 52–63.

Huang, K.. (2026). A survey on hallucination in large language models. *ACM Computing Surveys*, *59*(1), 1–38.

International Electrotechnical Commission. (2015). IEC 62304:2006+AMD1:2015—Medical device software: Software life cycle processes. https://webstore.iec.ch/en/publication/22794

Islam, H.. (2024). Federated learning and distributed applications for electronic health records and structured medical data: A scoping review. *Journal of the American Medical Informatics Association : JAMIA*, *30*(12), 2041–2049.

Jacobs, M.. (2021). The value of interpretability in machine learning for medicine. *Communications of the ACM*, *64*(1), 57–65. DOI: 10.1145/3348485

Jain, J., & Jaiswal, U. K. (2025). Revolutionizing Medicine: The Impact of Artificial Intelligence in Healthcare. In *Generative Intelligence in Healthcare* (pp. 176-209). CRC Press.

Jaiswal, U. K., Chauhan, A., & Gupta, R. (2023). Brain Tumor Recognition Leveraging Machine Learning and CNN. In International Conference on Artificial-Business Analytics, Quantum and Machine Learning (pp. 53-65). Singapore: Springer Nature Singapore.

Javed, H., Ali, F., Shah, B., Dilshad, N., & Kwak, D. (2025). MediGuard: Protecting Sensitive Healthcare Data with Privacy-Preserving Language Models. *IEEE Journal of Biomedical and Health Informatics*, •••, 1–14. DOI: 10.1109/JBHI.2025.3602983 PMID: 40864576

Jiang, F., Jiang, Y., & Zhi, H.. (2021). Artificial intelligence in healthcare: Past, present and future. *Stroke and Vascular Neurology*, *6*(2), 230–243. PMID: 29507784

Jiang, H., Liu, X., Wang, Q., Chen, Z., Zhao, J., & Li, M. (2025). EHR-Bench: End-to-end evaluation of LLMs in electronic health record simulation environments. *Journal of the American Medical Informatics Association : JAMIA, 32*(5), e201–e213.

Jindal, M., ... (2025). SAGE: A generic framework for large language model safety evaluation. *Proceedings of the EMNLP Industry Track.* https://aclanthology.org/2025.emnlp-industry.2/

Jin, Q.. (2021). *PubMedQA: A dataset for biomedical research question answering.* EMNLP., DOI: 10.18653/v1/2021.emnlp-main.784

Ji, Z., Lee, N., Frieske, R., Yu, T., Su, D., Xu, Y., Ishii, E., Bang, Y., Madotto, A., & Fung, P. (2023). Survey of hallucination in natural language generation. *ACM Computing Surveys, 55*(12), 1–38. DOI: 10.1145/3571730

Johannssen, A., & Chukhrova, N. (2025). The crucial role of explainable artificial intelligence (XAI) in improving health care management. *Health Care Management Science, 28*(3), 565–570. DOI: 10.1007/s10729-025-09720-y PMID: 41026402

Johnson, D., Kumar, V., & Lee, S. (2022). Balancing innovation and patient data protection in healthcare AI. *IEEE Transactions on Medical Systems, 38*(4), 555–569.

Johri, S., Jeong, J., Tran, B. A., Schlessinger, D. I., Wongvibulsin, S., Barnes, L. A., Zhou, H.-Y., Cai, Z. R., Van Allen, E. M., Kim, D., Daneshjou, R., & Rajpurkar, P. (2025). An evaluation framework for clinical use of large language models in patient interaction tasks. *Nature Medicine, 31*(1), 77–86. DOI: 10.1038/s41591-024-03328-5 PMID: 39747685

Jung, J., Kang, S., Choi, J., El-Kareh, R., & Kim, H. (2024). *Evaluating the Impact of Explainable Ai on Clinicians' Decision-Making: A Study on Icu Length of Stay Prediction. SSRN.* DOI: 10.2139/ssrn.5017467

Jung, K. H. (2025). Large language models in medicine: Clinical applications, technical challenges, and ethical considerations. *Healthcare Informatics Research, 31*(2), 114–124. DOI: 10.4258/hir.2025.31.2.114 PMID: 40384063

Kalodanis, K., Feretzakis, G., Rizomiliotis, P., Verykios, V. S., Papapavlou, C., Skrekas, A. C., & Anagnostopoulos, D. (2025). Evaluating the Impact of the EU AI Act on Medical Device Regulation. In *Envisioning the Future of Health Informatics and Digital Health* (pp. 40–44). IOS Press., DOI: 10.3233/SHTI250045

Kamel Rahimi, A., Pienaar, O., Ghadimi, M., Canfell, O. J., Pole, J. D., Shrapnel, S., van der Vegt, A. H., & Sullivan, C. (2024). Implementing AI in hospitals to achieve a learning health system: Systematic review of current enablers and barriers. *Journal of Medical Internet Research, 26*, e49655. DOI: 10.2196/49655 PMID: 39094106

Kao, J.-P., & Kao, H.-T. (2025). Large Language Models in radiology: A technical and clinical perspective. *European Journal of Radiology Artificial Intelligence*, *2*, 100021. DOI: 10.1016/j.ejrai.2025.100021

Karayanni, N., Awwad, A., Hsiao, C.-L., & Shanmugam, S. P. (2024). Keeping experts in the loop: Expert-guided optimization for clinical data classification using large language models. *arXiv preprint arXiv:2412.02173*.

Kassirer, J. P. (2024). Practicing principled medicine. In *Masterclass in medicine: Lessons from the experts*. DOI: 10.1201/9781003409373-8

Kellogg, K. C.. (2017). Patient safety incident reporting systems. *BMJ Quality & Safety*, *26*(2), 96–105. DOI: 10.1136/bmjqs-2015-004386 PMID: 29217696

Kelly, C. J., Karthikesalingam, A., Suleyman, M., Corrado, G., & King, D. (2021). Key challenges for delivering clinical impact with artificial intelligence. *BMC Medicine*, *19*(1), 1–9. PMID: 33390155

Khan, S. D., Hoodbhoy, Z., Raja, M. H. R., Kim, J. Y., Hogg, H. D. J., Manji, A. A. A., Gulamali, F., Hasan, A., Shaikh, A., Tajuddin, S., Khan, N. S., Patel, M. R., Balu, S., Samad, Z., & Sendak, M. P. (2024). Frameworks for procurement, integration, monitoring, and evaluation of artificial intelligence tools in clinical settings: A systematic review. *PLOS Digital Health*, *3*(5), e0000514. DOI: 10.1371/journal.pdig.0000514 PMID: 38809946

Kim, Y., Jeong, H., Chen, S., Li, S. S., Park, C., Lu, M., . . . Breazeal, C. (2025). Medical hallucinations in foundation models and their impact on healthcare. arXiv preprint arXiv:2503.05777. https://doi.org//arXiv.2503.05777DOI: 10.1101/2025.02.28.25323115

Kim, M., Sohn, H., Choi, S., & Kim, S. (2023). Requirements for trustworthy artificial intelligence and its application in healthcare. *Healthcare Informatics Research*, *29*(4), 315–322. DOI: 10.4258/hir.2023.29.4.315 PMID: 37964453

Kim, S. C., & Yoon, H. J. (2025, August). uestioning Our uestions: How Well Do Medical A Benchmarks Evaluate Clinical Capabilities of Language Models? In *Proceedings of the 24th Workshop on Biomedical Language Processing* (pp. 274-296). https://doi.org/DOI: 10.18653/v1/2025.bionlp-1.24

Kirk, H. R., Jun, Y., Volpin, F., Iqbal, H., Benussi, E., Dreyer, F., Shtedritski, A., & Asano, Y. (2021). Bias out-of-the-box: An empirical analysis of intersectional occupational biases in popular generative language models. In *Advances in Neural Information Processing Systems* (pp. 2611–2624).

Kiseleva, A., Kotzinos, D., & De Hert, P. (2022). Transparency of AI in healthcare as a multilayered system of accountabilities: Between legal requirements and technical limitations. *Frontiers in Artificial Intelligence, 5*, 879603. Advance online publication. DOI: 10.3389/frai.2022.879603 PMID: 35707765

Kleebayoon, A., & Wiwanitkit, V. (2024). Re: Investigating the impact of innovative AI chatbot on post-pandemic medical education and clinical assistance: a comprehensive analysis. *ANZ Journal of Surgery, 94*(3), 492. DOI: 10.1111/ans.18717 PMID: 37749857

Kocaman, V. (2025). Clinical large language model evaluation by expert review. *Journal of Medical Artificial Intelligence*. PMID: 41343765

Kocaman, V., Kaya, M. A., Feier, A. M., & Talby, D. (2025). Clinical large language model evaluation by expert review (CLEVER): Framework development and validation. *JMIR AI, 4*, e72153. DOI: 10.2196/72153 PMID: 41343765

Kocbek, S.. (2020). Text mining electronic hospital records to automate clinical coding. *Journal of Biomedical Informatics, 102*, 103374. DOI: 10.1016/j.jbi.2019.103374

Kreuzberger, D., Kühl, N., & Hirschl, S. (2023). Machine learning operations (MLOps): Overview and challenges. *IEEE Access : Practical Innovations, Open Solutions, 11*, 30920–30938. DOI: 10.1109/ACCESS.2023.3262138

Krishna, A., & Gupta, M. (2025). Next-gen 3rd party cybersecurity risk management practices. In Advancing IT Audits Through Integrative Approaches and Emerging Technologies (pp. 1–30). IGI Global Scientific Publishing. DOI: 10.4018/979-8-3373-3078-5.ch001

Krittanawong, C.. (2023). ChatGPT in cardiovascular medicine. *Nature Reviews. Cardiology, 20*, 593–594. DOI: 10.1038/s41569-023-00819-8

Kumar, S., Nargund, A. A., & Sridhar, V. (2025, July). CourtEval: A courtroom-based multi-agent evaluation framework. In *Findings of the Association for Computational Linguistics: ACL 2025* (pp. 25875-25887). https://doi.org/DOI: 10.18653/v1/2025.findings-acl.1327

Kumar, P., Adams, J., & Li, Y. (2024). Data anonymization and de-identification challenges in clinical NLP: A review. *Journal of Biomedical Informatics, 139*, 104–136.

Kumar, P., Li, Y., & Adams, J. (2023). Re-identification risks in clinical NLP models. *Frontiers in Artificial Intelligence, 6*(3), 1–9.

Kung, T. H., Cheatham, M., Medenilla, A., Sillos, C., De Leon, L., Elepaño, C., Madriaga, M., Aggabao, R., Diaz-Candido, G., Maningo, J., & Tseng, V. (2023). Performance of ChatGPT on USMLE: Potential for AI-assisted medical education. *PLOS Digital Health, 2*(2), e0000198. DOI: 10.1371/journal.pdig.0000198 PMID: 36812645

Kurita, K., Belova, A., & Anastasopoulos, A. (2019). Towards robust toxic content classification. arXiv preprint arXiv:1912.06872.

Lacerda, A. (2025). Evaluation of medical large language models: Taxonomy and structured assessment framework. In *Proceedings of the Thirty-Fourth International Joint Conference on Artificial Intelligence (IJCAI)*.

Laukamp, K. R., Terzis, R. A., Werner, J.-M., Galldiks, N., Lennartz, S., Maintz, D., Reimer, R., Fervers, P., Gertz, R. J., Persigehl, T., Rubbert, C., Lehnen, N. C., Deuschl, C., Schlamann, M., Schönfeld, M. H., & Kottlors, J. (2024). Monitoring Patients with Glioblastoma by Using a Large Language Model: Accurate Summarization of Radiology Reports with GPT-4. *Radiology, 312*(1), e232640. Advance online publication. DOI: 10.1148/radiol.232640 PMID: 39041936

Lawrence, H. R., Schneider, R. A., Rubin, S. B., Matarić, M. J., McDuff, D. J., & Jones Bell, M. (2024). The opportunities and risks of large language models in mental health. *JMIR Mental Health, 11*, e59479. DOI: 10.2196/59479 PMID: 39105570

LeCun, Y., Bengio, Y., & Hinton, G. (2021). Deep learning. *Nature, 521*(7553), 436–444. DOI: 10.1038/nature14539 PMID: 26017442

Lee, J., Park, S., Shin, J., & Cho, B. (2024). Analyzing evaluation methods for large language models in the medical field: A scoping review. *BMC Medical Informatics and Decision Making, 24*(1), 366. DOI: 10.1186/s12911-024-02709-7 PMID: 39614219

Lee, J., Wu, A. S., Li, D., & Kulasegaram, K. M. (2024). Artificial intelligence in undergraduate medical education: A systematic review. *Academic Medicine : Journal of the Association of American Medical Colleges, 99*(8), 916–925. DOI: 10.1097/ACM.0000000000005685

Lee, P., Bubeck, S., & Petro, J. (2023). Benefits, limits, and risks of GPT-4 as an AI chatbot for medicine. *The New England Journal of Medicine, 388*(13), 1233–1239. DOI: 10.1056/NEJMsr2214184 PMID: 36988602

Leivaditis, V., Maniatopoulos, A. A., Lausberg, H., Mulita, F., Papatriantafyllou, A., Liolis, E., Beltsios, E., Adamou, A., Kontodimopoulos, N., & Dahm, M. (2025). Artificial Intelligence in Thoracic Surgery: A Review Bridging Innovation and Clinical Practice for the Next Generation of Surgical Care. *Journal of Clinical Medicine*, *14*(8), 2729. DOI: 10.3390/jcm14082729 PMID: 40283559

Leslie, D. (2019). *Understanding artificial intelligence ethics and safety*. The Alan Turing Institute. https://doi.org/DOI: 10.5281/zenodo.3240529

Leslie, D. (2022). *Understanding artificial intelligence ethics and safety*. Alan Turing Institute.

Levine, D. M.. (2023). Monitoring deployed clinical AI systems. *NPJ Digital Medicine*, *6*, 55. DOI: 10.1038/s41746-023-00760-9

Leypold, T., Lingens, L. F., Beier, J. P., & Boos, A. M. (2024). Integrating AI in lipedema management: Assessing the efficacy of GPT-4 as a consultation assistant. *Life (Basel, Switzerland)*, *14*(5), 646. DOI: 10.3390/life14050646 PMID: 38792666

Liao, Y., Meng, Y., Liu, H., Wang, Y., & Wang, Y. (2023). An automatic evaluation framework for multi-turn medical consultations of large language models. *arXiv*. https://arxiv.org/abs/2309.02077

Li, C., Meng, Y., Dong, L., Ma, D., Wang, C., & Du, D. (2025). Ethical Privacy Framework for Large Language Models in Smart Healthcare: A Comprehensive Evaluation and Protection Approach. *IEEE Journal of Biomedical and Health Informatics*, •••, 1–14. DOI: 10.1109/JBHI.2025.3576579 PMID: 40465443

Li, D., Jin, Z., Guan, C., Ji, L., Zhang, Y., Xu, Z., & Zhang, J. (2026). KACNet: Enhancing CNN feature representation with Kolmogorov-Arnold networks for medical image segmentation and classification. *Information Sciences*, *726*, 122760. DOI: 10.1016/j.ins.2025.122760

Li, H., Tan, M., & Chang, Y. (2024). Ethical frameworks for trustworthy medical AI. *Bioethics and Data Science Review*, *12*(1), 33–47.

Li, J., Zhou, Z., Lyu, H., & Wang, Z. (2025). Large language models-powered clinical decision support: Enhancing or replacing human expertise? *Intelligent Medicine*, *5*(1), 1–4. DOI: 10.1016/j.imed.2025.01.001

Lim, E., He, Y. V., & Joselowitz, J.. (2025). MATRIX: Multi-agent simulation framework for safe interactions and contextual clinical conversational evaluation. *arXiv*. https://arxiv.org/abs/2508.19163

Lin, C. C., Huang, A. Y., & Lu, O. H. (2023). Artificial intelligence in intelligent tutoring systems toward sustainable education: A systematic review. *Smart Learning Environments*, *10*(1), 41. DOI: 10.1186/s40561-023-00260-y

Lin, C., & Kuo, C.-F. (2025). Roles and potential of large language models in healthcare: A comprehensive review. *Biomedical Journal*, *48*(5), 100868. DOI: 10.1016/j.bj.2025.100868 PMID: 40311872

Lindner, G., & Ravioli, S. (2025). Performance of the artificial intelligence-based Swiss medical assessment system versus Manchester triage system in the emergency department: A retrospective analysis. *The American Journal of Emergency Medicine*, *94*, 46–49. DOI: 10.1016/j.ajem.2025.04.023 PMID: 40273637

Li, S.. (2023). A review of privacy-enhancement methods for federated learning in healthcare systems. *International Journal of Environmental Research and Public Health*, *20*(15), 6539. DOI: 10.3390/ijerph20156539

Li, S., & Paik, H. (2023). A systematic review of federated learning from clients' perspective: Challenges and solutions. *Artificial Intelligence Review*, *56*(S2, Suppl 2), 1773–1827. DOI: 10.1007/s10462-023-10563-8

Liu, Y., Wang, Z., Li, Y., Liang, X., Liu, L., Wang, L., & Zhou, L. (2024). MRScore: Evaluating radiology report generation with LLM-based reward system. *arXiv preprint arXiv:2404.17778.*

Liu, L.. (2024). Towards automatic evaluation for LLMs' clinical capabilities: Metric, data, and algorithm. *arXiv*. https://arxiv.org/abs/2403.16446 DOI: 10.1145/3637528.3671575

Li, Y.. (2026). Large language models in healthcare: Opportunities and challenges. *Journal of Biomedical Informatics*, *139*, 104312.

Long, J.. (2023). Evaluating AI systems under real-world clinical conditions. *Nature Medicine*, *29*, 202–210. DOI: 10.1038/s41591-022-02043-7

López-Pérez, B., Chen, Y., Li, X., Cheng, S., & Razavi, P. (2025). Exploring the potential of large language models to understand interpersonal emotion regulation strategies from narratives. *Emotion (Washington, D.C.)*, *25*(7), 1653–1667. DOI: 10.1037/emo0001528 PMID: 40244995

Lu, H., Lin, Y., Li, Z., Yiu, M. L., Gao, Y., & Uddin, S. (2025). Toward fair medical advice: Addressing and mitigating bias in large language model-based healthcare applications. *Artificial Intelligence in Medicine*, *168*, 103216. DOI: 10.1016/j.artmed.2025.103216 PMID: 40680485

Lu, J.. (2022). Learning under concept drift: A review. *IEEE Transactions on Knowledge and Data Engineering*, *34*(9), 4287–4312. DOI: 10.1109/TKDE.2020.3042330

Luxton, D. D. (2021). Artificial intelligence in psychological practice: Current and future applications and implications. *Professional Psychology, Research and Practice*, *45*(5), 332–339. DOI: 10.1037/a0034559

Lwakatare, L. E.. (2020). DevOps in practice: A multiple case study. *Information and Software Technology*, *114*, 106–118. DOI: 10.1016/j.infsof.2019.06.009

Macmillan-Scott, O., & Musolesi, M. (2024). (Ir)rationality and cognitive biases in large language models. *Royal Society Open Science*, *11*(6), 240255. DOI: 10.1098/rsos.240255 PMID: 39100158

Macrae, C. (2025, April). Managing risk and resilience in autonomous and intelligent systems: Exploring safety in the development, deployment, and use of artificial intelligence in healthcare. *Risk Analysis : An Official Publication of the Society for Risk Analysis*, *45*(4), 910–927. DOI: 10.1111/risa.14273 PMID: 38246857

Madden, M. G., McNicholas, B. A., & Laffey, J. G. (2023). Assessing the usefulness of a large language model to query and summarize unstructured medical notes in intensive care. *Intensive Care Medicine*, *49*(8), 1018–1020. DOI: 10.1007/s00134-023-07128-2 PMID: 37338549

Maity, S. (2025). Large language models in healthcare and medical applications: A survey and future directions. *Bioengineering (Basel, Switzerland)*, *12*(6), 631. DOI: 10.3390/bioengineering12060631 PMID: 40564447

Manakul, P., Liusie, A., & Gales, M. (2023). SelfCheckGPT: Zero-resource black-box hallucination detection for generative large language models. In *Proceedings of the 2023 Conference on Empirical Methods in Natural Language Processing* (pp. 9004–9017). DOI: 10.18653/v1/2023.emnlp-main.557

Mathur, Y., Rangreji, S., Kapoor, R., Palavalli, M., Bertsch, A., & Gormley, M. R. (2023). SummQA at MEDIQA-Chat 2023: In-context learning with GPT-4 for medical summarization. *arXiv preprint arXiv:2306.17384*. DOI: 10.18653/v1/2023.clinicalnlp-1.51

Matthew, G., & Hicks, Y. (2025). Enhancing Clinical Decision Support with LLMs: A Feasibility Study Integrating CoT, RAG, and QLoRA. *Procedia Computer Science*, *270*, 4946–4956. DOI: 10.1016/j.procs.2025.09.621

Maurya, S., Asudani, D. S., Jain, J., Jaiswal, U. K., Jain, E., & Malviya, K. (2025). Evaluating the effectiveness of regression algorithms in predicting cancer progression. In Parul University International Conference on Engineering and Technology 2025 (PiCET 2025) (Vol. 2025, pp. 1367-1373). IET. DOI: 10.1049/icp.2025.1593

Mehandru, N., Miao, B. Y., Almaraz, E. R., Sushil, M., Butte, A. J., & Alaa, A. (2024). Evaluating large language models as agents in the clinic. *NPJ Digital Medicine*, *7*(1), 84. DOI: 10.1038/s41746-024-01083-y PMID: 38570554

Mehrabi, N., Morstatter, F., Saxena, N., Lerman, K., & Galstyan, A. (2021). A survey on bias and fairness in machine learning. *ACM Computing Surveys*, *54*(6), 1–35. DOI: 10.1145/3457607

Melas, N., Amin, R., Gyllemark, P., Younes, A. H., & Almer, S. (2021). Whipple's disease: The great masquerader—A high level of suspicion is the key to diagnosis. *BMC Gastroenterology*, *21*(1), 128. DOI: 10.1186/s12876-021-01664-1 PMID: 33743602

Meng, X., Yan, X., Zhang, K., Liu, D., Cui, X., Yang, Y., Zhang, M., Cao, C., Wang, J., Wang, X., Gao, J., Wang, Y.-G.-S., Ji, J., Qiu, Z., Li, M., Qian, C., Guo, T., Ma, S., Wang, Z., & Tang, Y.-D. (2024). The application of large language models in medicine: A scoping review. *iScience*, *27*(5), 109713. DOI: 10.1016/j.isci.2024.109713 PMID: 38746668

Meskó, B. C., & Topol, E. J. (2023). The imperative for regulatory oversight of large language models (or generative AI) in healthcare. *NPJ Digital Medicine*, *C*(1), 120. DOI: 10.1038/s41746-023-00873-0 PMID: 37414860

Meunier, P.-Y., Raynaud, C., Guimaraes, E., Gueyffier, F., & Letrilliart, L. (2023). Barriers and facilitators to the use of clinical decision support systems in primary care: A mixed-methods systematic review. *Annals of Family Medicine*, *21*(1), 57–69. DOI: 10.1370/afm.2908 PMID: 36690490

Miller, T. (2021). Explanation in artificial intelligence: Insights from the social sciences. *Artificial Intelligence*, *267*, 1–38. DOI: 10.1016/j.artint.2018.07.007

Ministry of Health of the Republic of Indonesia. (2021). Minister of Health Regulation No. 14 of 2021 on standards for health service digital technology.

Ministry of Health of the Republic of Indonesia. (2024). Minister of Health Regulation No. 17 of 2024 on data governance and interoperability in the national digital health ecosystem. Kemenkes RI.

Ministry of Health of the Republic of Indonesia. (2025). Minister of Health Regulation No. 11 of 2025 on business licensing in the health sub-sector.

Mishra, V., Lurie, Y., & Mark, S. (2025). Accuracy of LLMs in medical education: Evidence from a concordance test with medical teacher. *BMC Medical Education*, *25*(1), 443. DOI: 10.1186/s12909-025-07009-w PMID: 40140805

Moëll, B., Farestam, F., & Beskow, J. (2025). Swedish Medical LLM Benchmark: Development and evaluation of a framework for assessing large language models in the Swedish medical domain. *Frontiers in Artificial Intelligence*, *8*(1557920), 1557920. DOI: 10.3389/frai.2025.1557920 PMID: 40718621

Moëll, B., Sand Aronsson, F., & Akbar, S. (2025). Medical reasoning in LLMs: An in-depth analysis of DeepSeek R1. *Frontiers in Artificial Intelligence*, *8*, 1616145. DOI: 10.3389/frai.2025.1616145 PMID: 40607450

Moëll, B., Sand, C., & Aronsson, F. (2025). Harm reduction strategies for thoughtful use of large language models in the medical domain: Perspectives for patients and clinicians. *Journal of Medical Internet Research*, *27*, e75849. DOI: 10.2196/75849 PMID: 40712151

Mohammed, S., & Malhotra, N. (2025). Ethical and regulatory challenges in machine learning-based healthcare systems: A review of implementation barriers and future directions. *BenchCouncil Transactions on Benchmarks. Standards and Evaluations*, *5*(1), 100215. DOI: 10.1016/j.tbench.2025.100215

Momani, A. (2025). Implications of artificial intelligence on health data privacy and confidentiality. arXiv. https://arxiv.org/abs/2501.01639

Morley, J., Morton, C., Karpathakis, K., Taddeo, M., & Floridi, L. Towards a Framework for Evaluating the Safety, Acceptability and Efficacy of Ai Systems for Health: An Initial Synthesis. SSRN Electron J. Published online 2021. DOI: 10.2139/ssrn.3826358

Morley, J., Machado, C. C., Burr, C., Cowls, J., Joshi, I., Taddeo, M., & Floridi, L. (2020). The ethics of AI in health care: A mapping review. *Social Science & Medicine*, *260*, 113172. DOI: 10.1016/j.socscimed.2020.113172 PMID: 32702587

Mount Sinai Health System. (2025). AI safety red-teaming report: Chatbot elaboration of fabricated illnesses. Icahn School of Medicine Research Reports. https://icahn.mssm.edu/research/ai-safety-2025

Mourby, M., Ó Cathaoir, K., & Collin, C. B. (2021). Transparency of machine-learning in healthcare: The GDPR & European health law. *Computer Law & Security Review*, *43*, 105611. DOI: 10.1016/j.clsr.2021.105611

Muhammad, D., & Bendechache, M. (2024). Unveiling the black box: A systematic review of Explainable Artificial Intelligence in medical image analysis. *Computational and Structural Biotechnology Journal*, *24*, 542–560. DOI: 10.1016/j.csbj.2024.08.005 PMID: 39252818

Murdoch, B. (2021). Privacy and artificial intelligence: Challenges for protecting health information in a new era. *BMC Medical Ethics*, *22*(1), 122. DOI: 10.1186/s12910-021-00687-3 PMID: 34525993

Nangia, N., Vania, C., Bhalerao, R., & Bowman, S. R. (2020). CrowS-Pairs: A challenge dataset for measuring social biases in masked language models. arXiv preprint arXiv:2010.00133. DOI: 10.18653/v1/2020.emnlp-main.154

Natali, A., Mosca, N., & Zucco, R. (2025). Clinical deskilling in the age of AI: Reconsidering Klein's Second Singularity. *BMJ Open*, *15*(3), e092345.

Neha, F., Bhati, D., & Shukla, D. K. (2025). Retrieval-augmented generation (RAG) in healthcare: A comprehensive review. *AI*, *6*(9), 226. DOI: 10.3390/ai6090226

Nguyen, G.. (2022). Machine learning lifecycle management. *IEEE Software*, *39*(2), 42–49. DOI: 10.1109/MS.2021.3135619

NHS England. (2023). DCB0129: Clinical risk management—its application in the manufacture of health IT systems. https://digital.nhs.uk/data-and-information/information-standards/information-standards-and-data-collections-including-extractions/publications-and-notifications/standards-and-collections/dcb0129-clinical-risk-management-its-application-in-the-manufacture-of-health-it-systems

Nori, H., King, N., McKinney, S. M., Carignan, D., & Horvitz, E. (2023). Capabilities of GPT-4 on medical challenge problems. *arXiv preprint arXiv:2303.13375.*

Nori, H.. (2023). Capabilities of GPT-4 in medicine. *NPJ Digital Medicine*, *6*, 98. DOI: 10.1038/s41746-023-00788-x

Nurfadhilah, E., Santosa, A., & Putra, P. K. (2025). Retrieval-augmented large language models for a chronic kidney disease patient education chatbot. 2025 International Conference on Computer, Control, Informatics and its Applications (IC3INA). DOI: 10.1109/IC3INA68387.2025.11325127

Obermeyer, Z.. (2019). Dissecting racial bias in health algorithms. *Science*, *366*(6464), 447–453. DOI: 10.1126/science.aax2342 PMID: 31649194

Obermeyer, Z., & Emanuel, E. J. (2020). Predicting the future—Big data and machine learning in clinical medicine. *The New England Journal of Medicine*, *375*(13), 1216–1219. DOI: 10.1056/NEJMp1606181 PMID: 27682033

Odera, D. (2023). Federated learning and differential privacy in clinical health: Extensive survey. *World Journal of Advanced Engineering Technology and Sciences*, *8*(02), 305–329. DOI: 10.30574/wjaets.2023.8.2.0113

Omiye, J. A., Gui, H., Rezaei, S. J., Zou, J., & Daneshjou, R. (2024). Large language models in medicine: The potentials and pitfalls: A narrative review. *Annals of Internal Medicine*, *177*(2), 210–220. DOI: 10.7326/M23-2772 PMID: 38285984

Omiye, J. A., Lester, J. C., Spichak, S., Rotemberg, V., & Daneshjou, R. (2023). Large language models propagate race-based medicine. npj. *Digital Medicine*, *6*(1), 195. DOI: 10.1038/s41746-023-00939-z PMID: 37864012

Osheroff, J. A., Teich, J. M., Levick, D., Saldana, L., Velasco, F., Sittig, D. F., & Rogers, K. M. (2012). *Improving outcomes with clinical decision support: An implementer's guide*. HIMSS. DOI: 10.4324/9781498757461

Osheroff, J. A., Teich, J. M., Middleton, B., Steen, E. B., Wright, A., & Detmer, D. E. (2007). A roadmap for national action on clinical decision support. *Journal of the American Medical Informatics Association : JAMIA*, *14*(2), 141–145. DOI: 10.1197/jamia.M2334 PMID: 17213487

Ousidhoum, N., Zhao, X., Fang, T., Song, Y., & Yeung, D. Y. (2021). Probing toxic content in large pre-trained language models. In *Proceedings of the 59th Annual Meeting of the Association for Computational Linguistics*. DOI: 10.18653/v1/2021.acl-long.329

Owoyemi, A., Osuchukwu, J., Salwei, M. E., & Boyd, A. (2025). Checklist approach to developing and implementing AI in clinical settings: Instrument development study. *JMIRx Med*, *6*, e65565. DOI: 10.2196/65565 PMID: 39977249

Palomo, G. M., Pose-Boirazian, T., Naumann-Winter, F., Costa, E., Duarte, D. M., Kalland, M. E., Malikova, E., Matusevicius, D., Vitezic, D., Larsson, K., Magrelli, A., Stoyanova-Beninska, V., & Mariz, S. (2023). The European landscape for gene therapies in orphan diseases: 6-year experience with the EMA Committee for Orphan Medicinal Products. *Molecular Therapy : The Journal of the American Society of Gene Therapy*, *31*(12), 3414–3423. DOI: 10.1016/j.ymthe.2023.09.020 PMID: 37794679

Pan, X., Zhang, M., Ji, S., & Yang, M. (2020). Privacy risks of general-purpose language models. In *IEEE Symposium on Security and Privacy* (pp. 1314–1331).

Parish, S. T., Aschner, M., Casey, W., Corvaro, M., Embry, M. R., Fitzpatrick, S., Kidd, D., Kleinstreuer, N. C., Lima, B. S., Settivari, R. S., Wolf, D. C., Yamazaki, D., & Boobis, A. (2020). An evaluation framework for new approach methodologies (NAMs) for human health safety assessment. *Regulatory Toxicology and Pharmacology : RTP, 112*, 104592. DOI: 10.1016/j.yrtph.2020.104592 PMID: 32017962

Park, Y. J., Pillai, A., Deng, J., Guo, E., Gupta, M., Paget, M., & Naugler, C. (2024). Assessing the research landscape and clinical utility of large language models: A scoping review. *BMC Medical Informatics and Decision Making*, *24*(1), 72. DOI: 10.1186/s12911-024-02459-6 PMID: 38475802

Pashangpour, S., & Nejat, G. (2024). The future of intelligent healthcare: A systematic analysis and discussion on the integration and impact of robots using large language models for healthcare. *Robotics (Basel, Switzerland), 13*(8), 112. DOI: 10.3390/robotics13080112

Pavlopoulos, J., Sorensen, J., Dixon, L., Thain, N., & Androutsopoulos, I. (2020). Toxicity detection: Does context really matter? In *Proceedings of the 58th Annual Meeting of the Association for Computational Linguistics* (pp. 4296–4305). DOI: 10.18653/v1/2020.acl-main.396

Pedersen, T., Pakhomov, S. V., Patwardhan, S. C., & Chute, C. G. (2007). Measures of semantic similarity and relatedness in the biomedical domain. *Journal of Biomedical Informatics*, *40*(3), 288–299. DOI: 10.1016/j.jbi.2006.06.004 PMID: 16875881

Poitras, M. E., Gauvin, F., Bhosrekar, S., & Morin, S. N. (2025). Socioeconomic bias in clinical AI: Evidence from simulated patient scenarios. *Journal of General Internal Medicine*, *40*(1), 78–85.

Poursabzi-Sangdeh, F.. (2021). Manipulating and measuring model interpretability. *CHI Conference*. DOI: 10.1145/3411764.3445315

Prenosil, G., Hügli, R., Brönnimann, M., Sendi, P., & Kluckert, T. (2025). Neurosymbolic hybrid AI for clinical decision support: Architecture and evaluation. *JAMIA Open*, *8*(1), ooae123.

Preti, L. M., Ardito, V., Compagni, A., Petracca, F., & Cappellaro, G. (2024). Implementation of machine learning applications in health care organizations: Systematic review of empirical studies. *Journal of Medical Internet Research*, *26*, e55897. DOI: 10.2196/55897 PMID: 39586084

Price, W. N.II, & Cohen, I. G. (2019). Privacy in the age of medical big data. *Nature Medicine*, *25*(1), 37–43. DOI: 10.1038/s41591-018-0272-7 PMID: 30617331

Prosper, A. E., Kammer, M. N., Maldonado, F., Aberle, D. R., & Hsu, W. (2023). Expanding Role of Advanced Image Analysis in CT-detected Indeterminate Pulmonary Nodules and Early Lung Cancer Characterization. *Radiology, 309*(1), e222904. Advance online publication. DOI: 10.1148/radiol.222904 PMID: 37815447

Putra, P. K., Nurfadhilah, E., Pebiana, S., & Prakasa, E. (2025). Towards a safe and trustworthy LLM-RAG chatbot for hemodialysis patient education: Design, implementation, and preliminary evaluation. 2025 International Conference on Computer, Control, Informatics and its Applications (IC3INA). DOI: 10.1109/IC3INA68387.2025.11325125

Qiu, P., Wu, C., Liu, S., Fan, Y., Zhao, W., Chen, Z., Gu, H., Peng, C., Zhang, Y., Wang, Y., & Xie, W. (2025). Quantifying the reasoning abilities of LLMs on clinical cases. *Nature Communications, 16*(1), 9799. DOI: 10.1038/s41467-025-64769-1 PMID: 41198657

Raeini, M. (2023). The Evolution of Language Models: From N-Grams to LLMs, and Beyond. SSRN *Electronic Journal.* DOI: 10.2139/ssrn.4625356

Rahav Koren, R., Suriu, C., Yakir, O., Akria, L., Barhoum, M., & Braester, A. (2017). Physicians' lack of knowledge - a possible reason for red blood cell transfusion overuse? *Israel Journal of Health Policy Research, 6*(1), 49. Advance online publication. DOI: 10.1186/s13584-017-0173-0 PMID: 29228989

Raji, I. D., Smart, A., White, R. N., Mitchell, M., Gebru, T., Hutchinson, B., Smith-Loud, J., Theron, D., & Barnes, P. (2020). Closing the AI accountability gap: Defining an end-to-end framework for internal algorithmic auditing. In *Proceedings of the 2020 ACM Conference on Fairness, Accountability, and Transparency* (pp. 33–44). DOI: 10.1145/3351095.3372873

Rajkomar, A., Dean, J., & Kohane, I. (2019). Machine Learning in Medicine. *The New England Journal of Medicine, 380*(14), 1347–1358. DOI: 10.1056/NEJMra1814259 PMID: 30943338

Rajkomar, A., Hardt, M., Howell, M. D., Corrado, G., & Chin, M. H. (2018). Ensuring fairness in machine learning to advance health equity. *Annals of Internal Medicine, 169*(12), 866–872. DOI: 10.7326/M18-1990 PMID: 30508424

Rajpurkar, P., Irvin, J., Ball, R. L., Zhu, K., Yang, B., Mehta, H., Duan, T., Ding, D., Bagul, A., Langlotz, C. P., Patel, B. N., Yeom, K. W., Shpanskaya, K., Blankenberg, F. G., Seekins, J., Amrhein, T. J., Mong, D. A., Halabi, S. S., Zucker, E. J., & Lungren, M. P. (2021). Deep learning for chest radiograph diagnosis: A retrospective comparison of the CheXNeXt algorithm to practicing radiologists. *PLoS Medicine, 15*(11), e1002686. DOI: 10.1371/journal.pmed.1002686 PMID: 30457988

Ramprasad, S., Ferracane, E., & Lipton, Z. C. (2024, August). Analyzing LLM behavior in dialogue summarization: Unveiling circumstantial hallucination trends. In *Proceedings of the 62nd Annual Meeting of the Association for Computational Linguistics (*Volume 1*: Long Papers)* (pp. 12549-12561). DOI: 10.18653/v1/2024.acl-long.677

Ravikumar, A. Olimbaevich, I. R., Mashkhura, S., & Musayeva, S. (2025). Transforming Healthcare with Large Language Models and AI agents. In Advances in Computational Intelligence and Robotics (pp. 51–82). IGI Global Scientific Publishing. DOI: 10.4018/979-8-3373-2008-3.ch003

Ravikumar, A. S., Atamuratova, Z., Ashirova, A., Jurayev, K., & Hayitova, M. (2025). Comprehensive evaluation of AI-driven systems in modern hospital environments. In Advances in Computational Intelligence and Robotics (pp. 61–88). IGI Global Scientific Publishing. DOI: 10.4018/979-8-3373-2787-7.ch003

Ravikumar, R. S., Manujakshi, Aarthi, S., Urazbaeva, Y., & Tamilselvi, S. (2025). Navigating data privacy, security, and regulatory challenges in healthcare AI ensuring fairness, bias mitigation, interpretability, and trust. In Transformative Role of Transformer Models in Healthcare (pp. 25–54). IGI Global Scientific Publishing. DOI: 10.4018/979-8-3373-2038-0.ch002

Ravikumar, R. N., & Aarthi, S. (2025). AI-powered synergistic robotics and IoT ecosystems for predictive and preventive healthcare. In *Robotics and IoT Synergy in Next-Generation Healthcare* (pp. 1–32). IGI Global Scientific Publishing., DOI: 10.4018/979-8-3373-5447-7.ch001

Ray, P. P. (2025). Toward Transparent AI-Enabled Patient Selection in Cosmetic Surgery by Integrating Reasoning and Medical LLMs. *Aesthetic Plastic Surgery*, *49*(19), 5641–5642. DOI: 10.1007/s00266-025-05038-w PMID: 40563006

Reddy, S. (2023). Evaluating large language models for use in healthcare. *Patterns (New York, N.Y.)*, *4*(8), 100796.

Reddy, S., Allan, S., Coghlan, S., & Cooper, P. (2020). A governance model for the application of AI in health care. *Journal of the American Medical Informatics Association : JAMIA*, *27*(3), 491–497. DOI: 10.1093/jamia/ocz192 PMID: 31682262

Reddy, S., Lebrun, A., Chee, A., & Kalogeropoulos, D. (2024). Discussing the role of explainable AI and evaluation frameworks for safe and effective integration of large language models in healthcare. *Telehealth and Medicine Today*, *9*(2). Advance online publication. DOI: 10.30953/thmt.v9.485

Reddy, S., Rogers, W., Makinen, V. P., Coiera, E., Brown, P., Wenzel, M., Weicken, E., Ansari, S., Mathur, P., Casey, A., & Kelly, B. (2021). Evaluation framework to guide implementation of AI systems into health care settings. *BMJ Health & Care Informatics*, *28*(1), e100444. DOI: 10.1136/bmjhci-2021-100444 PMID: 34642177

Ribeiro, J., Lima, R., Eckhardt, T., & Paiva, S. (2021). Robotic process automation and artificial intelligence in industry 4.0—A literature review. *Procedia Computer Science*, *181*, 51–58. DOI: 10.1016/j.procs.2021.01.104

Ríos-Hoyo, A., Shan, N. L., Li, A., Pearson, A. T., Pusztai, L., & Howard, F. M. (2024). Evaluation of large language models as a diagnostic aid for complex medical cases. *Frontiers in Medicine*, *11*, 1380148. DOI: 10.3389/fmed.2024.1380148 PMID: 38966538

Rogler, G., Singh, A., Kavanaugh, A., & Rubin, D. T. (2021). Extraintestinal manifestations of inflammatory bowel disease: Current concepts, treatment, and implications for disease management. *Gastroenterology*, *161*(4), 1118–1132. DOI: 10.1053/j.gastro.2021.07.042 PMID: 34358489

Roselló Atanet, I., Tomova, M., Sieg, M., Sehy, V., Mäder, P., & März, M. (2025). Generating learning guides for medical education with LLMs and statistical analysis of test results. *BMC Medical Education*, *25*(1), 458. DOI: 10.1186/s12909-025-06978-2 PMID: 40158187

Roshanov, P. S., Misra, S., Gerstein, H. C., Garg, A. X., Sebaldt, R. J., Mackay, J. A., Weise-Kelly, L., Navarro, T., Wilczynski, N. L., & Haynes, R. B. (2011). Computerized clinical decision support systems for chronic disease management: A decision-maker-researcher partnership systematic review. *Implementation Science : IS*, *6*(1), 1–16. DOI: 10.1186/1748-5908-6-92 PMID: 21824386

Ross, T. J. (2010). *Fuzzy logic with engineering applications* (3rd ed.). Wiley. DOI: 10.1002/9781119994374

Roustan, D., & Bastardot, F. (2025). The clinicians' guide to large language models: A general perspective with a focus on hallucinations. *Interactive Journal of Medical Research*, *14*(1), e59823. DOI: 10.2196/59823 PMID: 39874574

Rudin, C. (2020). Stop explaining black box machine learning models for high stakes decisions and use interpretable models instead. *Nature Machine Intelligence*, *1*(5), 206–215. DOI: 10.1038/s42256-019-0048-x PMID: 35603010

Rudin, C., Chen, C., Chen, Z., Huang, H., Semenova, L., & Zhong, C. (2022). Interpretable machine learning: Fundamental principles and 10 grand challenges. *Statistics Surveys*, *16*(none), 1–85. DOI: 10.1214/21-SS133

Sallam, M. (2023). ChatGPT utility in healthcare education, research, and practice: Systematic review on the promising perspectives and valid concerns. *Health Care, 11*(6), 887. DOI: 10.3390/healthcare11060887 PMID: 36981544

Salvi, S., Vu, G., Gurupur, V., & King, C. (2025). Digital Convergence in Dental Informatics: A Structured Narrative Review of Artificial Intelligence, Internet of Things, Digital Twins, and Large Language Models with Security, Privacy, and Ethical Perspectives. *Electronics (Basel), 14*(16), 3278. DOI: 10.3390/electronics14163278

Samek, W., Montavon, G., Vedaldi, A., Hansen, L. K., & Müller, K. R. (Eds.). (2021). *Explainable AI: Interpreting, explaining and visualizing deep learning*. Springer Nature.

Savage, T., Nayak, A., Gallo, R., Rangan, E., & Chen, J. H. (2024). Diagnostic reasoning prompts reveal the potential for large language model interpretability in medicine. *NPJ Digital Medicine, 7*(1), 20. DOI: 10.1038/s41746-024-01010-1 PMID: 38267608

Schick, T., Udupa, S., & Schütze, H. (2021). Self-diagnosis and self-debiasing: A proposal for reducing corpus-based bias in NLP. *Transactions of the Association for Computational Linguistics, 9*, 1408–1424. DOI: 10.1162/tacl_a_00434

Seh, A. H., Zarour, M., Alenezi, M., Sarkar, A. K., Agrawal, A., Kumar, R., & Ahmad Khan, R. (2020). Healthcare Data Breaches: Insights and Implications. *Health Care, 8*(2), 133. DOI: 10.3390/healthcare8020133 PMID: 32414183

Selivanov, A., Rogov, O. Y., Chesakov, D., Shelmanov, A., Fedulova, I., & Dylov, D. V. (2023). Medical image captioning via generative pretrained transformers. *Scientific Reports, 13*(1), 4171. DOI: 10.1038/s41598-023-31223-5 PMID: 36914733

Sendak, M. P.. (2020). A path for translation of machine learning products into healthcare delivery. *NPJ Digital Medicine, 3*, 109. DOI: 10.1038/s41746-020-00349-5

Sendak, M. P., D'Arcy, J., Kashyap, S., Gao, M., Nichols, M., Corey, K., Ratliff, W., & Balu, S. (2020). *A path for translation of machine learning products into healthcare delivery*. EMJ Innovations.

Seyyed-Kalantari, L., Zhang, H., McDermott, M., Chen, I. Y., & Ghassemi, M. (2021). Underdiagnosis bias of AI algorithms applied to chest radiographs. *Nature Medicine*, 27(12), 2176–2182.World Health Organization (WHO). (2021). *Ethics and governance of artificial intelligence for health*. WHO.

Sharma, S., Zahir, A., & Lee, S. W. (2024). Trustworthy privacy-preserving hierarchical ensemble and federated learning in Healthcare 4.0 with blockchain. arXiv. https://arxiv.org/abs/2305.09209

Sheng, E., Chang, K.-W., Natarajan, P., & Peng, N. (2021). Societal Biases in Language Generation: Progress and Challenges. *Proceedings of the 59th Annual Meeting of the Association for Computational Linguistics and the 11th International Joint Conference on Natural Language Processing (*Volume 1*: Long Papers)*, 4275–4293. DOI: 10.18653/v1/2021.acl-long.330

Shen, Y.. (2023). Large language models in medicine: Evaluation and deployment. *Nature Medicine*, *29*, 26–36. DOI: 10.1038/s41591-022-02116-7

Shen, Y., Heacock, L., Elias, J., Hentel, K. D., Reig, B., Shih, G., & Moy, L. (2023). ChatGPT and Other Large Language Models Are Double-edged Swords. *Radiology*, *307*(2), e230163. Advance online publication. DOI: 10.1148/radiol.230163 PMID: 36700838

Shi, X.. (2023). LLM-Mini-CEX: Automatic evaluation of large language model for diagnostic conversation. *arXiv*. https://arxiv.org/abs/2308.07635

Shool, S., Adimi, S., Saboori Amleshi, R., Bitaraf, E., Golpira, R., & Tara, M. (2025). A systematic review of large language model evaluations in clinical medicine. *BMC Medical Informatics and Decision Making*, *25*(1), 54. DOI: 10.1186/s12911-025-02954-4 PMID: 40055694

Shortliffe, E. H., & Sepúlveda, M. J. (2018). Clinical decision support in the era of artificial intelligence. *Journal of the American Medical Association*, *320*(21), 2199–2200. DOI: 10.1001/jama.2018.17163 PMID: 30398550

Singhal, P., Goyal, T., Xu, J., & Durrett, G. (2024). *A Long Way to Go: Investigating Length Correlations in RLHF* (arXiv:2310.03716). arXiv. https://doi.org//arXiv.2310.03716DOI: 10.48550

Singhal, K.. (2023). Towards expert-level medical question answering with large language models. *arXiv*. https://arxiv.org/abs/2305.09617

Singhal, K., Azizi, S., Tu, T., Mahdavi, S. S., Wei, J., Chung, H. W., Scales, N., Tanwani, A., Cole-Lewis, H., Pfohl, S., Payne, P., Seneviratne, M., Gamble, P., Kelly, C., Babiker, A., Schärli, N., Chowdhery, A., Mansfield, P., Demner-Fushman, D., & Natarajan, V. (2023). Large language models encode clinical knowledge. *Nature*, *620*(7972), 172–180. DOI: 10.1038/s41586-023-06291-2 PMID: 37438534

Singhal, K., Tu, T., Gottweis, J., Sayres, R., Wulczyn, E., Amin, M., Hou, L., Clark, K., Pfohl, S. R., Cole-Lewis, H., Neal, D., Rashid, Q. M., Schaekermann, M., Wang, A., Dash, D., Chen, J. H., Shah, N. H., Lachgar, S., Mansfield, P. A., & Natarajan, V. (2025). Toward expert-level medical question answering with large language models. *Nature Medicine*, *31*(3), 943–950. DOI: 10.1038/s41591-024-03423-7 PMID: 39779926

Singh, P., & Rao, T. (2024). Blockchain as a privacy enabler in clinical AI systems. *International Journal of Digital Health*, *8*(1), 88–104.

Smith, R., O'Brien, J., & Patel, A. (2023). Data governance and patient rights under HIPAA and GDPR. *Health Policy and Research*, *19*(3), 144–160.

Song, C., & Raghunathan, A. (2020). Information leakage in embedding models. In *ACM SIGSAC Conference on Computer and Communications Security* (pp. 377–390).

Sorich, M. J., Menz, B. D., & Hopkins, A. M. (2024). Quality and safety of artificial intelligence generated health information. *BMJ (Clinical Research Ed.)*, *384*, q596. DOI: 10.1136/bmj.q596 PMID: 38508683

Steybe, D., Poxleitner, P., Aljohani, S., Herlofson, B. B., Nicolatou-Galitis, O., Patel, V., Fedele, S., Kwon, T.-G., Fusco, V., Pichardo, S. E. C., Obermeier, K. T., Otto, S., Rau, A., & Russe, M. F. (2025). Evaluation of a context-aware chatbot using retrieval-augmented generation for answering clinical questions on medication-related osteonecrosis of the jaw. *Journal of Cranio-Maxillo-Facial Surgery*, *53*(4), 355–360. DOI: 10.1016/j.jcms.2024.12.009 PMID: 39799075

Suenghataiphorn, K.. (2025). Bias detection in healthcare AI systems. *IEEE Access : Practical Innovations, Open Solutions*, *13*, 55678–55690.

Sujan, M., White, S., Habli, I., & Reynolds, N. Stakeholder Perceptions of the Safety and Assurance of Artificial Intelligence in Healthcare. SSRN Electron J. Published online 2022.

Sun, Z., Yim, W.-W., Uzuner, Ö., Xia, F., & Yetisgen, M. (2025). A scoping review of natural language processing in addressing medically inaccurate information: Errors, misinformation, and hallucination. *Journal of Biomedical Informatics*, *169*, 104866. DOI: 10.1016/j.jbi.2025.104866 PMID: 40706945

Sutton, R. T., Pincock, D., Baumgart, D. C., Sadowski, D. C., Fedorak, R. N., & Kroeker, K. I. (2020). An overview of clinical decision support systems: Benefits, risks, and strategies for success. *NPJ Digital Medicine*, *3*(1), 17. DOI: 10.1038/s41746-020-0221-y PMID: 32047862

Tam, T. Y. C., Sivarajkumar, S., Kapoor, S., Stolyar, A. V., Polanska, K., McCarthy, K. R., Osterhoudt, H., Wu, X., Visweswaran, S., Fu, S., Mathur, P., Cacciamani, G. E., Sun, C., Peng, Y., & Wang, Y. (2024). A framework for human evaluation of large language models in healthcare derived from literature review. *NPJ Digital Medicine*, *7*(1), 258. DOI: 10.1038/s41746-024-01258-7 PMID: 39333376

Tang, K. S., Cheng, D. L., Mi, E., & Greenberg, P. B. (2020). Augmented reality in medical education: A systematic review. *Canadian Medical Education Journal*, *11*(1), e81. DOI: 10.36834/cmej.61705 PMID: 32215146

Tan, T. F., Thirunavukarasu, A. J., Quek, C., & Ting, D. S. W. (2025). Evaluation of ophthalmic large language models: Quantitative vs. qualitative methods. *Current Opinion in Ophthalmology*, *36*(6), 466–471. DOI: 10.1097/ICU.0000000000001171 PMID: 40910897

Tan, Y., Zhang, Z., Li, M., Pan, F., Duan, H., Huang, Z., Deng, H., Yu, Z., Yang, C., Shen, G., Qi, P., Yue, C., Liu, Y., Hong, L., Yu, H., Fan, G., & Tang, Y. (2024). MedChatZH: A tuning LLM for traditional Chinese medicine consultations. *Computers in Biology and Medicine*, *172*, 108290. DOI: 10.1016/j.compbiomed.2024.108290 PMID: 38503097

Temsah, O., Khan, S. A., Chaiah, Y., Senjab, A., Alhasan, K., Jamal, A., Aljamaan, F., Malki, K. H., Halwani, R., Al-Tawfiq, J. A., Temsah, M.-H., & Al-Eyadhy, A. (2023). Overview of early ChatGPT's presence in medical literature. *Cureus*, *15*(4), e37281. DOI: 10.7759/cureus.37281 PMID: 37038381

Teo, Z. L., Jin, L., Liu, N., Li, S., Miao, D., Zhang, X., Ng, W. Y., Tan, T. F., Lee, D. M., Chua, K. J., Heng, J., Liu, Y., & Goh, R. S. M. (2024). Federated machine learning in healthcare: A systematic review on clinical applications and technical architecture. *Cell Reports Medicine*, *5*(3), 101481. DOI: 10.1016/j.xcrm.2024.101481

Thirunavukarasu, A. J., Ting, D. S. J., Elangovan, K., Gutierrez, L., Tan, T. F., & Ting, D. S. W. (2023). Large language models in medicine. *Nature Medicine*, *29*(8), 1930–1940. DOI: 10.1038/s41591-023-02448-8 PMID: 37460753

Thirupathi, L., Kaashipaka, V., Dhanaraju, M., & Katakam, V. (2025). AI and IoT in Mental Health Care: From Digital Diagnostics to Personalized, Continuous Support. In Joshi, H., Kumar Reddy, C., Ouaissa, M., Hanafiah, M., & Doss, S. (Eds.), *Intelligent Systems and IoT Applications in Clinical Health* (pp. 271–294). IGI Global Scientific Publishing., DOI: 10.4018/979-8-3693-8990-4.ch012

Thirupathi, L., Srinivasulu, B., Khanapurkar, U., Rambabu, D., & Preeti, C. M. (2023). Heart Disease Prediction in Healthcare Communities by Machine Learning Over Big Data. In Bhateja, V., Sunitha, K. V. N., Chen, Y. W., & Zhang, Y. D. (Eds.), *Intelligent System Design. Lecture Notes in Networks and Systems* (Vol. 494). Springer., DOI: 10.1007/978-981-19-4863-3_38

Thrasher, J., Devkota, A., Siwakotai, P., Chivukula, R., Poudel, P., Hu, C., Bhattarai, B., & Gyawali, P. (2023). Multimodal federated learning in healthcare: A review. arXiv. https://arxiv.org/abs/2310.09650

Tonekaboni, S., Joshi, S., McCradden, M. D., & Goldenberg, A. (2023). What clinicians want: Contextualizing explainable machine learning for clinical end use. In *Machine Learning for Healthcare Conference* (pp. 359–380).

Topol, E. (2019). *Deep medicine: how artificial intelligence can make healthcare human again.*

Topol, E. (2019). High-performance medicine: The convergence of human and artificial intelligence. *Nature Medicine*, *25*(1), 44–56. DOI: 10.1038/s41591-018-0300-7 PMID: 30617339

Tripathi, S., Sukumaran, R., & Cook, T. S. (2024). Efficient healthcare with large language models: Optimizing clinical workflow and enhancing patient care. *Journal of the American Medical Informatics Association : JAMIA*, *31*(6), 1436–1440. DOI: 10.1093/jamia/ocad258 PMID: 38273739

Tsoutsanis, P., & Tsoutsanis, A. (2024). Evaluation of Large language model performance on the Multi-Specialty Recruitment Assessment (MSRA) exam. *Computers in Biology and Medicine*, *168*, 107794. DOI: 10.1016/j.compbiomed.2023.107794 PMID: 38043471

Tu, T.. (2024). Towards conversational diagnostic AI. *arXiv*. https://arxiv.org/abs/2401.05654

Tu, T.. (2025). Towards conversational diagnostic AI (AMIE). *Nature*. Advance online publication. DOI: 10.1038/s41586-025-08866-7

U.S. Food and Drug Administration. (2021). Good machine learning practice for medical device development: Guiding principles. https://www.fda.gov/medical-devices/software-medical-device-samd/good-machine-learning-practice-medical-device-development-guiding-principles

U.S. Food and Drug Administration. (2023). *Artificial intelligence and machine learning in medical devices.*

Ueda, D., Mitsuyama, Y., Takita, H., Horiuchi, D., Walston, S. L., Tatekawa, H., & Miki, Y. (2023). Diagnostic Performance of ChatGPT from Patient History and Imaging Findings on the Diagnosis Please Quizzes. *Radiology*, *308*(1), e231040. Advance online publication. DOI: 10.1148/radiol.231040 PMID: 37462501

Ui-Haq, Z., Causin, L., Kamalati, T., Kahol, D., Vaikunthanathan, T., Wong, C., & Arebi, N. (2024). Health-care resource use and costs associated with inflammatory bowel disease in northwest London: A retrospective linked database study. *BMC Gastroenterology*, *24*(1), 480. DOI: 10.1186/s12876-024-03559-3 PMID: 39736541

Ukwuoma, C. C., Cai, D., Eziefuna, E. O., Oluwasanmi, A., Abdi, S. F., Muoka, G. W., Thomas, D., & Sarpong, K. (2025). Enhancing histopathological medical image classification for Early cancer diagnosis using deep learning and explainable AI – LIME & SHAP. *Biomedical Signal Processing and Control*, *100*, 107014. DOI: 10.1016/j.bspc.2024.107014

UNESCO. (2024). *Ethics of Artificial Intelligence in Healthcare: Policy Guidance Report*. UNESCO Press.

Vaezi, A. (2025). Legal Challenges in the Deployment of Large Language Models: A Comparative Analysis under the GDPR and EU AI Act. *Available at SSRN* 5285174. https://dx.doi.org/DOI: 10.2139/ssrn.5285174

Van De Sijpe, G., Quintens, C., Walgraeve, K., Van Laer, E., Penny, J., De Vlieger, G., Schrijvers, R., De Munter, P., Foulon, V., Casteels, M., Van der Linden, L., & Spriet, I. (2022). Overall performance of a drug–drug interaction clinical decision support system: Quantitative evaluation and end-user survey. *BMC Medical Informatics and Decision Making*, *22*(1), 48. DOI: 10.1186/s12911-022-01783-z PMID: 35193547

van der Vegt, A. H., Campbell, V., Mitchell, I., Malycha, J., Simpson, J., Flenady, T., Flabouris, A., Lane, P. J., Mehta, N., Kalke, V. R., Decoyna, J. A., Es'haghi, N., Liu, C.-H., & Scott, I. A. (2024). Systematic review and longitudinal analysis of implementing Artificial Intelligence to predict clinical deterioration in adult hospitals: What is known and what remains uncertain. *Journal of the American Medical Informatics Association : JAMIA*, *31*(2), 509–524. DOI: 10.1093/jamia/ocad220 PMID: 37964688

Van Dort, B. A., Zheng, W. Y., Sundar, V., & Baysari, M. T. (2021). Optimizing clinical decision support alerts in electronic medical records: A systematic review of reported strategies adopted by hospitals. *Journal of the American Medical Informatics Association : JAMIA*, *28*(1), 177–183. DOI: 10.1093/jamia/ocaa279 PMID: 33186438

Van Melle, W. (1978). MYCIN: A knowledge-based consultation program for infectious disease diagnosis. *International Journal of Man-Machine Studies*, *10*(3), 313–322. DOI: 10.1016/S0020-7373(78)80049-2

van Nuland, M., Lobbezoo, A.-F. H., van de Garde, E. M. W., Herbrink, M., van Heijl, I., Bognàr, T., Houwen, J. P. A., Dekens, M., Wannet, D., Egberts, T., & van der Linden, P. D. (2024). Assessing accuracy of ChatGPT in response to questions from day to day pharmaceutical care in hospitals. *Exploratory Research in Clinical and Social Pharmacy*, *15*(100464), 100464. DOI: 10.1016/j.rcsop.2024.100464 PMID: 39050145

van Tongeren, J. M. Z., Harkes-Idzinga, S. F., van der Sijs, H., Atiqi, R., van den Bemt, B. J. F., Draijer, L. W., Hiel, D., Kerremans, A., Kremers, B., de Leeuw, M., Olthoff, M. V., Pham, T. K.-L., Valentijn-Robertz, R., Tsoi, K., Wichers, I., de Wit, M., & Borgsteede, S. D. (2020). The development of practice recommendations for drug-disease interactions by literature review and expert opinion. *Frontiers in Pharmacology*, *11*, 707. DOI: 10.3389/fphar.2020.00707 PMID: 32499701

Veale, M., & Binns, R. (2024). Fairer machine learning in the real world: Mitigating discrimination without collecting sensitive data. *Big Data & Society*, *4*(2). DOI: 10.1177/2053951717743530

Verghese, A., Shah, N. H., & Harrington, R. A. (2023). What this computer needs is a physician: Humanism and artificial intelligence. *Journal of the American Medical Association*, *319*(1), 19–20. DOI: 10.1001/jama.2017.19198 PMID: 29261830

Vieujean, S., Jairath, V., Peyrin-Biroulet, L., Dubinsky, M., Iacucci, M., Magro, F., & Danese, S. (2025). Understanding the therapeutic toolkit for inflammatory bowel disease. *Nature Reviews. Gastroenterology & Hepatology*, *22*(6), 371–394. DOI: 10.1038/s41575-024-01035-7

Vorisek, C. N., Lehne, M., Klopfenstein, S. A., Mayer, P. J., Bartschke, A., Haase, P., & Prasser, F. (2022). Fast healthcare interoperability resources (FHIR) for interoperability in health research: Systematic review. *JMIR Medical Informatics*, *10*(7), e35724. DOI: 10.2196/35724 PMID: 35852842

Vrdoljak, J., Boban, Z., Vilović, M., Kumrić, M., & Božić, J. (2025). A review of large language models in medical education, clinical decision support, and healthcare administration. *Health Care*, *13*, 603. PMID: 40150453

Wadden, J. J. (2021). Defining the undefinable: The black box problem in healthcare artificial intelligence. *Journal of Medical Ethics*. PMID: 34290113

Waheed, N., Ur Rehman, A., Nehra, A., Farooq, M., Tariq, N., Jan, M. A., Alalmaie, A. Z., & Nanda, P. (2023). FedBlockHealth: A synergistic approach to privacy and security in IoT-enabled healthcare through federated learning and blockchain. arXiv. https://arxiv.org/abs/2304.07668 DOI: 10.1109/GLOBECOM54140.2023.10437356

Wang, H., Gao, C., Dantona, C., Hull, B., & Sun, J. (2024). DRG-LLaMA: Tuning LLaMA model to predict diagnosis-related group for hospitalized patients. *NPJ Digital Medicine*, *7*(1), 16. DOI: 10.1038/s41746-023-00989-3 PMID: 38253711

Wang, L., Yan, Y., He, K., Wu, Y., & Xu, W. (2021). Dynamically Disentangling Social Bias from Task-Oriented Representations with Adversarial Attack. *Proceedings of the 2021 Conference of the North American Chapter of the Association for Computational Linguistics: Human Language Technologies*, 3740–3750. DOI: 10.18653/v1/2021.naacl-main.293

Wang, M. H. (2025). Explainable artificial intelligence framework for predicting treatment outcomes in age-related macular degeneration. *Sensors (Basel)*, *25*(22), 6879. DOI: 10.3390/s25226879 PMID: 41305085

Wang, Q., Torres, L., & Chen, M. (2024). Explainable AI for clinical decision support: Current status and prospects. *Computers in Biology and Medicine*, *170*, 108–120.

Wang, S.. (2025). A novel evaluation benchmark for medical large language models illuminating safety and effectiveness. *npj. Digital Medicine*.

Wang, S., Tang, Z., Yang, H., Gong, Q., Gu, T., Ma, H., Wang, Y., Sun, W., Lian, Z., Mao, K., Jiang, Y., Huang, Z., Ma, L., Shen, W., Ji, Y., Tan, Y., Wang, C., Gao, Y., Ye, Q., & Wu, J. (2025). A novel evaluation benchmark for medical LLMs illuminating safety and effectiveness in clinical domains. npj. *Digital Medicine*, *9*(1), 91. Advance online publication. DOI: 10.1038/s41746-025-02277-8 PMID: 41454006

Wang, X., Zhang, N. X., He, H., Nguyen, T., Yu, K.-H., Deng, H., Brandt, C., Bitterman, D. S., Pan, L., Cheng, C.-Y., Zou, J., & Liu, D. (2024). Safety challenges of AI in medicine in the era of large language models. arXiv. https://arxiv.org/abs/2409.18968

Warm, E. (2025, August 26). Deskilling and automation bias: A cautionary tale for health professions educators. ICE Blog. https://icenet.blog/2025/08/26/deskilling-and-automation-bias-a-cautionary-tale-for-health-professions-educators/

Warraich, H. J., Tazbaz, T., & Califf, R. M. (2025). FDA perspective on the regulation of artificial intelligence in health care and biomedicine. *Journal of the American Medical Association*, *333*(3), 241–247. DOI: 10.1001/jama.2024.21451 PMID: 39405330

Wawra-Hehenberger, K., Pencelli, V., Pardo, J. A., Tremmel, L., Ataher, Q., & Waschbusch, M. (2025). A visual safety risk evaluation tool in early clinical phases. *Contemporary Clinical Trials, 154*, 107953. DOI: 10.1016/j.cct.2025.107953 PMID: 40381907

Welbl, J., Glaese, A., Uesato, J., Dathathri, S., Mellor, J., Hendricks, L. A., Anderson, K., Kohli, P., Coppin, B., & Huang, P. S. (2021). Challenges in detoxifying language models. arXiv preprint arXiv:2109.07445. DOI: 10.18653/v1/2021.findings-emnlp.210

Widmer, G., & Kubat, M. (1996). Learning in the presence of concept drift. *Machine Learning, 30*(1), 69–101. DOI: 10.1023/A:1018046501280

Wiens, J., Saria, S., Sendak, M., Ghassemi, M., Liu, V. X., Doshi-Velez, F., & Goldenberg, A. (2019). Do no harm: A roadmap for responsible machine learning for health care. *Nature Medicine, 25*(9), 1337–1340. DOI: 10.1038/s41591-019-0548-6 PMID: 31427808

Williams, C. Y., Bains, J., Tang, T., Patel, K., Lucas, A. N., Chen, F., Miao, B. Y., Butte, A. J., & Kornblith, A. E. (2025). Evaluating large language models for drafting emergency department encounter summaries. *PLOS Digital Health, 4*(6), e0000899. DOI: 10.1371/journal.pdig.0000899 PMID: 40526634

Williams, C. Y., Subramanian, C. R., Ali, S. S., Apolinario, M., Askin, E., Barish, P., Cheng, M., Deardorff, W. J., Donthi, N., Ganeshan, S., Huang, O., Kantor, M. A., Lai, A. R., Manchanda, A., Moore, K. A., Muniyappa, A. N., Nair, G., Patel, P. P., Santhosh, L., & Rosner, B. I. (2025). Physician- and large language model–generated hospital discharge summaries. *JAMA Internal Medicine, 185*(7), 818. DOI: 10.1001/jamainternmed.2025.0821 PMID: 40323616

Williams, R., Kantilal, K., Man, K. K. C., Blandford, A., & Jani, Y. (2025). Barcode medication administration system use and safety implications: A data-driven longitudinal study supported by clinical observation. *BMJ Health & Care Informatics, 32*(1), e101214. DOI: 10.1136/bmjhci-2024-101214 PMID: 39832825

Wong, R., Ming, L., & Raja Ali, R. (2023). The Intersection of ChatGPT, Clinical Medicine, and Medical Education. *JMIR Medical Education, 9*, e47274. https://mededu.jmir.org/2023/1/e47274. DOI: 10.2196/47274 PMID: 37988149

Woo, B. F. Y., Song, J., Middleton, E., Fijačko, N., & Cato, K. (2025). Teaching critical thinking in the age of AI: Safeguarding clinical reasoning in healthcare documentation. *International Nursing Review, 72*(3), e70102. DOI: 10.1111/inr.70102 PMID: 40845221

World Health Organization. (2021). *Ethics and governance of artificial intelligence for health*. WHO.

World Health Organization. (2023). *Guidance on Ethics and Governance of Artificial Intelligence for Health*. World Health Organization.

World Health Organization. (2024). Ethics and governance of artificial intelligence for health: Guidance on large multi-modal models. https://www.who.int/publications/i/item/9789240084759

Wright, A., & Sittig, D. F. (2008). A four-phase model of the evolution of clinical decision support architectures. *International Journal of Medical Informatics*, *77*(10), 641–649. DOI: 10.1016/j.ijmedinf.2008.01.004 PMID: 18353713

Wu, X., Huang, Y., Liu, Z., Lai, W., Long, E., Zhang, K., Jiang, J., Lin, D., Chen, K., Yu, T., Wu, D., Li, C., Chen, Y., Zou, M., Chen, C., Zhu, Y., Guo, C., Zhang, X., Wang, R., & Lin, H. (2019). Universal artificial intelligence platform for collaborative management of cataracts. *The British Journal of Ophthalmology*, *103*(11), 1553–1560. DOI: 10.1136/bjophthalmol-2019-314729 PMID: 31481392

Xiong, G., Jin, Q., Lu, Z., & Zhang, A. (2024). Benchmarking retrieval-augmented generation for medicine. In *Findings of the Association for Computational Linguistics* (pp. 6233–6251). ACL.

Xompero, C., Rossi, L., Amoroso, F., Bechara Ghobril, A., Ionita, D. E., Souied, E. H., & Mehanna, C.-J. (2025). Pilot study of ASSORT (AI-based Symptom Stratification in Ophthalmology for Rapid Triage): A triage tool for ophthalmic emergencies. *AJO International*, *2*(3), 100159. DOI: 10.1016/j.ajoint.2025.100159

Xu, D., Zhang, Z., Zhu, Z., Lin, Z., Liu, Q., Wu, X., Xu, T., Zhao, X., Zheng, Y., & Chen, E. (2024). Mitigating hallucinations of large language models in medical information extraction via contrastive decoding. /arXiv.2410.15702DOI: 10.18653/v1/2024.findings-emnlp.456

Xu, H., Ji, J., & Jin, H.. (2026). Ethical risks of large language models in medical consultation: An assessment based on reproductive ethics. *arXiv*. https://arxiv.org/abs/2601.22621

Yang, L., Xu, C., & Wang, X. (2025). Cost-Effective Medical Dialogue Summarization with Fine-Tuned Compact LLMs. In Mahmud, M., Doborjeh, M., Wong, K., Leung, A. C. S., Doborjeh, Z., & Tanveer, M. (Eds.), *Neural Information Processing. ICONIP 2024. Communications in Computer and Information Science* (Vol. 2287). Springer., DOI: 10.1007/978-981-96-6963-9_18

Yarram, S., Dasari, N., Seshagani, S. B., & Ganguly, P. (2025). Privacy-Preserving Healthcare Data Security Using Large Language Models and Adaptive Access Control. *2025 IEEE World AI IoT Congress (AIIoT)*, 0854–0860. DOI: 10.1109/AIIoT65859.2025.11105296

Yasaka, K., Kanzawa, J., Kanemaru, N., Koshino, S., & Abe, O. (2025). Fine-Tuned Large Language Model for Extracting Patients on Pretreatment for Lung Cancer from a Picture Archiving and Communication System Based on Radiological Reports. *Journal of Imaging Informatics in Medicine*, *38*(1), 327–334. DOI: 10.1007/s10278-024-01186-8 PMID: 38955964

Yu, C., Jeoung, S., Kasi, A., Yu, P., & Ji, H. (2023). Unlearning Bias in Language Models by Partitioning Gradients. *Findings of the Association for Computational Linguistics: ACL, 2023*, 6032–6048. DOI: 10.18653/v1/2023.findings-acl.375

Yu, M., Ren, L., Zheng, M., Hong, M., & Wei, Z. (2022). Delayed diagnosis of Wilson's disease: Report from 179 newly diagnosed cases in China. *Frontiers in Neurology*, *13*, 884840. DOI: 10.3389/fneur.2022.884840 PMID: 35865642

Yu, P., Xu, H., Hu, X., & Deng, C. (2023). Leveraging generative AI and large language models: A comprehensive roadmap for healthcare integration. *Health Care*, *11*, 2776. PMID: 37893850

Yu, Y., Ying, H., & Jin, H.. (2025). MedKGEval: A knowledge graph-based multi-turn evaluation framework for open-ended patient interactions with clinical large language models. *arXiv*. https://arxiv.org/abs/2510.12224

Zack, T., Luhanga, M., Rajkomar, A., & Obermeyer, Z. (2024). Assessing the potential of GPT-4 to perpetuate racial and gender biases in health care. *The Lancet. Digital Health*, *6*(1), e12–e22. DOI: 10.1016/S2589-7500(23)00225-X PMID: 38123252

Zadeh, L. A. (1965). Fuzzy sets. *Information and Control*, *8*(3), 338–353. DOI: 10.1016/S0019-9958(65)90241-X

Zaki, N., Akor, A., & Aburuz, S. C ZainAlAbdin, S. (2025). Beyond Accuracy: An Efficiency-and Safety-Aware Framework for Evaluating Clinical AI with Large Language Models. medRxiv, 2025-10. https://doi.org/DOI: 10.1101/2025.10.14.25338039

Zakka, C., Chaurasia, A., Shad, R., Dalal, A. R., Kim, J. L., Moor, M., ... & Hiesinger, W. (2024). Almanac — Retrieval-augmented language models for clinical medicine. NEJM AI, 1(2), AIoa2300068. DOI: 10.1056/AIoa2300068

Zampieri, M., Malmasi, S., Nakov, P., Rosenthal, S., Farra, N., & Kumar, R. (2019). Predicting the type and target of offensive posts in social media. In *Proceedings of the 2019 Conference of the North American Chapter of the Association for Computational Linguistics: Human Language Technologies* (pp. 1415–1420). DOI: 10.18653/v1/N19-1144

Zanchi, M. G. (2024). Crafting the future of healthcare with LLMs. Medium. https://medium.com/ninacapital/crafting-the-future-of-healthcare-with-llms-01a3e6b92df9

Zanchi, M. G.. (2024). Generative AI in Medical Practice: In-Depth Exploration of Privacy and Security Challenges. *Journal of Medical Internet Research*, *26*, e53008. DOI: 10.2196/53008

Zanella-Béguelin, S., Wutschitz, L., Tople, S., Rühle, V., Paverd, A., Ohrimenko, O., Köpf, B., & Brockschmidt, M. (2020). Analyzing information leakage of updates to natural language models. In *Proceedings of the 2020 ACM SIGSAC Conference on Computer and Communications Security* (pp. 363–375). DOI: 10.1145/3372297.3417880

Zhang, B., Zhu, J., & Su, H. (2023). Toward the third generation artificial intelligence. *Science China. Information Sciences*, *66*(2), 121101. DOI: 10.1007/s11432-021-3449-x

Zhang, K., Li, Y., Wu, P., Li, Y., Zhang, C., & Zan, H. (2025). Knowledge Enhancement with LLMs for Few-Shot Medical Relation Extraction. In Zhang, Y. (Eds.), *Health Information Processing. CHIP 2024. Communications in Computer and Information Science* (Vol. 2433). Springer., DOI: 10.1007/978-981-96-3752-2_10

Zhang, R., & Patel, N. (2025). Privacy-preserving LLMs in medicine: Trends and challenges. *AI in Healthcare Journal*, *9*(2), 102–119.

Zhang, Y.. (2024). Real-time monitoring of large language models in healthcare. *IEEE Journal of Biomedical and Health Informatics*. Advance online publication. DOI: 10.1109/JBHI.2024.3341125

Zhao, X., Blotske, K., Cargile, M., Tilley, A., Murray, B., Gao, Y., . . . Sikora, A. (2025). Rx-LLM: a benchmarking suite to evaluate safe large language model performance for medication-related tasks. medRxiv, 2025-12. https://doi.org/DOI: 10.64898/2025.12.01.25341004

Zhen, J., & Gao, C. (2023). From challenges and pitfalls to recommendations and opportunities: Implementing federated learning in healthcare. *Journal of Healthcare Informatics Research*.

Zhong, X., Li, S., Chen, Z., Ge, L., Yu, D., Wang, S., You, L., & Shang, H. (2025). Considerations for Patient Privacy of Large Language Models in Health Care: Scoping Review. *Journal of Medical Internet Research, 27*, e76571. DOI: 10.2196/76571 PMID: 41269747

Zhou, H., Liu, F., Gu, B., Zou, X., Huang, J., Wu, J., ... A survey of large language models in medicine: progress, application, and challenge. ArXiv Preprint. 2023;arXiv:231105112.

Zhou, C., Rahman, A., & Liu, D. (2024). Secure federated architectures for health data. *Journal of Medical AI Security, 7*(1), 65–80.

Zhou, S., Luo, X., Chen, C., Jiang, H., Yang, C., Ran, G., Yu, J., & Yin, C. (2024). The performance of large language model-powered chatbots compared to oncology physicians on colorectal cancer queries. *International Journal of Surgery, 110*(10), 6509–6517. DOI: 10.1097/JS9.0000000000001850 PMID: 38935100

Zhu, Q., Hou, B., Mathai, T. S., Mukherjee, P., Jin, Q., Chen, X., Wang, Z., Cheng, R., Summers, R. M., & Lu, Z. (2025). How well do multimodal LLMs interpret CT scans? An auto-evaluation framework for analyses. *Journal of Biomedical Informatics, 168*, 104864. DOI: 10.1016/j.jbi.2025.104864 PMID: 40578543

Zou, J., & Schiebinger, L. (2022). AI can be sexist and racist—It's time to make it fair. *Nature, 559*(7714), 324–326. DOI: 10.1038/d41586-018-05707-8 PMID: 30018439

About the Contributors

Fernando Ortiz-Rodriguez is a Full Professor and Head of the Artificial Intelligence and Innovation Lab at Tamaulipas Autonomous University. He was the Executive Director at the International Institute of Studies (IIES). He created the First Business School in Tamaulipas, Mexico. He worked as the Information Technology Manager at Emerson Electric, where he developed more than 40 pieces of software, some of them used globally in Emerson, and he achieved technology convergence by implementing the first efforts on IoT and Industry 4.0. Fernando is a member of National Systems Researchers (SNI) Level 1 of the National Council of Science and Technology (CONACYT) and INDEX IT Advisor

Mrignainy Kansal is a Ph.D. researcher in Computer Science and Engineering at Netaji Subhas University of Technology (NSUT), New Delhi, India. She previously served as an Assistant Professor in the Department of Information Technology at Ajay Kumar Garg sEngineering College (AKGEC), Ghaziabad, where she contributed to teaching, research, and academic development. She brings over six years of academic experience in higher education. Her research lies at the intersection of software engineering and artificial intelligence, with a primary focus on software defect prediction, explainable AI, and intelligent data-driven systems. She has an extensive publication record, with contributions in reputed journals and conferences including Springer, IEEE, Wiley, and IGI Global. Her work emphasizes the development of robust, interpretable, and scalable solutions for real-world software quality challenges. She has also made notable contributions through edited volumes, book chapters, and active participation in international conferences, including serving as a Conference Program Committee Member. She is the recipient of multiple Best Paper Awards and holds several published and granted patents in emerging domains such as artificial intelligence, blockchain, and smart systems. She is an IEEE member and remains actively engaged in advancing research, innovation, and scholarly collaboration in intelligent software engineering.

Rajesh Kumar Dhanaraj is a distinguished Professor at Symbiosis International (Deemed University) in Pune, India. Prior to this, he served as a Professor at the School of Computing Science & Engineering at Galgotias University in Greater Noida, India. His exceptional academic and research contributions have placed him among the top 2% of scientists globally, an honor recognized by Elsevier and Stanford University. Dr. Dhanaraj completed his B.E. in Computer Science and Engineering from Anna University Chennai, followed by an M.Tech from Anna University Coimbatore. He earned his Ph.D. in Computer Science from Anna University, Chennai. His prolific career includes authoring and editing over 100 books on advanced technologies and holding 27 patents. He has published over 200 articles in esteemed journals and international conferences, including six papers in IEEE Transactions. As a mentor, Dr. Dhanaraj has guided four PhD candidates to completion, with eight more currently under his supervision. He is renowned for delivering insightful tech talks on disruptive technologies and has established valuable collaborations with professors from top QS-ranked universities globally. Dr. Dhanaraj's research interests include Applied AI, Cyber-Physical Systems, and Wireless Sensor Networks. His expertise in these areas has led to numerous research talks at esteemed institutions. He is a Senior Member of the IEEE, and a member of the CSTA and IAENG. Additionally, he serves as an Associate Editor and Guest Editor for several prestigious journals and is an Expert Advisory Panel Member of Texas Instruments Inc., USA.

Firoz Khan is an academic and researcher with a distinguished Ph.D. in Computer Science from the British University in Dubai. He also holds a Master's in Information Technology from the University of Southern Queensland (USQ) and a Master's in Information, Network, and Computer Security from the New York Institute of Technology (NYIT). His research interests include IoT applications in agriculture, automotive cybersecurity, and the integration of AI with cybersecurity in healthcare. He is also exploring advanced topics such as precision farming techniques, privacy-preserving models, and liquid neural networks for time-series prediction in healthcare. As an educator, Firoz specializes in teaching IoT security, cybersecurity, and advanced networking. He emphasizes a hands-on, active learning approach to equip students with practical skills and foster innovation, preparing them for challenges in an ever-evolving technological landscape.

***

Ravi Aavula working as an Associate Professor in the Department of Data Science, Anurag University, has about 21 years of teaching experience. He received his B.Tech degree in Computer Science and Engineering with distinction and

M.Tech. degree in Software Engineering with distinction from JNTUH University, HYDERABAD. He received Ph.D degree in Computer Science and Engineering from GITAM University, Andhra Pradesh state. He has published 20 research papers in refereed International journals and 10 research papers in the proceedings of various International conferences. He has received several best paper awards for his research papers at various International conferences. His areas of research include Machine Learning, Artificial Intelligence, Data Mining, Computer Networks, Deep Learning, Cloud Computing. He is an active member of CSE, ISTE.

Maheswaran C. P. has more than 17 years of expertise in teaching. He completed his under graduation in Manonmaniam Sundaranar University and post graduation in Anna University. Dr. Maheswaran C. P. obtained his Doctorate of Philosophy in Faculty of Information and Communication Engineering at 2017 from Noorul Islam Centre for Higher Education. He is a supervisor in Anna University. He started his career in 2006 and worked in few institutions. His areas of interest constitute the study of wireless networks, cloud computing, mobile networks, and information security. He has published 75 research papers in SCI-indexed journals, UGC and Scopus-indexed journals. He has written ten book chapters and two books. He filed five patents to demonstrate the potential of his studies and four of them were published and a few patents under examination. He has extensive experience in guiding students in a variety of national and international activities. He was also influential in industry academic collaboration. Dr. Maheswaran C.P. is a reviewer in 6 of the IEEE conferences held at various places in India. Currently, He is a working as Professor and Head at Department of Artificial Intelligenc

Radhiyatul Fajri, S.Kom., M.Pd.T., M.Kom. is a First Engineer at the National Research and Innovation Agency (BRIN), Indonesia. She is a data-driven researcher with expertise in analyzing both structured and unstructured data using programming and statistical tools. Her academic and applied research focuses on Natural Language Processing (NLP), sentiment analysis, and computer vision. She has extensive experience in data cleaning, exploratory data analysis, and machine learning model development, as well as working with survey data in social and educational contexts. Her work also involves data visualization and translating analytical findings into actionable insights for non-technical stakeholders. Her research contributions are indexed in major academic databases, including Scopus (Author ID: 57956375200), ORCID (0000-0003-2812-1077), Web of Science (ResearcherID: OYD-4394-2025), and Google Scholar. She is committed to advancing AI-driven research and leveraging data science for real-world impact, particularly in education and interdisciplinary applications.

G. Loganayaki is an Assistant Professor in the Department of English at SRC, SASTRA Deemed University. With over 18 years of teaching experience, she has published around 25 research papers and contributed several book chapters. Her areas of specialization include Ecocriticism, Spatial Theory, and Hauntology. She also serves as a research supervisor for Ph.D. scholars and has led projects integrating literature, indigenous knowledge systems, and environmental sustainability.

Shashi Kant Gupta is a distinguished academic and researcher in the field of Computer Science and Engineering, with a prolific career spanning over a decade. His extensive contributions to academia and industry are marked by his roles in various prestigious institutions and his leadership in innovative research projects. Prof. Gupta's work primarily focuses on Cloud Computing, Big Data Analytics, IoT, and Computational Intelligence with multidisciplinary areas in which he has made significant advancements. Prof. Gupta is currently serving as a Post-Doctoral Fellow and Researcher at Eudoxia Research University, USA, where he is involved in cutting-edge research in Computer Science and Engineering. In addition, he holds the position of Adjunct Faculty, Faculty of Information Technology, Victorian Institute of Technology, Level 14,123 Queen Street, Melbourne VIC 3000, Australia. And an Adjunct Professor at Lincoln University College, Malaysia, contributing to the academic development of students in the region. His role as a Research Fellow at Inti International University, Malaysia, further underscores his commitment to fostering research and innovation.

Vishal Jain currently serves as a Professor and Dean of Accreditation, Statutory Compliances & Institutional Development at the School of Engineering & Technology, Vivekananda Institute of Professional Studies - Technical Campus, New Delhi. His previous roles include Professor at Sharda University, Greater Noida, and Associate Professor at Bharati Vidyapeeth's Institute of Computer Applications and Management (BVICAM), New Delhi. Dr. Jain has actively participated in various academic governance bodies, including the Faculty Board, Board of Planning and Management, Executive Council, Academic Council, Curriculum Development and Review Committee, and Academic Audit across multiple higher education institutions. He collaborates with Kuala Lumpur University of Science and Technology (KLUST), Malaysia, Lincoln University College, Malaysia and the Research Institute of IoT Cybersecurity at National Kaohsiung University of Science and Technology in Taiwan for research initiatives. He has supervised three Ph.D. candidates, with two additional scholars currently pursuing their degrees under his guidance.

Kruthika K is a student from the Department of Computer Science and Engineering at Ramaiah University of Applied Sciences, India. Her research interests include Artificial Intelligence, Generative AI, and healthcare applications.

Vijetha Katakam is currently working as an Analyst role for an organization Visa Inc., having 10+ years of experience in the IT industry. She completed her B.Tech at JITS Karimnagar with the specialization of Computer Science and Information Technology. She worked for more than 2 organizations and was exposed to different software platforms.She played key roles in her area of interest. She worked for Dover Fueling Solutions as a QA Analyst, Applause (formally uTest) and Walmart eCommerce companies at USA.

Kokoy Siti Komariah is a researcher at the National Research and Innovation Agency (BRIN) in Indonesia. She completed her Doctor of Engineering in Artificial Intelligence Convergence at Pukyong National University in South Korea. Currently, she work at BRIN in the Research Center for Data and Information Science and joined the Natural Language Processing (NLP) research group at BRIN. Her research focuses on text processing, machine learning, NLP technologies, and information retrieval.

R. Felista Sugirtha Lizy is employed as an Assistant Professor in the PG Department of Computer Science at A.P.C. Mahalaxmi College for Women, Thoothukudi, Tamil Nadu, India. With more than 17 years of academic and research experience, she actively engages in research in cryptography, artificial intelligence, cybersecurity, cloud computing, blockchain technologies, and data-driven sustainable systems. She has published extensively in reputed Scopus-indexed, UGC-approved, and international peer-reviewed journals, with notable contributions to the performance enhancement of Elliptic Curve Cryptography (ECC) and RSA using innovative approaches such as Runge–Kutta and Game Theory models for secure digital identity applications. Dr. Felista has authored over 20 academic books spanning Python programming, cloud computing, data science, generative AI, big data technologies, and research methodologies, and has contributed several international book chapters published by Springer, IEEE, and other global publishers in areas including AI-driven sustainability, reinforcement learning, IoT–cloud integration, and smart urban systems. She holds two patents in machine learning–based data security and AR/VR application development. In addition to her research contributions, she serves as a reviewer and editorial board member for international journals and has chaired sessions, delivered invited talks, and coordinated national and international conferences, FDPs, and academic workshops. Her current research focuses on AI-enabled intelligent systems, cybersecurity frameworks for smart environments, and sustainable digital ecosystems.

M. Praveen is currently pursuing his Ph.D. from Visvesvaraya Technological University (VTU). He is presently working as an Assistant Professor in the Department of Data Science at Vignana Bharathi Institute of Technology (VBIT), Hyderabad. With a strong academic foundation and a passion for emerging technologies, he is dedicated to advancing both teaching and research in the field of Data Science. His professional interests span Machine Learning, Artificial Intelligence, Data Analytics, and Cloud-Based Data Engineering. He is actively engaged in research aimed at developing intelligent, data-driven solutions to real-world problems. Throughout his academic career, he has demonstrated a consistent commitment to high-quality education, student mentoring, and the integration of industry-relevant practices into the curriculum. He is also involved in academic responsibilities including curriculum design, laboratory development, and guiding students in projects and research activities. His long-term vision is to contribute meaningful research outcomes to the scientific community and to foster innovation in data-centric technologies.

Archan Mitra is an Assistant Professor at School of Media Studies (SOMS) at Presidency University, Bangalore. He is the author of two book "Cases for Classroom Media and Entertainment Business" and "Multiverse and Media", he also has other several edited books to his credit. He has done his doctorate from Visva-Bharati Santiniketan, West Bengal in the field of "environmental informatics and communication for sustainability". In addition to that he is a certified Science Communicator and Journalism from Indian Science Communication Society (ISCOS), certified Corporate Trainer with Amity Institute of Training and Development, Certified Social Media Network Analyst. He has a strong interest in environmental communication. He was awarded certificate of merit by PRSI, Kolkata Chapter and Medal of Honor by Journalistic Club of Kolkata. He was working as a research assistant with the World Bank's "Environmental Capacity Building in Southeast Asia" project at IIM Kashipur. He was instrumental in launching the World Bank's Green MBA MOOC, he has also assisted in the research project on Uttarakhand disaster mitigation by ICSSR, the leading research on Uttarakhand disaster.

M. Jeya Pandian is currently working as Assistant Professor in Srinivasa Ramanujan Centre, SASTRA Deemed University, Kumbakonam, India. He received his Bachelor of Engineering from Madurai Kamaraj University and Master of Engineering from Anna University, Chennai and pursuing Ph.D. from SASTRA

Deemed University, Thanjavur, India. He has more than 16 years of teaching experience. His area of research includes, data mining, internet of things and machine learning. He published good number of publications in the peer reviewed journals and conferences.

P. Saranraj holds a Ph.D. in Microbiology from Annamalai University, Chidambaram, India, and is NET (ASRB–ICAR) qualified in Microbiology. He is currently serving as Assistant Professor and Head, Department of Microbiology, at Sacred Heart College (Autonomous), Tirupattur, Tamil Nadu, India. In addition, he is the Proprietor and Managing Director of JPS Scientific Publications, contributing actively to academic publishing and research dissemination. Dr. Saranraj has over 15 years of research experience and 10 years of teaching experience in the fields of Environmental Microbiology, Agricultural Microbiology, Industrial Microbiology, Bioremediation, Microbial Biotechnology, and Sustainable Ecosystem Management. His research work has focused on Microbial degradation of pollutants, Effluent treatment, Soil health improvement, Plant–microbe interactions, and Applied environmental sustainability. He has an extensive publication record, with more than 240 international research articles, over 90 books (international and national), and 70+ book chapters published with reputed academic publishers.

Umamaheswari Purushothaman holds a B.E. in Information Technology from Periyar Maniammai College of Engineering and Technology (2003), an M.B.A. from Alagappa University, Karaikudi, Tamil Nadu (2006), and an M.Tech in Computer Science from SASTRA Deemed University, Thanjavur, Tamil Nadu (2011). She earned her Ph.D. in Computer Science and Engineering from SASTRA Deemed University. With two decades of experience, she has taught both undergraduate and postgraduate courses in Computer Science. She is currently an Assistant Professor in the Department of Computer Science and Engineering at SRC Campus, SASTRA University, Kumbakonam. Her research interests focus on Data Mining, Machine Learning, and Deep Learning. She has published numerous research papers in international conferences, SCI-indexed journals, Scopus, and book chapters.

Sahana P Shankar, for three years. She holds a US Patent in the field so software testing. She has worked with RIT as a Teaching Assistant for 6 months under the TEQIP-II scholarship program. She has published papers in various international journals and conferences. She has also authored several book chapters. She is an ISTQB certified software tester. She is pursuing her PhD from VTU, Belgaum. She is currently working with Ramaiah University of Applied Sciences, Bangalore as an Assistant Professor in the Department of Computer Science and Engineering since 2018. She was awarded as "Annual Exemplary Faculty Member" on occassion of Teacher's Day in September 2023 for her overall contribution to teaching and learning. Through her industry connections, she has been able to get placement and paid internship opportunities to the students of RUAS every year. She also actively participates in all the university events and always strives for the well being and betterment of the students.

Siska Pebiana is a researcher specializing in Natural Language Processing and artificial intelligence. Her work focuses on large language models, AI safety, and responsible AI applications for public-sector.

Dhanalakshmi P is a Pharm.D graduate currently pursuing her Ph.D. She has over three years of experience in teaching and research. Her academic interests include clinical pharmacy, pharmacovigilance, and community pharmacy practice. She is actively involved in research activities and is committed to contributing to pharmaceutical education and patient care through evidence-based practice.

Ravikumar R. N. is currently a Postdoctoral researcher at Universiti Malaysia Perlis, Malaysia. Also, working as an Associate Professor in the department of Computer Engineering at Marwadi University, Rajkot, Gujarat. He has 12+ years of national and international teaching experience. He completed his PhD at Amity University, Rajasthan, M.E at VMRF Deemed University, B.E at Anna University, Chennai. He is the co-founder of the Research Activities Club at Marwadi University and trains students on research activities, which leads to the publication of 7 Scopus/SCI journals, 20 Book chapters, 25 Conference papers, and 10 patents. His specialization is ML, DL, Federated Learning, Recommendation Systems, and Optimization Techniques.

Sujarani Rajendran obtained M.Tech and Ph.D. degrees in Computer Science from SASTRA Deemed University, Thanjavur, Tamil Nadu, India in the years of 2010 and 2021, respectively. She obtained her M.C.A. degree from Annamalai University in 2008. She is currently working as an Assistant Professor in the Department of Computer Science at SASTRA Deemed University, Kumbakonam. Her research interests include Chaotic Cryptography, Steganography, Wireless Sensor Networks, Machine Learning, and Deep Learning. She published many articles in SCIE and SCOPUS indexed journals and also presented articles in different international conferences.

Aarthi S is a dedicated Assistant Professor in Computer Science with over six years of teaching experience. She is currently pursuing her Ph.D. at Marwadi University, Gujarat, and holds an M.Phil. and MCA from Bharathiar University, Tamil Nadu. Throughout her academic career, Aarthi has specialized in programming languages such as C++, Java, and C, and contributed to research in recommender systems and AI-related data privacy. She has published journal articles, contributed to book chapters, and actively participated in technical workshops. Known for her student mentorship and engagement in academic events, Aarthi remains committed to fostering innovation and excellence in computer science education.

Pradeepa Sampath is currently working as an Assistant Professor in the Department of Information Technology at SASTRA Deemed University, Thanjavur. She received her Ph.D. in Computer Science and Engineering in 2021. Her research interests include deep learning, machine learning, hypergraph neural networks, and data analytics, with a focus on medical image analysis and smart healthcare systems. She has authored 20 SCI papers and 10 Scopus papers. Her academic contributions reflect her commitment to advancing AI-driven solutions in the healthcare domain.

Agung Santosa received the BSEE from University of Toledo, USA, in 1992 and Master of Computer Science from University of Indonesia, Indonesia, in 2015. He is an associate researcher at the Research Center for Data and Information Sciences, affiliated with the National Research and Innovation Agency (BRIN) in Indonesia. Since 2021, he has been an active researcher in the domain of artificial intelligence, specifically focusing on speech and natural language processing. His research includes speech recognition, speech analytics, sentiment analysis, and natural language processing.

Sayali Kishan Somwanshi is a Quality Analyst who has a professional experience of more than three years working in the field of software testing in Telecom and Retail spheres. She is a specialist in Manual Testing, Functional and Non-Functional Testing, API Testing and in Automation Testing with Selenium WebDriver and Java. Her knowledge of SDLC, STLC, defect life cycle management, regression testing, and end to end validation of web applications is high. Sayali is also well-acquainted with practical experience of MySQL, Adobe campaign, Cosmos DB and Azure storage platforms. She received SRTMUN University, Nanded Bachelor of Engineering (Computer) first class. Her work is based on a high level of quality assurance, constant learning, and provision of best software solutions to organizational objectives.

Ravshan Sultanov is affiliated with the Department of Medical Fundamental Sciences at Termez University of Economics and Service, Termez, Uzbekistan. His academic interests focus on fundamental medical sciences, biomedical education, and the development of foundational scientific knowledge essential for medical and healthcare training. He is actively involved in teaching and academic activities that support students in building strong theoretical and practical understanding of core medical concepts. His work emphasizes evidence-based learning, interdisciplinary collaboration, and the integration of modern scientific approaches in medical education. Ravshan Sultanov also contributes to academic discussions related to biomedical sciences, health education, and the advancement of contemporary teaching methodologies in medical studies. Through his scholarly engagement and teaching practice, he aims to promote high-quality medical education and support the preparation of competent healthcare professionals capable of addressing modern health challenges.

A. Sumathi is working as an Assistant Professor in the Department of Computer Science and Engineering, SRC, SASTRA Deemed to be University, Kumbakonam, TN, India. Research areas include Data Mining, Machine Learning, Data Science, and Healthcare applications.

Ruthiwik T is a dedicated undergraduate student currently pursuing a B.Tech in Artificial Intelligence and Machine Learning at Sreenidhi Institute of Science and Technology, India. With a strong foundation in AI and ML, he is actively involved in both academic and research activities. At Sreenidhi, Ruthiwik has distinguished himself through his exceptional academic performance and his commitment to advancing his field of study. His passion for machine learning has driven him to explore various research areas, including data science and natural language processing. Ruthiwik is actively involved in research, currently working on a paper focused on the applications of machine learning in healthcare revolution. His research explores the potential of AI/ML technologies to drive innovations and improve healthcare practices, leveraging advanced techniques to analyze complex medical data and develop intelligent decision support systems.

Aman Suresh T is an Assistant Professor in Pharmacy Practice, currently serving at the Faculty of Pharmacy, Dr. M.G.R. Educational and Research Institute, Chennai. With a Pharm.D and ongoing PhD in Pharmacy Practice from SIMATS, he brings academic depth and clinical insight to his teaching and research. His teaching repertoire includes subjects such as pharmacotherapeutics, biostatistics, and pharmacoepidemiology for undergraduate and doctoral pharmacy programs. Dr. Aman is an active contributor to scholarly literature with multiple publications in Scopus and Web of Science-indexed journals, including research on diabetes, nephrology, and pharmacovigilance. His work has earned recognition such as subject-wise ranks at RGUHS and a prestigious ASCPT LMIC Travel Grant. Beyond academia, Dr. Aman has reviewed over 200 manuscripts and serves on editorial boards of reputed journals like Acta Scientific Pharmaceutical Sciences, PLOS ONE, and Cureus. He is also a frequent workshop resource person and guest lecturer on clinical pharmacy and regulatory topics. With strong skills in academic mentorship, interdisciplinary collaboration, and public health education, he actively bridges class

Lingala Thirupathi is a seasoned academician and researcher with over 18 years of experience spanning teaching and industry, specializing in Artificial Intelligence, Cybersecurity, and the Internet of Things. He is currently serving as an Assistant Professor at SNIST, Hyderabad. A Gold Medalist in M.Tech (Software Engineering) from JNTUH, he also holds a B.Tech in CSIT and multiple professional certifications, including Cisco Instructor, Oracle Certified Associate, and Salesforce Ranger. With over 60 research publications in reputed journals such as Scopus, IEEE, Elsevier, and Springer, he also holds one Australian and three Indian patents. Mr. Thirupathi has authored three textbooks and contributed to over 30 book chapters. He actively participates in academic and technical communities as a reviewer, committee member, and SPOC for Smart India Hackathons, and is affiliated with professional bodies like CSTA, TERA, and ICSES. His dedication to innovation and excellence has earned him accolades, including the Expert Instructor Award from Cisco Networking Academy.

Doniyor Umarov holds a PhD and is affiliated with the Department of Clinical Sciences at Mamun University, Khiva, Uzbekistan. His academic and research interests focus on clinical medicine, medical sciences, and healthcare education. He is actively involved in teaching and research activities that support the advancement of clinical knowledge and evidence-based medical practices. His work emphasizes the integration of modern medical research, diagnostic approaches, and clinical training to improve healthcare outcomes. Doniyor Umarov also contributes to academic discussions related to patient care, clinical research methodologies, and medical education development. Through his scholarly engagement and professional activities, he aims to strengthen clinical education and promote research that supports the improvement of healthcare systems and medical practice.

Deepak Varadam holds a Masters Degree in Microsystems Engineering from Heriot-Watt University, Edinburgh (Scotland), U.K. and P.G.Diploma in ECE from Napier University, U.K. He worked as a Postgraduate Masters Research Scientist under Biomedical Microengineering Group (BMG) at Heriot-Watt University. He is currently working as an Assistant Professor in Faculty of Engineering and Technology, Computer Science and Engineering Department at Ramaiah University of Applied Sciences (RUAS) since 2010. He has been actively participating in delivering corporate trainings, seminars and have publications in national, international journals and conferences. His research interests is in MEMS, Embedded

Systems, Software Engineering, Computer Graphics, AI, Blockchain, and IoT. He is currently an ExeCom Member of the IEEE RUAS Student Chapter.

S. Srinivasan is an Assistant Professor in the Department of Humanities and Social Sciences at Graphic Era (Deemed to be University), with 16 years of teaching and field expertise. He has served in the Ministry of Health and Family Welfare, as a Guest Faculty, and as a Mobilization Training Specialist with the State Government. Recently, he contributed to a tuberculosis project funded by GFATM and USAID. He has published 90 papers, with more under peer review in UGC-CARE and SCOPUS journals.

Index

A

B

C

D

E

F

G

H

L

M

N

P

Q

R

S

T

U

www.ingramcontent.com/pod-product-compliance
Lightning Source LLC
LaVergne TN
LVHW062335300926
849161LV00007B/1706